New Insights into Cardiac Arrhythmias

New Insights into Cardiac Arrhythmias

Edited by **Ruth Brown**

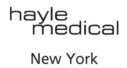

New York

Published by Hayle Medical,
30 West, 37th Street, Suite 612,
New York, NY 10018, USA
www.haylemedical.com

New Insights into Cardiac Arrhythmias
Edited by Ruth Brown

© 2015 Hayle Medical

International Standard Book Number: 978-1-63241-297-3 (Hardback)

Contents

Preface

Irregular heartbeat or cardiac arrhythmias is a severe medical condition. The close mechanisms of cardiac arrhythmias remain unidentified to experts. Genetic researches on ionic modifications, the electrocardiographic characteristics of cardiac rhythm and multiple diagnostic tests have achieved more in the last few years than in the history of cardiology. Similarly, treatments to avoid or cure such disorders are rising speedily. This book discusses uncommon heart rhythm disorders and various miscellaneous topics related to cardiac arrhythmias. It also elucidates various aspects related to cardiac electrophysiology. This book is a compilation of several well conducted researches accomplished by experts all over the world and will provide valuable insights to its readers.

The information shared in this book is based on empirical researches made by veterans in this field of study. The elaborative information provided in this book will help the readers further their scope of knowledge leading to advancements in this field.

Finally, I would like to thank my fellow researchers who gave constructive feedback and my family members who supported me at every step of my research.

Editor

Part 1

Uncommon Heart Rhythm Disorders

Bradycardia in Children During General Anaesthesia

Judith A. Lens[1], Jeroen Hermanides[1], Peter L. Houweling[1],
Jasper J. Quak[2] and David R. Colnot[2]
[1]Diakonessenhuis Utrecht, Departments of Anaesthesiology
[2]Otolaryngology/Head and Neck Surgery
The Netherlands

1. Introduction

Bradycardia in association with anaesthesia may lead to insufficient cardiac output and decreased delivery of oxygen to vital organs. In children the heart rate is the dominant factor for cardiac output, since the developing heart is less compliant and contractile and stroke volume cannot increase much. Thus, when bradycardia occurs in children during anaesthesia, cardiac output falls and may lead to serious cardiac arrhythmias and even cardiac arrest. In this chapter, the incidence, causes and risk factors, as well as the consequences and possible treatment of bradycardia in children during general anaesthesia are described and discussed. A focus is made on the incidence and causes of bradycardia in children undergoing adenotonsillectomy under general anaesthesia.

2. Bradycardia and general anaesthesia in children

2.1 Physiology

The normal heart rate decreases with increasing age in children (Figure 1). Therefore, a heart rate less then 100 beats per minute in very young children is a bradycardia by definition. For children 3 years of age, this means a heart rate less then 65 beats per minute. In the first months after birth, the risk for bradycardia is even higher as a result of an autonomic imbalance in the heart innervation (Rothrock, 2004).

Causes for bradycardia can be either intrinsic (e.g. cardiac abnormalities), or extrinsic (e.g. medication). During general anaesthesia children are at an increased risk of bradycardia in case of hypoxemia or hypervagotonia. Hypoxemia can be caused by administration of anaesthetics or other medication. Hypervagotonia can be evoked by oesophageal or nasal stimulation as a consequence of anaesthesia, for example in case of endotracheal intubation. However, surgery can also cause hypervagotonia by manipulation of the head or neck region, which is especially the case in otolaryngology. Among otolaryngology surgical procedures, adenotonsillectomy is a procedure likely to be responsible for direct stimulation of the vagal nerve. This stimulation is caused by placement of the mouth gag and the instruments used during the surgical procedure and the manipulation in the mouth and oropharynx. Together with placement of ventilation tubes, adenotonsillectomy is one of the most frequently performed types of surgery in children worldwide.

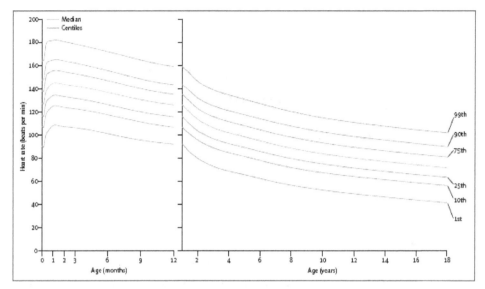

Fig. 1. Heart rate values in centiles from birth to age 18. (Fleming et al, 2011)

2.2 Aetiology

Bradycardia during general anaesthesia can have different causes, and depending on patient characteristics and conditions, the sequelae can be serious. Especially in children, bradycardia can lead to failure of cardiac output and may also lead to serious cardiac arrhythmias and even cardiac arrest. In a study performed by the Australian Patient Safety Foundation, the first 4000 incidents reported to the Australian Incident Monitoring Study (AIMS) were analysed for the incident bradycardia. A total of 265 reports describing bradycardia in both adults and children during anaesthesia were extracted and studied (Watterson et al., 2005). In general, bradycardia was associated with hypotension in 51% of cases, cardiac arrest in 25% of cases and hypertension in one case. In 22% of reports apparent desaturation or an abnormality of ventilation was described. The authors concluded that cardiopulmonary events causing bradycardia are more likely than other causes to be associated with cardiac arrest. The causes of bradycardia were drug events in 28% of cases, airway related events in 16%, autonomic reflexes in 14%, and regional anaesthesia in 9% of the cases. Most episodes of bradycardia occurred during surgery (61%), whereas 20% was observed before and during induction.

In 43 of these 265 reports, bradycardia occurred in children under the age of 14 years. The distribution of ASA grading in children was similar to that of adults, but the haemodynamic profile was different for children as compared to adults. Whereas in adults airway and drug events together were responsible for 44% of causes, in children up to 75% of bradycardias were associated with airway and drug events. Airway events were the predominant cause of bradycardia in children (47%). In 51% of children studied there was no abnormality of blood pressure, which was attributed to the high incidence of airway events, in which hypoxaemia was associated with rapid deterioration in heart rate. Hypotension was present in 21% of the cases, but cardiac arrest was described in 32% of the cases. Whereas a good outcome was reported in 63% of both adults and children, in only 48% of incidents concerning children a good outcome was reported. This might indicate that an incident during general anaesthesia with bradycardia in children has an important risk of poor outcome.

An epidemiologic study by Keenan and co-workers on bradycardia during anaesthesia concluded from data abstracted from almost 8,000 anaesthetic records of children 0-4 years of age that the frequency of bradycardia was 1.27% in the age group 0-1 years of age. This was considerably less in the older age groups, that is 0.65% and 0.16% in the 3rd and 4th year of age, respectively (Keenan et al., 1994). Causes of bradycardia included disease or surgery in 35%, inhalation anaesthetics in 35%, and hypoxaemia in 22% of children. Hypotension was observed in 10% of patients, whereas asystole of ventricular fibrillation occurred in 10%. All children underwent non-cardiac surgery and brdaycardia was defined as heart rate lower than 100 beats per minute. The study population was considerably younger than in the study described by Watterson. The authors concluded that bradycardia was more frequent in very young children aged 0-1 years undergoing anaesthesia, and that it was associated with substantial morbidity such as hypotension and asystole.

2.3 Airway related

The laryngeal reflex prevents foreign substances from entering into the lower airway and maintaining upper airway integrity. However, in some circumstances the laryngeal reflexes can induce cardiorespiratory events, that can even lead to life-threatening events such as apnea or even death. Gastroesophageal and pharyngolaryngeal refluxes are associated with both bradycardia and apnea, and may play a role in acute life threatening events (ALTE) or sudden infant death syndrome (SIDS). In airway management during general anaesthesia the laryngeal reflex can cause bradycardia by vagal stimulation and apnoea (Reix et al., 2007). In procedures especially during induction of anaesthesia, such as intubation, bradycardia and apnoea can be provoked. Other manoeuvres, like inserting a nasal feeding tube or head manipulation after endotracheal intubation, can induce bradycardia in a later phase of anaesthesia. In newborns and infants the upper airway sensitivity is even increased due to the immaturity of the chemo- and mechanoreceptors in the larynx. The innervation of the larynx is displayed in Figure 2.

In airway management during anaesthesia, the incidence of bradycardia is reported to be 0.5-4.2%, and the risk is increased when children are younger (Keenan et al., 1994, Fastle and Roback, 2004; Gencorelli et al., 2010). In an analysis of bradycardia incidents during anaesthesia, 20% of bradycardia events occurred in the pre-induction or induction phase (Watterson et al. 2005). In a large study population of 1070 children aged 3–12 years who underwent rapid sequence induction for intubation, bradycardia was observed in 5 patients (0.5%). Bradycardia was defined as a heart rate lower than 60 beats per minute. In the same study group, moderate hypoxemia with SaO_2 of 80-89% was observed in 20 patients (1.9%) and 18 patients (1.7%) developed severe hypoxemia with SaO_2 lower than 80%. The risk for hypoxemia was increased when the weight was below 20 kg (Gencorelli et al., 2010). In another group of 163 children undergoing rapid sequence induction for intubation, the incidence of bradycardia was 4%. The median age was 12 months (range 3 months to 19 years), which might explain the higher incidence of bradycardia. Definition of bradycardia was a heart rate falling two standard deviations below normal for age as described by the American Heart Association (Table 1).

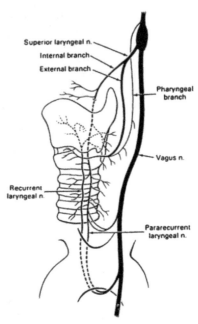

Fig. 2. Innervation of the larynx, reproduced from Reix et al, 2007

Age	Heart Rate
0-3 months	85-205
3 months to 2 years	100-190
2-10 years	60-140
>10 years	60-100

Table 1. The 95% confidence interval for normal heart rates in children (American Heart Association).

Analysis of the children with bradycardia showed hypoxemia prior to the bradycardia in 4 out of 6 patients. Most of the patients were intubated for respiratory disease (45%), trauma (19%), or seizures (12%). All bradycardia episodes resolved with ventilation or after endotracheal intubation (Fastle and Roback, 2004). In a series of 475 children (aged 1–22 years) who underwent operative intervention for post-tonsillectomy haemorrhage, bradycardia during rapid sequence induction was observed in 20 (4.2%) of patients. Bradycardia was defined as a heart rate lower than 60 beats per minute, appearing in at least two consecutive recorded vital signs, 15 seconds apart. In total 9.9% of the studied cohort had a moderate or severe hypoxemic event. Moderate hypoxemia was defined as $SaO_2 <$ 90%, and severe hypoxemia was defined as $SaO_2 <$ 80%. All bradycardia events resolved without pharmacological intervention (Fields et al., 2010).

2.4 Medication related
Many drugs used in the operating theatre can cause bradycardia. Calcium-channel blockers and ß-blockers are specifically used to slow heart rate. Also amiodarone has calcium channel

and ß-blocking properties. Most anaesthetics used during general anaesthesia have the potential of inducing bradycardia. In an extensive meta-analysis, propofol was associated with increased risk of bradycardia, also when compared to other anaesthetics (Tramèr et al., 1997), an odds ratio of 2.3 is thereby reported. Although it is difficult to compare the different trials, it seems clear that propofol carries an evident risk of bradycardia. The risk of death after bradycardia during propofol anaesthesia was 1.4/100.000. However, propofol is often administered together with opioids and muscle relaxants, which are also associated with bradycardia. By stimulation of the muscarinic receptors of the heart, suxamethonium (a depolarizing muscle relaxant) can cause bradycardia. Case reports on the occurrence of bradycardia or even asystole with the use of succinylcholine have been published (Delphin et al., 1987). However, incidence numbers are lacking. Also other non-depolarizing muscle relaxants and opioids like fentanyl or remifentanil have been associated with development of bradycardia in a meta-analysis of 85 randomised, controlled trials (Komatsu et al., 2007). Clonidine, an α-2-receptoragonist which is frequently used in addition to local anaesthesia, can also elicit bradycardia (Pöpping et al., 2009). From the vapour anaesthetics, halothane has been associated with the most cardiovascular changes, including bradycardia especially in adenotonsillectomy (van Nouhuys, 1973; Slappendel & Rutten, 1989). Data on bradycardia and the use of sevoflurane, isoflurane and desflurane is scarce. Thus, many drugs used in the perioperative period have been more or less associated with bradycardia. It is however difficult to elucidate which drugs contribute most to this risk, as randomized trials are lacking and most drugs are administered simultaneously.

2.5 Premedication with atropine

As discussed before, children that need endotracheal intubation commonly develop bradycardia. In literature there is discussion about the effect of premedication with atropine in children under the age of 5. Some authors advise atropine as pretreatment in all children under 1 year of age receiving succinylcholine and all patient with profound bradycardia during intubation. As stated earlier, bradycardia during intubation is probably due to combined vagal response and hypoxia. During intubation the vagal nerve is activated and because the parasympathetic-sympathetic imbalance in young children, this reaction is more profound in children. This imbalance disappears at the age of one year (Rothrock and Pagane, 2005). By administrating atropine, or other anticholinergic medication, the incidence of bradycardia could decrease. Atropine inhibits the binding of acetylcholine on the muscarinereceptors, thereby diminishing the vagal response and bradycardia. On the other hand, atropine can induce dysrhythmias, such as tachycardia. It has some side-effects that could be unwanted, such as malignant hyperthermia, seizure and an increased risk of aspiration by relaxation of the lower oesophageal sphincter. In case of underdosing of atropine, there is a chance of provoking bradycardia. In case of overdosing, ventricular dysrhythmias and tachyarrhythmia may occur.

The review of Fleming and co-workers is a good overview of the evidence pro and contra the use of atropine. Most evidence for the use of atropine as a standard in all children under the age of 18 is from before 1990. Halothane and repeated succinylcholine was often used in that period. Therefore there was an increased risk for bradycardia. Nowadays, incidence of bradycardia is decreased because other anaesthetics showing less side-effects are used. Considering the disadvantage of atropine, it can be stated that standard premedication is not advised (Fleming et al., 2005).

2.6 Physical status

Infants with a poor physical status have an increased risk for bradycardia. A higher ASA score is associated with more bradycardia, especially with an ASA score higher than 3. Infants with congenital diseases, especially heart disease may develop bradycardia easier and more prominent. Formally pre-mature infants have considerably more risk for apnoea and bradycardia. This can be associated with cardiac arrest and death. To reduce this risk, elective surgery should be postponed until after 55 weeks of post conceptual age. For explanation of ASA score, see Table 2.

ASA score	
1	A normal healthy patient
2	A patient with mild systemic disease
3	A patient with severe systemic disease
4	A patient with severe systemic disease that is a constant threat to life
5	A moribund patient who is not expected to survive without the operation
6	A declared brain-dead patient whose organs are being removed for donor purposes

Table 2. ASA classification system according to the American Society of Anaesthesiologists.

Children with Down syndrome have an increased risk of developing bradycardia during anaesthesia. Up to 50% of them have congenital cardiac abnormalities. But irrespective of the presence or absence of congenital heart disease, bradycardia as well as hypotension during anaesthetic induction in children with Down syndrome (n=567) occurred more frequently as compared to controls (Kraemer et al., 2010). Although patients with Down syndrome develop bradycardia at the same time after induction, the decrease in heart rate from baseline was greater in patients with Down syndrom as compared to healthy children (Bai et al., 2010).

The presence of obstructive sleep apnea-hyppopnea syndrome (OSAS) can influence the heart rate in children. Bradycardia is a common feature in children with OSAS during overnight sleep (Huang et al., 2008). Children woth OSAS undergoing adenotonsillectomy had more respiratory complications (Sanders et al., 2006).

2.7 Age

Cardiovascular and respiratory factors are the major causes of cardiopulmonary arrest in the pediatric population during anesthesia. Data from the American Society of Anesthesiologist Closed Claims Project showed that cardiopulmonary arrest during anesthesia in the pediatric population was different than in the adult population. In the pediatric population, cardiopulmonary arrest during anesthesia was commonly caused by respiratory events (inadequate ventilation with cyanosis and/or bradycardia proceding the cardiac arrest) and is more likely to result in mortality than in the adult cases. As known from the in 1994 founded Pediatric Perioperative Cardiac Arrest (POCA) registry anesthesia related cardiopulmonary arrest is fortunately an uncommon event, that is 1.4 per 10,000. It must, however, be emphasized that although cardiac arrest is rare significant, bradyarrhythmias must be treated immediately to prevent an irreversible cardiac arrest which occurs in 26% and have a mortality rate of 72% (Morray, 2010). Special precaution measurement should be considered in patients less than 1 year with severe underlying or concurrent disease having emergency surgery as they are the most at risk for a fatal outcome. In patients who are ASA 1 or 2, 64% of the cardiac arrests are medication-related arrests. In these patients conservative management includes removing or reducing the dose of drugs known to inhibit the sinus atrial node or removing the surgical stimulus (i.e oculocardia reflex). If this is not effective or possible, anticholinergics like atropine or sympathicomimetics (i.e. ephedrine, epinephrine, isoproterenol) must be considered. The risk of bradycardia and cardiovascular complications in children is inversely proportional to age.

2.8 Temperature
Lowering temperature is a risk for developing bradycardia, in children as well as in adults. In extreme cases of hypothermia (less than 32 °C), extreme bradycardia with a heart rate of less than 40 beats per minute may occur. In a case report concerning a child with an extreme bradycardia of 30 beats per minute at a temperature of 24.8°C, no serious effects in neurological outcome were observed (Balagna et al., 1999). In adults hypothermia is often deliberately used in patients after cardiac arrest to protect their brain. These patients have a better neurological outcome. In these adults, bradycardia is often monitored. Usually there is no decreased myocardial contractility (Polderman and Herold, 2009).

3. The incidence of bradycardia in children undergoing adenotonsillectomy

3.1 Incidence and surgical technique
Adenotonsillectomy is one of the most frequently performed types of surgery in children worldwide. The surgical rate in United States and England is approximately 50-65 per 10,000, respectively. In the Netherlands the surgical rate in 1998 was 115, and was even higher in the decades before (Van den Akker et al., 2004). In the last decade, the incidence of adenotonsillectomy has decreased to a surgical rate of 110 per 10,000 in 2008 (Prismant, 2010). In The Netherlands, the most frequently used surgical technique for adenotonsillectomy is the guillotine technique as described by Sluder in 1911. One of the advantages of the guillotine technique as compared to traditional dissection is a shorter duration of surgery (Mulder et al., 1995). Moreover, several studies have shown that the guillotine technique is less painful (Homer et al., 2000). Finally, there is less blood loss during surgery, and the incidence of postoperative haemorrhage is lower (Wake et al., 1989; Ünlü et al., 1992; Scheenstra et al., 2007; Lowe et al., 2007). The guillotine technique can be performed intubated and nonintubated under inhalation anaesthesia. A nonintubated adenotonsillectomy can be performed either in supine of sitting position.

Whereas the traditional dissection technique for adenotonsillectomy is the dominant technique worldwide, in The Netherlands guillotine adenotonsillectomy is most frequently performed, and in the majority of patients the surgery is performed nonintubated under inhalation anaesthesia (Tjon Pian Gi et al., 2010). For several years, there has been discussion about the ideal anaesthesia technique for adenotonsillectomy, either intubated or nonintubated. Those in favor of the intubated technique, claim that the most important reason to use endotracheal intubation is that the airway is secured, thus allowing the administration of inhalation anaesthetics and/or oxygen. Moreover, intubation could decrease the incidence of aspiration of blood or tissue, for example of the adenoid or tonsils. However, there is no evidence whether intubation indeed decreases the risk of aspiration of, for example, blood. In the nonintubated child, the short duration of anaesthesia and the fact that no intravenous muscle relaxantia are used, may allow the child to recover more quickly and thus decrease the risk of aspiration of blood, since laryngeal reflexes will be earlier as compared to intubated patients due to the use of more anaesthetics. This, among others, may be in favor of performing adenotonsillectomy nonintubated under inhalation anaesthesia. As already mentioned, the duration of surgery is substantially shorter. Moreover, the amount of inhalated anaesthetics administered to the child is less as compared to children undergoing adenotonsillectomy intubated. Only inhalation anaesthetics (sevoflurane) are necessary, whereas for the intubated technique muscle relaxantia are required. In a Dutch study performed by Mulder, it was found that the incidence of postoperative fever and pain was lower in children undergoing adenotonsillectomy under inhalation anaesthesia and nonintubated as compared to those undergoing the adenotonsillectomy intubated (Mulder et al., 1995). An explanation for this observation could be that intubation through an infection upper airway (tonsils) might facilitate spread of microorganisms to the lower respiratory tract. Another explanation was that the children undergoing adenotonsillectomy nonintubated had better laryngeal and tracheal reflexes, thus allowing a more effective removal of aspirated fluids by coughing direct postoperatively.

3.2 Hypoxemia and bradycardia in children undergoing adenotonsillectomy

Cardiac arrhythmias as a consequence of bradycardia have been described in children undergoing adenotonsillectomy with inhalation anaesthesia (Van Nouhuys, 1973; Slappendel and Rutten, 1989). The inhalation anaesthetics used in these studies were nitrous oxide, halothane and trichloroethylene. Although nitrous oxide is still used nowadays, the used of trichloroethylene and halothane has been decreased significantly. The different types of inhalation anaesthetics, and the specific type of surgery may well contribute to the occurrence of bradycardia. Only few studies have compared different anaesthesia techniques, nonintubated versus intubated, and comparison of the supine versus sitting position. In a prospective, randomised trial three groups of patients were compared (Knape, 1988). The first group of patients (n=42) underwent adenotonsillectomy with Sluder technique nonintubated, in a sitting position. In a second group of patients (n=42), the adenotonsillectomy was performed intubated. The third group (n=38) underwent circumcision nonintubated. Oxygen levels were registered using pletysmography. In this study, the pulse rate was not assessed. The incidence of hypoxemia was measured for each group. Hypoxemia was defined as SaO_2 lower than 90% and severe hypoxemia as SaO_2 lower than 75%. Nitrous oxide was used as inhalation anaesthetic, together with halothane, for all patients including those undergoing adenotonsillectomy intubated. The number of episodes per 100 patients was calculated for hypoxemia. In the nonintubated group undergoing adenotonsillectomy in a sitting position, the number of hypoxemia episodes was 331 per 100 patients, which was significantly higher than the incidence of hypoxemia in the group undergoing adenotonsillectomy with intubation, 29 per 100 patients. The incidence of hypoxemia in the control group undergoing circumcision was 32 per 100 patients. Severe hypoxemia with SaO_2 lower than 75% was only observed in the patients undergoing adenotonsillectomy in a sitting position and nonintubated. The incidence of severe hypoxemia was 117 per 100 patients. Hypoxemia occurred at the end of surgery and direct postoperatively in the nonintubated group undergoing adenotonsillectomy in a sitting position, whereas hypoxemia in the intubated group was seen after extubation. In the control group undergoing circumcision nonintubated hypoxemia was observed at the time the child got awake, indicating laryngospasm. In the study by van der Werff, a total of four groups were compared with different anaesthesia techniques (van der Werff et al., 1991). Children underwent adenotonsillectomy with Sluder technique nonintubated (n=20), adenoidectomy (n=20), adenotonsillectomy with Sluder technique nonintubated with placement of grommets (n=20), or only placement of grommets (n=20). All patients underwent surgery in a supine position. In none of the patient groups severe hypoxemia with SaO_2 lower than 75% was observed. In the group of patients undergoing adenotonsillectomy with Sluder technique nonintubated with placement of grommets, the mean SaO_2 was 94% versus 97% for the other groups. Wagemans performed continuous SaO_2 registration and assessment of pulse rate in 37 children undergoing adenotonsillectomy or placement of grommets under inhalation anaesthesia (Wagemans et al., 1991). Adenotonsillectomy was performed nonintubated, in a sitting position. Both groups received nitrous oxide and halothane as inhalation anaesthetics. Hypoxemia was defined as SaO_2 lower than 90% and bradycardia was defined as a heart frequency under 70 beats per minute. In the patients undergoing adenotonsillectomy, a mean SaO_2 of 94.7% was found, as compared to a mean SaO_2 of 96.5% in the patient group undergoing placements of grommets. This was not significantly different. In only one patient (5.3%) undergoing adenotonsillectomy a single SaO_2 lower than 90% was observed. The time of hypoxemia was 35 seconds and the lowest registration value of SaO_2 was 74%. Bradycardia was not observed in both groups. These findings were considerably different from those described by Knape, who found in 80% of patients hypoxemia with a SaO_2 lower than 90%. The authors concluded that the duration of surgery was increasingly shorter in their study population for adenotonsillectomy: 24 seconds versus 80 seconds in the patients studies by Knape. They concluded that the interaction between the anaesthesiologist and otolaryngologist was of great importance, resulting in a shorter duration of surgery. This leads to their conclusion that performing adenotonsillectomy under inhalation anaesthesia nonintubated in a sitting position, is a safe procedure. Based on these studies the Dutch Association of Otolaryngology and Head & Neck Surgery, in cooperation with the Dutch Institute for Healthcare Improvement (CBO) published the practice guideline 'Adenoid and tonsil disorders in secondary care' in 2008 (CBO, 2008). In this practice guideline, the advice was given to perform adenotonsillectomy using guillotine technique according to Sluder in a supine position if nonintubated inhalation anaesthesia is given.

In a study recently performed by our departments, we retrospectively analysed the incidence of hypoxemia and bradycardia in children undergoing adenotonsillectomy (Kretzschmar et al., 2010). Analysis was performed on a total of 2963 children who underwent adenotonsillectomy nonintubated in a sitting position. Hypoxemia was defined as a SaO_2 lower than 85% with a duration longer than 60 seconds. Incidental desaturation was defined as SaO_2 lower than 90%, with a duration shorter than 60 seconds. Bradycardia was defined as a heart frequency under 60 beats per minute, for longer than 30 seconds. Incidental bradycardia was defined as a heart frequency lower than 60 beats per minute for a duration shorter than 30 seconds. For both incidental desaturation and bradycardia, the incidence per 100 patients was calculated in order to compare our data with earlier studies described above. Sevoflurane was used as inhalation anaesthetic. Hypoxemia occurred in 132 patients (4.5%) and the incidence of incidental desaturations (SaO_2 lower than 90%) was 217 per 100 patients. In 1724 patients no incidental desaturations at all were seen. In 280 patients (9.4%) bradycardia was observed. The incidence of incidental bradycardia, a heart frequency lower than 60 beats per second but shorter than 30 seconds, was 234 per 100 patients. In 2683 patients (90.6%) bradycardia with a heart rate lower than 60 and a duration of more than 30 seconds did not occur. In 25 patients (0.8%) bradycardia and hypoxemia both occurred. The bradycardia was registered at the same moment or directly after hypoxemia in 3 of these 25 patients. All episodes were reversible and in none of the patients peri-operative complications due to hypoxemia or bradycardia were observed.

	No Hypoxemia	Hypoxemia	Total
No Bradycardia	2576 (86.9%)	107 (3.6%)	2683 (90.6%)
Bradycardia	255 (8.6%)	25 (0.8%)	280 (9.4%)
Total	2831 (95.5%)	132 (4.5%)	2963 (100%)

Table 3. Incidence of hypoxemia and bradycardia in patients undergoing adenotonsillectomy. Hypoxemia was defined as a SaO_2 lower than 85% with a duration longer than 60 seconds. Bradycardia was defined as a heart frequency under 60 beats per minute, for longer than 30 seconds.

Different explanations for the occurrence of bradycardia can be given. Bradycardia as a direct consequence of hypoxemia is one of these, and can indicate severe problems during anesthesia. This was only observed in 3 of the patients (0.001%), and was reversible in all of them. It seems that the specific type of surgery is more likely to cause the bradycardia. Due to the placement of the mouth gag and guillotine procedure with manipulation of the tissue of the pharyngeal wall it is likely that the vagus nerve is stimulated leading to a reflex of lowering the heart rate.

We concluded that bradycardia and hypoxemia both occur during adenotonsillectomy nonintubated in a sitting position. Both bradycardia and hypoxemia have shown to be reversible and do not lead to perioperative complications. The incidence of bradycardia directly during or after an episode of hypoxemia is extremely rare, in our study the incidence was 0.001%. However, bradycardia does occur relatively often, that is in 9.5% of patients. One of the most important explanations is the specific kind of surgery, where stimulation of the vagal nerve leads to bradycardia.

4. Discussion

Cardiac output is determined by the product of heart rate and left ventricular stroke volume. Bradycardia may result in an insufficient rate to sustain cardiac output and hence oxygen delivery to tissue beds. This is particularly so in the case of young children in whom cardiac output is more affected by changes in heart rate than stroke volume. A prompt appropriate response to bradycardia under anaesthesia is important as some causes are rare and/or obscure and homeostatic mechanisms may be impaired by anaesthetic agents. Hamilton and co-workers suggest in a recent meta-analysis that a preemptive targeted approach to the management of hemodynamics in the perioperative period may reduce morbidity and mortality for high-risk surgical patients (Hamilton et al., 2011). Flick et al reported that postoperative cardiac arrest occurred most often in children with congenital heart disease as a result of factors not related to anesthesia. While cardiac surgery accounted for only 5% of all procedures, 87.5% of all arrests occurred in patients with congenital heart disease, usually during cardiac surgery as a result of failure to wean from cardiopulmonary bypass. Anesthesia factors were related in only 7.5% of all arrests, with an incidence of 0.65 per 10,000 anesthetics. Only six anesthesia-related arrests occurred in noncardiac cases during the 17-yr study period (Flick et al., 2007).

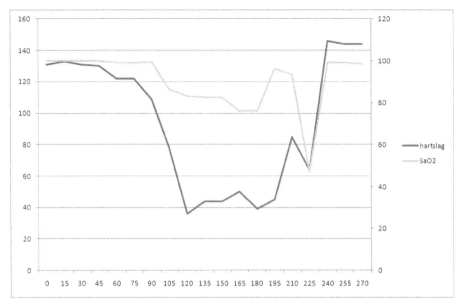

Fig. 3. Registration results of SaO_2 (green line, right axis, SaO_2 in %) and heart rate (red line, left axis, in beats per minute) as measured in time (horizontal-axis, in seconds) during inhalation anaesthesia in a 6-years old child undergoing adenotonsillectomy in sitting position.

During adenotonsillectomy under inhalation anaesthesia, bradycardia and hypoxemia both occur. In our study on children undergoing adenotonsillectomy in a sitting position nonintubated, both bradycardia and hypoxemia have shown to be reversible and do not lead to perioperative complications. The incidence of bradycardia directly during or after an episode of hypoxemia was extremely rare (0.001%). However, bradycardia does occur relatively often, in 9.5% of patients undergoing adenotonsillectomy in a sitting position nonintubated. An explanation might be a combination of study population, relatively young children, as well as the anaesthetics used, and the specific type of surgery leading to stimulation of the vagal nerve. Further research is necessary to compare different anesthesia techniques for adenotonsillectomy, with and without intubation.

5. Conclusion

Both bradycardia and hypoxemia occur relatively often during adenotonsillectomy, performed nonintubated in a sitting position under inhalation anaesthesia. The incidence of bradycardia in these children is 9.5%. Both bradycardia and hypoxemia are reversible and do not lead to perioperative complications. The incidence of bradycardia directly during or after an episode of hypoxemia is extremely rare. In general, in the pediatric population cardiovascular and respiratory factors are the major causes of cardiopulmonary arrest during anesthesia. The major causes of anesthesia-related cardiac arrest in the pediatric population are hypovolemia, preoperative anemia, pharmacological toxicity, hypoventilation and airway obstruction. Cardiopulmonary arrest during anesthesia in the pediatric population is different as compared to the adult population. In children, cardiopulmonary arrest during anesthesia is commonly caused by respiratory events and is more likely to result in mortality than in the adults. Anesthesia related cardiopulmonary arrest is fortunately an uncommon event, but it must be emphasized that significant bradyarrhythmias must be treated immediately to prevent an irreversible cardiac arrest. Special precaution measurement should be considered in patients less than 1 year with severe underlying or concurrent disease having emergency surgery as they are the most at risk for a fatal outcome. Finally, it must be clear that children should be cared for in facilities with adequate skilled medical and nursing staff and appropriately sized equipment.

6. References

Bai W., Voepel-Lewis, T., Malviya S. (2010) Hemodynamic changes in children with Down syndrome during and following inhalation induction of anesthesia with sevoflurane. *Journal of Clinical Anesthesia,* Vol 22, pp. 592-597

Balagna, R., Abbo, D., Ferrero, F., Valori, A., Peruzzi, L. (1999) Accidental hypothermia in a child. *Paediatric Anaesthesia,* Vol. 9: 342-244

CBO Kwaliteitsinstituut voor de gezondheidszorg (2008) Richtlijn Ziekten van Adenoïd en Tonsillen in de Tweede lijn. Utrecht:
    http://www.cbo.nl/thema/Richtlijnen/Overzicht-richtlijnen/KNO

Fastle, R.K. and Roback, M.G. (2004) Pediatric rapid sequence intubation. Incidence of reflex bradycardia and effects of pretreatment with atropine. *Pediatric Emergency Care,* Vol. 20 (10), pp. 651-655

Field, R.G., Gencorelli F.J., Litman, R.S. (2010) Anesthetic management of the pediatric bleeding tonsil. *Pediatric Anaesthesia,* Vol. 20, pp. 982-986

Fleming, B., McCollough, M., Henderson, S.O. (2005) Myth: atropine should be administered before succinylcholine for neonatal and pediatric intubation. Can J Emerg Med, Vol. 7 (2), pp. 114-117

Flick R.P., Sprung J., Harrison T.E., Gleich S.J., Schroeder D.R., Hanson A.C., Buenvenida S.L., Warner D.O. (2007) Perioperative cardiac arrests in children between 1988 and 2005 at a tertiary referral center: A study of 92,881 patients. *Anesthesiology,* Vol. 106, pp. 226–237

Gencorelli F.J., Fields, R.G., Litman, R.S. (2010) Complications during rapid sequence induction of general anaesthesia in children: a benchmark study. *Pediatric Anaesthesia,* Vol. 20, pp. 421-424

Hamilton, M.A., Cecconi, M., Rhodes, A. (2011) A Systematic Review and Meta-Analysis on the Use of Preemptive Hemodynamic Intervention to Improve Postoperative Outcomes in Moderate and High-Risk Surgical Patients. *Anesth & Analg,* Vol. 112(6), pp. 1259-1521

Homer, J.J., Williams, B.T., Semple, P., Swanepoel, A. en Knight, L.C. (2000) Tonsillectomy by guillotine is less painful than by dissection. *Int J Pediatr Otorhinolaryngol,* Vol 52, pp. 25-29

Huang, Z., Liu, D., Zhong, J., Chen, Q., Zhou, L., Sun, C., Wang, J. (2008) *Lin Chung Er Bi Yan Hou Jing Wai Ke Za Zhi,* Vol 22 (21), pp. 984-986

Keenan, R.L., Shapiro, J.H., Kane, F.R., Simpson, P.M. (1994) Bradycardia during Anesthesia in Infants. An Epidemiologic Study. *Anesthesiology,* Vol 80, pp. 976-982

Kalkman, C.J., Peelen, L., Moons, K.G., Veenhuizen, M., Bruens, M., Sinnema, G., De Jong, T.P. (2009) Behavior and Development in Children and Age at the Time of First Anaesthetic Exposure. *Anesthesiology*, Vol 110, pp. 805-812

Knape, J.T.A. (1989) Het verloop van de arteriële zuurstofsaturatie bij twee anesthesietechnieken voor (adeno)tonsillectomie bij kinderen. *Ned Tijdschr Geneeskd*, Vol 132, pp. 919-922

Komatsu, R., Turan, A.M., Orhan-Sungur, M., McGuire, J., Radke, O.C., Apfel, C.C. (2007) Remifentanyl for general anaesthesia: a systematic review. *Anesthesiology*, Vol. 62 (12), pp. 1266-1280

Kraemer, F.W., Stricker, P.A., Gumaney, H.G., McClung, H., Meador, M.R., Sussman, E., Burgess, B.J., Ciampa, B., Mendelsohn, J., Rehman, M.A., Watcha, M.F. (2010) Bradycardia During Induction of Anaesthesia with Sevoflurane in Children with Down Syndrome. *Anesth Analg*, Vol. 111, pp. 1259-1263

Kretzschmar, M.J., Siccama, I., Houweling, P.L., Quak, J.J., Colnot, D.R. (2010) Hypoxemia and bradycardia in children during adenotonsillectomy without intubation. *Ned Tijdschr Geneesk*, Vol. 154, pp. 1715-1719

Lowe, D., van der Meulen, J., Cromwell, D., Lewsey, J., Copley, L., Browne, J., Yung, M., Brown, P. (2007) Key messages from the National Tonsillectomy Audit. *Laryngoscope*, Vol 117, pp. 717-724

Morray, J.P. (2010) Cardiac arrest in anesthetized children: recent advances and challenges for future. Pediatric Anesthesia, doi:10.1111/j.1460-9592.2010.03440.x

Mulder, J.J.S., Mönnink, J.P., De Grood, P.M.R.M. (1995) Adenotonsillectomie volgens Sluder: met of zonder endotracheale intubatie? *Ned Tijdschr Geneeskd*, Vol 139, pp. 2730-2732

O'Connell T. Update in paediatric cardiopulmonary resuscitation. In: Keneally J, ed. Australasian anaesthesia. Melbourne: ANZCA, 1994:27-37

Polderman, K.H., Herold, I. (2009) Therapeutic hypothermia and controlled normothermia in the intensive care unit: practical considerations, side effects, and cooling methods. *Crit Care Med*, Vol. 37 (3), pp. 1101-1120

Pöpping, D.M., Alia, N., Marret, E., Wenk, M., Tramèr, M.R. (2009) Clonidine as an adjuvant to local anaesthetics for peripheral nerve and plexus blocks: a meta-analysis of randomized trials. *Anesthesiology*, Vol. 111(2), pp. 406-415

Prismant (2010), Informatie-expertise, ziekenhuisstatistieken, verrichtingen. Available from: www.prismant.nl

Scheenstra, R.J., Hilgevoord, A.A.J. en Van Rijn, P.M. (2007) Ernstige nabloeding na klassieke (adeno)tonsillectomie: zeldzaam en meestal op de dag van de ingreep. *Ned Tijdschr Geneeskd*, Vol 151, pp. 598-601

Reix, P., St-Hilaire, M., Praud, J-P. (2007) Laryngeal sensitivity in the neonatal period: from bench to bedside. *Pediatric Pulmonology*, Vol. 42, pp. 674-682

Rothrock, S.G. and Pagane, J. (2005) Letter to the Editors. *Pediatric Emergency Medicine*, Vol. 21 (9), pp. 637-638

Sanders, J.C., King, M., Mitchell, M.A., Kelly, J.P. (2006) Perioperative complications of adenotonsillectomy in children with obstructive sleep apnea syndrome. *Anesth Analg*, Vol 103 (5), pp. 1115-1121

Slappendel, R. & Rutten, J.M.J. (1989) Hartritmestoornissen tijdens adenotomie en adenotonsillectomie. *Ned Tijdschr Anesthesiol*, Vol2, pp. 11-13

Tjon Pian Gi, R., Bliek, V., Borgstein, J. (2010) The Sluder method in the Netherlands and the incidence of postoperative haemorrhage in a pediatric hospital. *Int J Ped Otorhinolaryngol,* Vol 74, pp. 56-59

Tramèr, M.R., Moore, R.A., McQuay, H.J.M. (1997) Propofol and bradycardia: causation, frequency and severity. *Brit J Anaesthesia,* Vol. 78, pp. 642-651

Ünlü, Y, Tekalan, S.A, Cemiloglu, R., Ketenci, I., Kutluhan, A. (1992) Guillotine and Dissection Tonsillectomy in Children. *J Laryngol Otol,* Vol. 106, pp. 817-820

Van den Akker, E.H., Hoes, A.W., Burton, M.J., Schilder, A.G.M. (2004) Large International Differences in (adeno)tonsillectomy rates. *Clin Otolarynol,* Vol. 29, pp. 161-164

Van der Meulen, J. (2004) Tonsillectomy technique as a risk factor for postoperative haemorrhage. *Lancet,* Vol 364, pp. 697-702

Van Nouhuys, F. (1973) Afwijkingen in het elektrocardiogram tijdens adenotonsillectomie onder narcose. *Ned Tijdschr Geneeskd,* Vol 117, pp. 137-141

Wagemans, M.F.M., van Dijk, B., Bakker, N.C., Ten Voorde, B.J., Faes, Th.J.C., Zuurmond, W.W.A., van der Werff, D.B.M., Scheffer, G.J. (1991). Continue SaO$_2$-meting en ECG-registratie onder inhalatieanesthesie voor adenotonsillectomie bij kinderen in zittende houding. *Ned Tijdschr Anesth,* Vol 4, pp. 61-61

Wake, M. & Glossop, P. (1989). Guillotine and dissection tonsillectomy compared. *J Laryngol Otol,* Vol. 103, pp. 588-591

Watterson, L.M., Morris, R.W., Westhorpe, R.N., Williamson, J.A. (2005) Crisis management during anaesthesia: bradycardia. *Qual Saf Health Care,* Vol. 14: e7

The Variations in Electrical Cardiac Systole and Its Impact on Sudden Cardiac Death

F. R. Breijo-Marquez[1] and M. Pardo Ríos[2]
[1]Clinical and Experimental Cardiology,
School of Medicine, Commemorative Hospital, Boston, Massachusetts
[2]School of Medicine and Dentistry,
University Research Institute on Aging, University of Murcia,
[1]USA
[2]Spain

1. Introduction

Before anything else, is essential to define what is the **electrical cardiac systole**. Especially when there are so many discrepancies among different authors.

Includes cardiac electrical systole from the beginning of the P wave (atrial depolarization) to the end of the T wave (ventricular repolarization).

Would cover thus the P wave, PR interval, QRS complex, ST segment, T wave.

For other authors, this one only would include from the beginning of QRS complex to the end of the T wave.

There are several changes, especially in its length, that can cause a sudden death in case that they are not adequately diagnosed and, thus, with the properly treated.

2. Standard values (in length)

P-wave: 0.06-0.09 seconds in length.
PR- interval: 0.12 to 0.20 seconds in length.
QRS- complex: 0.06 to 0.10 seconds in length.
QT- interval (corrected): 0.40 to 0.44 seconds in length.
RR- interval: 0.60-1.00 seconds in length.
Normal duration of cardiac electric systole: 35-45% of total duration of the cardiac cycle (R-R interval)

(The length of cardiac electrical systole is considered normal until reaching 45% of the overall length of cardiac cycle: a greater value is considered as prolonged and lesser is considered as shortened)

The sudden death is defined for most authors as a natural death that happens very instantaneously or within the first hour from the beginning of the symptoms, in a patient with well-known previous disease or without her, but is unexpected totally. Although we do not agree with some nuances of such definition, we will give it as acceptable.

Consequently, any sudden death should be considered either of cardiac origin when the heart is the affected organ, structurally or without macroscopic alterations of its structure. The cardiac problems are the main cause of unexpected death. It is estimated that occurs about 1 case of sudden death for every 100,000 young athletes each year (under 35). Even though exercise is beneficial for health, sport of competition increases the risk of sudden death [Brignole M, et al 2004].

CARDIAC COMMOTION.
CORONARY ARTERY ANOMALY.
LEFT VENTRICULAR HYPERTROPHY OF UNDETERMINED CAUSE.
MYOCARDITIS.
RUPTURE OF AORTIC ANEURYSM.
ARRHYTHMOGENIC RIGHT VENTRICULAR CARDIOMYOPATHY.
BYPASS CORONARY ARTERY.
AORTIC VALVE STENOSIS.
ATHEROSCLEROTIC DISEASE OF THE CORONARY ARTERY.
DILATED CARDIOMYOPATHY.
MYXOMATOUS MITRAL DEGENERATION.
ASTHMA.
HEATSTROKE.
DRUG ABUSE.
OTHER CARDIOVASCULAR CAUSES.
LONG QT SYNDROME.
RUPTURED BRAIN ANEURYSM.
CARDIAC SARCOIDOSIS.
TRAUMATIC CARDIAC INJURY.

[Thijs, RD., 2005]

Table 1. The most frequent causes of sudden death in overall.

The three most common causes for sudden cardiac death are:
1.   Hypertrophic cardiomyopathy (HCM). [Figure 1]:
It is a disease of the myocardium in which a portion of the myocardium is hypertrophied (thickened) without any obvious cause. It is perhaps most well-known as a leading cause of sudden cardiac death in young athletes. The occurrence of Hypertrophic cardiomyopathy is a significant cause of sudden unexpected cardiac death in any age group and as a cause of disabling cardiac symptoms [Richardson P., 1996]. Younger people are likely to have a more severe form of Hypertrophic cardiomyopathy. HCM is frequently asymptomatic until sudden cardiac death, and for this reason, some suggest routinely screening certain populations for this disease [Doerer JJ., 2009].
A cardiomyopathy is a primary disease that affects the muscle of the heart. With Hypertrophic cardiomyopathy (HCM), the sarcomeres (contractile elements) in the heart replicate causing heart muscle cells to increase in size, which results in the thickening of the heart muscle. In addition, the normal alignment of muscle cells is disrupted, a phenomenon known as myocardial disarray. HCM also causes disruptions of the electrical functions of the heart. HCM is most commonly due to a mutation in one of 9 sarcomeric genes that results in a mutated protein in the sarcomere, the primary component of the myocyte (the muscle cell of the heart) [Maron BJ ., 2010].
While most literature so far focuses on European, American, and Japanese populations, HCM appears in all racial groups. The prevalence of HCM is about 0.2% to 0.5% of the general population [Kuller LH., 1980]

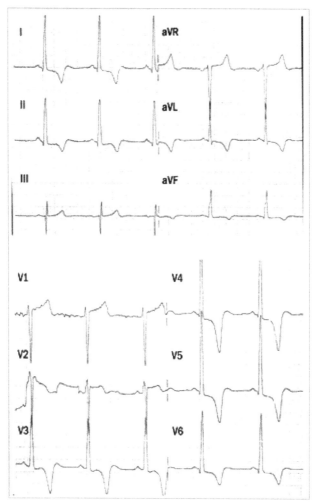

Fig. 1. ECG is abnormal., 80-90% of cases. Abnormal Q-waves in inferior leads. Increasing the voltage in medium or left precordial (V3-V6). ST segment depression, negative T- waves in precordial leads, middle and left. Less often: Increasing in the left atrium, left axis, Giant negative T waves, atrial fibrillation, ventricular extra-systoles, ventricular tachycardia in severe cases.

2.   Arrhythmogenic right ventricle cardiomyopathy (ARVD). [Figure 2]
Arrhythmogenic right ventricular dysplasia (ARVD), also called arrhythmogenic right ventricular cardiomyopathy (ARVC) or arrhythmogenic right ventricular dysplasia/cardiomyopathy (ARVD/C), is an inherited heart disease. ARVD is caused by genetic defects of the parts of heart muscle known as desmosomes, areas on the surface of heart muscle cells which link the cells together [Lahtinen, AM., 2011]. The desmosomes are composed of several proteins, and many of those proteins can have harmful mutations. The disease is a type of non-ischemic cardiomyopathy that involves primarily

the right ventricle. It is characterized by hypokinetic areas involving the free wall of the right ventricle, with fibro fatty replacement of the right ventricular myocardium, with associated arrhythmias originating in the right ventricle. ARVD is often found in association with diffuse palmo-plantar keratoderma, and woolly hair, because their genes are nearby and often inherited together. ARVC/D is an important cause of ventricular arrhythmias in children and young adults. It is seen predominantly in males, and 30-50% of cases have a familial distribution.

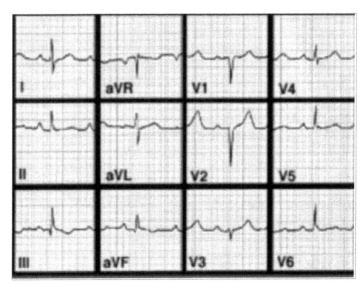

Fig. 2. 90% of individuals with ARVD have some EKG abnormality. The most common EKG abnormality seen in ARVD is T wave inversion in leads V_1 to V_3. However, this is a non-specific finding, and may be considered a normal variant in right bundle branch block (RBBB), women, and children under 12 years old. RBBB itself is seen frequently in individuals with ARVD. This may be due to delayed activation of the right ventricle, rather than any intrinsic abnormality in the right bundle branch. The **epsilon wave** is found in about 50% of those with ARVD. This is described as a terminal notch in the QRS complex. It is due to slowed intraventricular conduction. The epsilon wave may be seen on a surface EKG; however, it is more commonly seen on signal averaged EKGs. Ventricular ectopy seen on a surface EKG in the setting of ARVD is typically of left bundle branch block (LBBB) morphology, with a QRS axis of -90 to +110 degrees. The origin of the ectopic beats is usually from one of the three regions of fatty degeneration (the "triangle of dysplasia"): the RV outflow tract, the RV inflow tract, and the RV apex.

3.   Arrhythmogenic sudden death syndrome:
It is a generic name that includes many alterations in cardiac electrical conduction capable of produce instant death.
This syndrome includes all sudden cardiac deaths wherein the cause of death could not be diagnosed, even after the necropsy. It is the cause of more 5% of all sudden cardiac deaths.
That is, if we discard the non-cardiac causes and structural heart problems, this problem is denominated as arrhythmogenic sudden death syndrome from a generic form. As the

diagnostic techniques are being more appropriate each day, these numbers grows exponentially [Strickberger SA., 2006].

Here, would be included all events from our chapter proposal : Alterations in electrical cardiac systole and its impact on sudden cardiac death.

3. Other disorders in electrical cardiac systole as cause for sudden cardiac death

As we have said previously, the electrical cardiac systole originates from the beginning of the P wave (atrial depolarization) to the end of the descending branch of the T wave (ventricular repolarization). Are included, therefore, the succession of P-QRS-T and its corresponding intervals and segments: PQ, ST and QT. The mathematical possibilities in the variation on length of electrical systole of the heart may be several. It is well documented and demonstrated that such changes in length can cause that be more vulnerable and unstable all myocardial cells, and can also cause serious cardiac arrhythmias, several syncope episodes and even sudden death for this motive. Even today, many of these disorders are poorly understood and, too many times, its clinical manifestations are categorized as "episodes of epilepsy"; other times (most) are classified within a "common sack" called "channelopathies", when -actually- is the alteration from electrical cardiac systole the true etiology of them.

All these disorders can cause syncopal episodes and a sudden cardiac death.

The measures and lengths of the different components of electrical cardiac systole, considered for most authors as normal are these:

PR-interval: 0.120- 0.200 seconds.

QRS complex: 0.08-0.120 seconds.

QT-interval (corrected): 0.350-0.450 seconds. (Here, there is much disagreement among different authors). The most used methods for QT interval correction, since it is frequency-dependent, are Bazett, Fridericia.

When the PR-interval is lesser than 0.120 seconds, we call it a short PR-interval. In contrast, when is greater than 0,200 seconds, we call it a first-degree AV block. When the QRS complex is lesser than 0.08 seconds, we call it "narrow QRS" but when is greater than 0,120 seconds, we call it "wide QRS". Likewise, when the corrected QT- interval length is lesser than 0,350 seconds, we call it Short QT- interval and when is greater than 0,450 seconds, we call it a Long QTc- interval.

It is clear that there may be, in the same ECG recording, a combination of them all.

Some of these disorders, we will explain briefly below.

3.1 Wolff-Parkinson-White's syndrome (WPWS)

Wolff-Parkinson-White syndrome (WPWS) is a congenital heart disease (PRKAG2. Genetic map 7q36) characterized by a premature ventricular depolarization caused by an abnormal atrioventricular accessory pathway, between the atria and ventricles, known as Kent's bundle. However, even today, is called into question the real cause of Wolff-Parkinson-White, there are some authors who believe that, PRKAG2 mutations, are caused by a glycogen storage cardiomyopathy associated with WPWS, because the overwhelming majority of accessory pathways occur in individuals without structural heart disease, and probably without this mutation. The pathogenesis of accessory pathway formation in PRKAG2 may be completely different, and some authors believe it is due to an inflammation of myocardial cells that occur in the atrial-ventricular connections [L. Wolff., 1930].

In fact, do not even know if the accessory pathways are mediated genetically or due to environmental exposures or randomly.

A short PR interval, a delta wave, a wide QRS complex (greater than 120 ms) and, occasionally, alterations in the ventricular repolarization are its main electrocardiographic characteristics on the ECG. Its incidence varies between 0, 1% and 3% in the general population.

It is essential to achieve the right differential diagnosis between:

• Wolff-Parkinson-White's syndrome or real ventricular pre-excitation.
• Lown-Ganong-Levine syndrome or accelerated atrioventricular conduction.
• Mahaim's syndrome.
• "Short PR alongside short QT" intervals in the same person. (Breijo's Pattern).

3.1.1   Typical ECG image of the Wolff-Parkinson-White

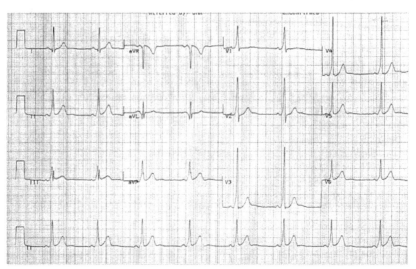

In this context of ECG recording, that has a normal heart rate, a short PR interval, a delta-wave and an early ventricular repolarization can be seen.

3.2 Lown-Ganong-Levine syndrome (LGL)

This syndrome was described in 1952 by Lown, Ganong, and Levine, forming the famous now used to describe it. It is considered a preexcitation syndrome [Lown B, Ganong WF, Levine SA., 1952].

We now know four types of pre-excitation syndrome:

• Wolff-Parkinson-White or ventricular preexcitation true.
• Lown-Ganong-Levine or accelerated atrioventricular conduction.
• Short PR alongside short QT" intervals in the same person. (Breijo's Pattern).
• Mahaim Syndrome.

LGL is a disease entity that is included within the more general condition called Short PR-Interval).

3.2.1 Etiology

- Acquired .
- Congenital :
  - Inherited.
  - Not inherited.

The familial form is inherited, as an autosomal dominant genetic trait has been associated with the PRKAG2 gene that encodes the activated AMP protein kinase, responsible for transport and store energy from the heart. A mutation in this gene could explain the susceptibility of the heart to the crises of tachycardia. Mutation has been identified on the long arm of chromosome 7 (7q34-q36).

The Lown-Ganong-Levine may affect approximately 1 in every 50,000 people.

Several structural abnormalities have been proposed as the possible basis for LGL, including the presence of James's fibbers, Mahaim's fibbers, Brechenmacher and underdeveloped anatomic sinus node (hypoplastic).

Each of these fibbers can only be identified histologically.

Thus, unless other studies demonstrate definitive- structural or functional -abnormalities, the diagnosis of LGL remains a clinical diagnosis.

In the absence of significant structural heart disease, the mortality rate appears to be very low.

Patients may present with an acute episode of tachycardia or a history of symptoms suggestive of paroxysmal tachycardia.

In diagnosis is necessary to make:

1. A standard test for tachycardia, including an ECG to document the rhythm.
2. Serum electrolytes, calcium, magnesium levels, and levels of serum thyroid hormone-stimulating hormone (TSH). Lithemy.
3. History suggestive of recurrent paroxysms of tachycardia,
4. A Holter monitor or event recorder may be useful to document the rhythm during acute symptomatic episodes.
5. An ergometric study.
6. In rare cases, an implantable monitor for pace may be helpful.
7. Family History. (Screening).

3.2.2 Differential diagnosis with Wolf-Parkinson-White

Although apparently similar, there are differences, which, in our opinion, are critical with respect to drug treatment elective. The key differences are:

- The LGL is a PR- interval shortened due to, the presence of accessory pathway, prevents the AV node but normal QRS because the accessory pathway (James fibbers) binds directly to the sinus and depolarizes the ventricles not directly, but does so by typical pathway, by the Hiss-Purkinje system.
- Not displayed "Delta waves -" in D1, aVL, V5 and V6.
- The QRS complexes tend to be narrow because there is usually no interventricular conduction disturbance.
- It is not be as frequent the association of atrial fibrillation during concomitant crisis.

3.2.3 Prognosis

No studies have shown an increased risk of sudden death or reduced survival for patients meeting the criteria for the diagnosis of LGL.

3.2.4 Current therapeutic bases

Rarely, the drug medical therapy can have failures usually, but there are patients in who there is not effective (for patients who continue to have recurrent and intolerable symptoms). In such extreme cases are used:

- Radiofrequency ablation (RF).
- The external pacemaker.
- The Implantable Cardioverter Defibrillators (ICDs).

This destroys the accessory pathway using a catheter (tube) inserted into the body to reach the heart. The success rate of this procedure ranges between 85 and 95% depending on the location of the extra or additional route.

Digoxin, verapamil and beta-blockers (other drugs commonly used to treat other types of tachycardia) can increase the frequency of episodes of tachycardia in some people with this syndrome. Beta-blockers may increase cardiac depression.

We can use drugs such as adenosine (Inpatient), and amiodarone to control or prevent episodes of tachycardia.

For the control of tachycardia is usually proceed according to the severity of the implementation of vagal maneuvers carotid massage type and Valsalva maneuver (forced expiratory made with the nose and mouth closed).

3.2.5 Typical ECG image of the Lown-Ganong-Levine

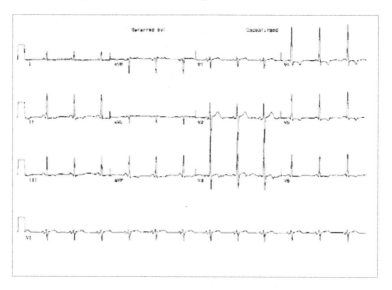

3.3 Short PR-interval alongside short QT-interval on the same person (Breijo's pattern)

In 2006, Breijo-Marquez, Pardo Ríos et al. evaluated a series of young patients, who had had, since childhood, many episodes of nocturnal palpitations, chest pain, full loss of consciousness (syncope), and which were accompanied by tonic-clonic seizures. All had been diagnosed and treated as epileptic episodes. Treatment outcomes were null. They were always considered as normal, in every cardiac studies performed absolutely [Breijo-Marquez, FR., 2008].

However, all these patients had an ECG recording common:
"A PR-interval lesser than 0,120 seconds with a QTc-interval equal to or lesser than 0.350 seconds".
That is, a pattern of short PR and QTc in the same person.
The correct treatment was begun (beta-blockers and, in some cases, an implantable cardio defibrillator, ICD.). Was removed all treatment from epilepsy.
The outcome to date is satisfactory.
Although we don't know, with certainty, the etiology of this pattern of ECG to date, we know that there were two important confusions:
First. - The physicians mistook to syncopal episode, with an epileptic episode.
Second. - The syncopal episodes are due to a cardiac disorder (was a cardiogenic syncope due to a cardiac electrical systole's alteration).
This ECG recording may be easily confused with a Lown-Ganong-Levine, since both have a short PR-interval. Nevertheless, in this type of ECG pattern there is also a short QTc-interval.
Unfortunately, both entities are confused with epileptic episodes too often.
Sudden cardiac death is extremely frequent in this type of event.

3.3.1 Typical ECG image of the "short PR alongside short QT" intervals in the same person (Breijo's Pattern)

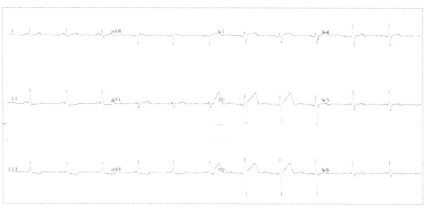

This ECG recording was the first with 12 leads that was obtained from our Hospital from Boston. MA. The patient was a 17 years-old male. We can see a shortening of the PR and QT intervals (Bazett), especially in inferior and left precordial leads. PR-interval length is lesser than 0.120 seconds and QTc length is lesser than 0.350 seconds. Patient had the symptoms exposed previously. He was also diagnosed for epileptic episodes. However, he had syncopal episodes and two cardiac arrests by cardiological disturbances.

3.4 Mahaim syndrome
Mahaim syndrome is characterized by:
The PR- interval with a standard length. Presence of pseudo-delta wave in the initial phase of the QRS complex because the sinus stimulus enters to AV node where physiological suffers a delay and then depolarizes the ventricles by an abnormal way: Mahaim fibers [Mahaim, I., 1937]

That is:
- PR-interval with a normal length.
- Wide QRS complexes.

3.4.1 Typical ECG image of the Mahaim's syndrome

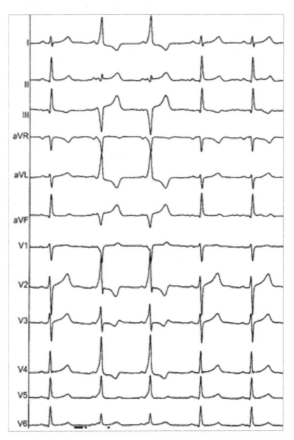

4. Differential diagnosis among various entities with alterations in electrical cardiac systole

ENTITY.	PR-interval	QRS complex	QTc -interval
W.P.W	Short.	Wide (δ-wave)	Normal
L.G.L	Short	Normal	Normal
Mahaim	Normal or Short	Normal or wide	Normal
Breijo's Pattern	Short	Normal	Short

Differential diagnosis, based on the characteristics from the different intervals and complex.

5. Some variations in electrical cardiac systole that can cause sudden death

(All these examples were discovered by Breijo-Marquez, FR. et al. They are still very underdiagnosed).

1. WOLFF-PARKINSON-WHITE AND PROLONGED"Q-T"PATTERNS IN THE SAME ELECTROCARDIOGRAPHIC RECORD [Breijo-Marquez, FR., 2011].

Wolff-Parkinson-White syndrome (WPWS) is a congenital heart disease (PRKAG2. Genetic map 7q36) characterised by a premature ventricular depolarisation caused by an abnormal atrioventricular accessory pathway known as Kent's bundle. Prolonged QT syndrome (PQTS) consists of an abnormal prolongation of the QT interval on the ECG, which can be both inherited and acquired. This anomaly is known to favour the occurrence of malign cardiac arrhythmias, above all polymorphic ventricular tachycardia, ventricular fibrillation and "torsade de pointes".

When taken separately, both syndromes have little incidence, which leads us to expect this incidence to be even lower when they are found on the same electrocardiogram. Incidentally, the current medical literature contains no publications on this topic. This clinical case aims to establish the existence of an electrocardiographic pattern characterised by WPW and a PQTS pattern on an ECG record. With a high susceptibility to crisis of tachycardia, especially at night, several episodes of syncope, even cardiac arrest and sudden cardiac death.

The patient is a 24 old- years man. Since childhood, he has suffered from more than four tachycardia attacks, three documented syncope episodes, as well as two cardiac arrests recovered, for which he was treated with electric discharges. Afterwards, he was treated with radiofrequency ablation of Kent's bundle, with permanent positive results so far.

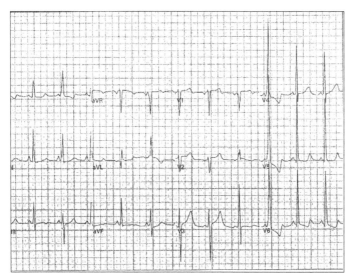

ECG' Image.

We can see a typical ECG recording of an intermittent WPW and a Long QT-interval together in a patient with several syncopal episodes and a recovered cardiac arrest.

2. ECG PATTERNS WITH SHORT PR INTERVAL TOGETHER TO A LONG QT (A) AND FIRST-DEGREE AV BLOCK ALONGSIDE A LONG QT (B: INCREASED OF CARDIAC ELECTRICAL SYSTOLE). [Breijo Marquez, FR., 2009].

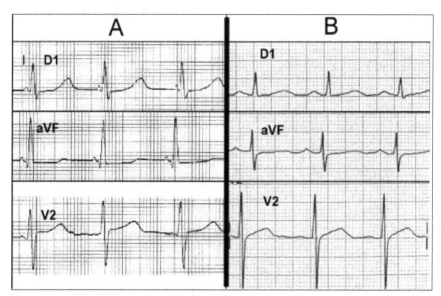

In this exposition, we present the ECG record of two patients with an obvious diversity and variability of alterations in the electrical system of heart. These electrical cardiac disturbances could explain completely the symptomatology from patients: nocturnal palpitations, several syncopal episodes.

In Figure A, we can see the presence of a short PR-interval together to a Long QT-interval. In Figure B, we can also see an ECG recording with a Long PR-interval alongside a Long QT-interval.

3.   PRESENCE OF A CRITICAL STENOSIS IN LEFT ANTERIOR DESCENDING CORONARY ARTERY ALONGSIDE A SHORT "P-R" AND "Q-T" PATTERN, IN THE SAME ELECTROCARDIOGRAPHIC RECORD [Breijo-Márquez, FR., 2010].

The knowledge of the heart and its functions is increasing every day. However, many cardiac dysfunctions remain undocumented.

One of them might be the presence of the Wellens' sign, minimally elevated or isoelectric ST segments, and inverted T waves in the precordial leads, without changes in the QRS complex, together with a shortened of "P-R and Q-T intervals" in the same electrocardiographic record. Both patterns are greatly underdiagnosed. The risk implied by the aforementioned underdiagnosis could have lethal consequences because the inherent problems in a short "P-R"-"Q-T" pattern could be added to those inherent in Wellens' sign.

Hereby, we set out to show both the description of the clinical case and the electrocardiogram (ECG) recording of a male having previously mentioned collection of symptoms.

The patient is a 42-year-old single man, previously diagnosed with unstable angina, who is an occasional smoker with arterial hypertension and who was prescribed a felodipine (5 mg/d) and ramipril (5 mg/d) treatment. The patient was complaining about an intense, oppressive, and progressive pain in the chest, which bore no relation to physical effort. The pain radiated toward both jaws and was accompanied by acute autonomic symptoms.

The sublingual administration of nitrates proved to be effective and led to a reduction of the pain as well as an improvement in the alterations the patient was showing. The ECG at presentation showed ST-segment elevations by more than 2 mm in all the precordial leads except lead one. The laboratory tests verified myocardial injury: L-lactate dehydrogenase, 1.220 UI/L (reference range, 230-460 UI/L);creatine kinase, 560 U/L (reference range, 37-290 U/L); creatine kinase], 1.85-14.45 U/L); aspartate transaminase, 376 U/L (reference range, 3-40 UI/L); alanine transaminase, 121 U/L (reference range, 5-37 UI/L); and troponin, 3.5 µg/L (Reference range, 0-0.1 ng/mL).

In spite of the elevated biochemical markers of myocardial injury, the case was classified as an unstable angina variant.

The patient made full recovery as well as radical improvement of the clinical manifestations after the administration of nitrates (b30 minutes). As soon as the patient was clinically stabilized and the enzymatic levels regained their stability, the patient was discharged. He was also given a medical appointment in the hospital 10 days later so that he could be submitted to a new evaluation (We must add that, we do not know why the patient was not studied according to international guidelines during his first cardiac evaluation: angiography study within 24 hours at least). The patient showed no symptoms whatsoever when he returned home.

However, the patient returned to the hospital before his appointment was scheduled, describing similar symptoms to those, he had previously been afflicted by, but complaining, they were more acute and persistent.

That is the reason why the patient was automatically transferred to intensive care, where he was diagnosed with Wellens' sign.

After the patient was clinically and hemodynamically stabilized, he underwent a battery of diagnostic tests, which included an angiographic study, an echocardiogram and a single-photon emission computed tomography (SPECT) study.

Interestingly enough, the patient was reported to have had 3 short syncope attacks, from which he had fully recovered. He also had several nocturnal palpitation episodes, which were diagnosed as idiopathic supraventricular tachycardia.

As far as his family clinical history is concerned, an uncle on his father's side is known to have died of sudden death at the age of 46. His father had a history of acute coronary syndrome with ECG changes confined to the anterolateral leads.

The Wellens' sign represents an evolutionary stage of ST elevation acute coronary syndrome. Today, most of the patients are classified as non-ST elevation myocardial infarction, as they will have elevated troponin levels. Some patients are classified as unstable angina. The patients have similar symptoms: severe oppressive chest pain and radiation of the pain to different segments over a short period, but they usually respond to the administration of nitrates very quickly. Electrocardiographically speaking, the patients have very characteristic patterns: T-wave symmetrical inversion, with occasionally very deep T waves in precordial derivations, especially in V3 to V4, although these characteristics may extend to all the precordial derivations.

The Wellens' sign is associated with a critical stenosis in the left anterior descending coronary artery. Before the widespread implementation of invasive cardiology and effective antithrombotic therapy, 3 of 4 patients with this ECG pattern developed a usually extensive anterior myocardial infarction within a few weeks of admission. Our patient had bypass surgery.

Breijo et al. described the pattern of short "P-R and Q-T" intervals in 2006. It is characterized by the presence of an ECG with a P-R interval lesser than 0.12 seconds and the Q-T interval lesser than 0.350 seconds and, which, in more than 80% of cases, is accompanied by syncope episodes, nocturnal tachycardia, and occasionally, by ventricular fibrillation and even sudden death.

The key to an accurate diagnosis of both dysfunctions must begin with a detailed analysis of all the symptoms reported by the patient. The ECG recording provides an almost definitive confirmation:

-    The T-wave characteristics in precordial derivations.
-    The duration of P-R and Q-T intervals.

5.1 Typical images of ECG recording (A: Crisis of myocardial infarction. B: Recovered)

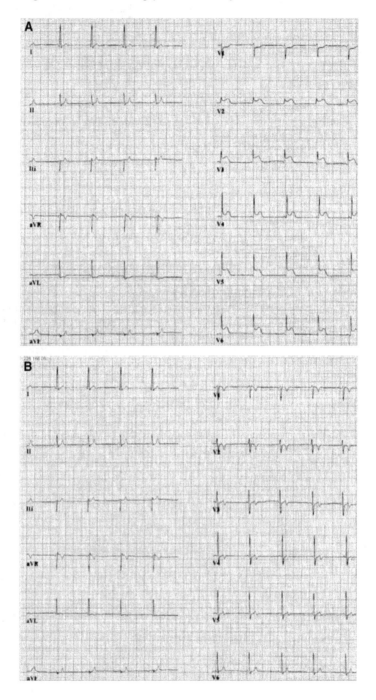

5.2 Thoughts about the patterns described above

All have a clear variation in the electrical cardiac systole.

All have a strong tendency to produce events of tachycardia / ventricular fibrillation.

Hence, all have a great capacity to produce cardiac arrest which, if not adequately diagnosed and treated, will inevitably occur sudden cardiac death.

6. Acknowledgements

To Lourdes and Alejandro Breijo, for their unselfishness collaboration from Miami. Florida. USA.
To Guadalupe Moreno Galisteo, whose smile always encouraged me to work.

7. References

Alboni P, Alboni M, Bertorelle G. (2008) The origin of vasovagal syncope: to protect the heart or to escape predation? *Clin Auton Res*, Vol.18, pp. 170-8.

Breijo Marquez, FR. Pardo Ríos, M. (2009). Variability and diversity of electrical cardiac systole. *BMJ Case Reports*, doi:10.1136/bcr.06.2008.0284.

Breijo Marquez, FR. Pardo Ríos, M. Alcaraz Baños, M. (2010). Association of Short PR Interval, Long QT Interval, and Sudden Cardiac Death in a Young Male. *Rev Esp Cardiol*, Vol. 63, pp. 362-4.

Breijo-Marquez, FR. (2008). Decrease of electrical cardiac systole. *Int J. Cardiol*, Vol. 126, pp. 36-8.

Breijo-Márquez, FR. Pardo Rios, M. (2010). Presence of a critical stenosis in left anterior descending coronary artery alongside a short "P-R" and "Q-T" pattern, in the same electrocardiographic record. *J Electrocardiology* , pp. 422-424.

Breijo-Marquez, FR. Pardo Ríos, M. (2010). Sudden cardiac death in a young adult with diagnosed with Tietze syndrome. *Rev. Esp. Dolor*, Vol. 56, pp. 321-6.

Breijo-Marquez, FR. Pardo Ríos, M. (2011). Wolff-Parkinson-White and Prolonged "Q-T" Patterns in the Same Electrocardiographic Record. *J Clinic Experiment Cardiol*, Vol. 2, pp. 118-20.

Brignole M, Alboni P, Benditt DG, Bergfeldt L, Blanc JJ, Bloch Thomsen PE, et al. (2004) Task Force on Syncope, European Society of Cardiology. Guidelines on management (diagnosis and treatment) of syncope — update 2004, *Europace*, Vol. 6, pp.467-537.

Brignole M, Gianfranchi L, Menozzi C, Raviele A, Oddone D, Lolli G, et al. (1993). Role of autonomic reflexes in syncope associated with paroxysmal atrial fibrillation. J *Am Coll Cardiol*, Vol. 22, pp 1123-9.

Consensus statement on the definition of orthostatic hypotension, pure autonomic failure, and multiple system atrophy. (1996). *J Neurol Sci*, Vol.144, pp. 218-9.

Ebert SN, Liu XK, Woosley RL. (1998). Female gender as a risk factor for drug-induced cardiac arrhythmias: evaluation of clinical and experimental evidence. J Womens Health, Vol.7, pp. 547-57.

Gibbons CH, Freeman R. (2006). Delayed orthostatic hypotension: a frequent cause of orthostatic intolerance. *Neurology*, Vol. 67, pp. 28-32.

Grubb BP, Kosinski DJ, Boehm K, Kip K. (1997). The postural orthostatic tachycardia syndrome: a neurocardiogenic variant identified during head-up tilt table testing. *Pacing Clin Electrophysiol*, Vol. 20, pp. 2205-12.

Hoefnagels WA, Padberg GW, Overweg J, Van der Velde EA, Roos RA. (1991) Transient loss of consciousness: the value of the history for distinguishing seizure from syncope. *J Neuro*, Vol. 238, pp. 39-43.

Leitch JW, Klein GJ, Yee R, Leather RA, Kim YH. (1992). Syncope associated with supraventricular tachycardia: an expression of tachycardia or vasomotor response? *Circulation*, Vol. 85, pp. 1064-71.

Lombroso CT, Lerman P. (1967). Breathholding spells (cyanotic and pallid infantile syncope). *Pediatrics*, Vol. 39, pp. 563-81.

Mathias CJ, Mallipeddi R, Bleasdale-Barr K. (1999). Symptoms associated with orthostatic hypotension in pure autonomic failure and multiple system atrophy. *J Neurol*, Vol. 246, pp. 893-8.

Naschitz J, Rosner I. (2007). Orthostatic hypotension: framework of the syndrome. *Postgrad Med J*, Vol. 83, pp. 568-74.

Podoleanu C, Maggi R, Brignole M, Croci F, Incze A, Solano A, et al. (2006). Lower limb and abdominal compression bandages prevent progressive orthostatic hypotension in the elderly. A randomized placebo-controlled study. *J Am Coll Cardiol*, Vol.48, pp. 1425-32.

Soteriades ES, Evans JC, Larson MG, Chen MH, Chen L, Benjamin EJ, Levy D. (2002). Incidence and prognosis of syncope, *N Engl J Med*, Vol. 347, pp.878-85.

Stephenson J. (1990) Fits and Faints. Oxford: Blackwell Scientific Publications. pp. 41-57.

Strickberger SA, Benson DW, Biaggioni I, Callans DJ, Cohen MI, Ellenbogen KA, et al. (2006). American Heart Association Councils on Clinical Cardiology, Cardiovascular Nursing, Cardiovascular Disease in the Young, and Stroke; Quality of Care and Outcomes Research Interdisciplinary Working Group; American College of Cardiology Foundation; Heart Rhythm Society. AHA/ACCF scientific statement on the evaluation of syncope. *J Am Coll Cardiol*, Vol. 47, pp. 473-84.

Tea SH, Mansourati J, L'Heveder G, Mabin D, Blanc JJ. (1996). New insights into the pathophysiology of carotid sinus syndrome. *Circulation*, Vol. 93, pp. 1411-6.

Thijs RD, Benditt DG, Mathias CJ, Schondorf R, Sutton R, Wieling W, et al. (2005) Unconscious confusion —a literature search for definitions of syncope and related disorders. *Clin Auton Res*, Vol .15, pp. 35-9.

Van Dijk JG, Sheldon R. (2008). Is there any point to vasovagal syncope? *Clin Auton Res*, Vol.18, pp. 167-9.

Verheyden B, Gisolf J, Beckers F, Karemaker JM, Wesseling KH, Aubert A, et al. (2007). Impact of age on the vasovagal response provoked by sublingual nitroglycerine in routine tilt testing. *Clin Sci (Lond)*, Vol.113, pp. 329-37.

Wieling W, Ganzeboom KS, Saul JP. (2004). Reflex syncope in children and adolescents. *Heart*, Vol.90, pp. 1094-100.

Wieling W, Krediet P, Van Dijk N, Linzer M, Tschakovsky M. (2007). Initial orthostatic hypotension: review of a forgotten condition. *Clin Sci (Lond)*, Vol. 112, pp.1 57-65.

Zareba W, Moss AJ, Le Cessie S, Locati EH, Robinson JL, Hall WJ, Andrews ML. (1995). Risk of cardiac events in family members of patients with Long QT syndrome. *J Am Coll Cardiol*, Vol. 26, pp.1685-91.

3

Spiral Waves, Obstacles and Cardiac Arrhythmias

Daniel Olmos-Liceaga
University of Sonora
México

1. Introduction

The propagation of electrical waves through cardiac tissue is a very important phenomenon to study since those waves activate the mechanisms for cardiac contraction, responsible to pump blood to the body. An electrical wave of excitation, called also an action potential wave, is initiated periodically at a place called the sinoatrial node, the natural pacemaker of the heart. This wave, propagates throughout the atria where it arrives at the atrioventricular node, where after some time delay, it propagates to the ventricles via the Purkinje fibers (Zaret et al., 1992). In normal conditions, this process is repeated approximately 70 to 100 times each minute and is commonly referred to as a heartbeat. The condition at which abnormal generation or propagation of excitation waves during the process described above, is termed as arrhythmia.

One of the proposed mechanisms involved in the development of certain type of arrhythmias, are spiral waves, a particular form of functional reentry (Fenton et al., 2002; Veenhuyzen et al., 2004). Spiral waves, are self sustained waves of excitation that rotate freely or around an obstacle, reactivating the same area of tissue at a higher frequency than the normal SA node would do, increasing the normal heartbeat rate. In the worst scenario, a spiral wave might break up into smaller spiral waves giving uncoordinated contractions of the heart in a phenomenon known as fibrillation. When this phenomenon occurs in the ventricles, the heart quivers and looses its strength to pump blood to the body leading to immediate cardiac arrest (Fenton et al., 2002; Zaret et al., 1992). Fibrillation, is the main cause of death in industrialized countries (Fenton et al., 2002; Priori et al., 2002; Tang et al., 2005; Zipes, 2005).

An important research area is the study of the interaction of spiral waves in cardiac tissue with obstacles. Obstacles in cardiac tissue can be partially excitable or non excitable. Examples of partially excitable obstacles are scar tissue (Starobin et al., 1996) or ionic heterogeneities (Starobin et al., 1996; Tusscher & Panfilov, 2002; Valderrábano et al., 2000), whereas examples of non excitable obstacles are arteries (Valderrábano et al., 2000) or the natural orifices in the atria (Azene et al., 2001).

It has been observed that an obstacle in cardiac tissue might act as a stabilizer of spiral wave dynamics (Davidenko et al., 1992; Ikeda et al., 1997; Kim et al., 1999; Lim et al., 2006; Pertsov et al., 1993; Valderrábano et al., 2000), as it provides a transition between meandering spiral waves (Ikeda et al., 1997) or multiple spiral waves (Shajahan et al., 2007; Valderrábano et al., 2000) into a simple rotation spiral, which is attached to the obstacle. This transition is clinically important because as it has been shown, fibrillation like activity changes to a tachycardia regime (Kim et al., 1999).

The interaction of spiral waves with obstacles and its relationship with the transition between different arrhythmic regimes has been experimentally and computationally studied by different researchers (Azene et al., 2001; Comtois & Vinet, 2005; Ikeda et al., 1997; Shajahan et al., 2007; 2009; Valderrábano et al., 2000). Valderrabano et al. (Valderrábano et al., 2000) studied in a cardiac tissue preparation the transition between ventricular fibrillation and ventricular tachycardia due to the presence of obstacles; Ikeda et al. (Ikeda et al., 1997), also considered the transition of different arrhythmic regimes due to the attachment of a spiral wave to an obstacle of minimum size. Shajahan et al. (Shajahan et al., 2007) used the Luo-Rudy and Panfilov models to study the transition of spiral turbulence to a simple rotating spiral wave due to the presence of an obstacle, which again provides a transition between different arrhythmic regimes; Xie et al. (Xie et al., 2001) presented a computational study of the effects of regional ischemia on the stability of a spiral wave; Azene et al. (Azene et al., 2001) carried out a computational study of the attachment and detachment of wavefronts to obstacles based on the Luo-Rudy model; Olmos (Olmos, 2010) studied the interaction of spiral waves in a particular case of the meandering regime, with rectangular obstacles. The aim in that work was to understand better necessary conditions in order to obtain attachment of the meandering spiral wave to the obstacle.

However, the interaction of spiral waves with obstacles and its relationship with transitions between different arrhythmic regimes, is a topic that has not been completely understood. For example, the interaction of a spiral wave in the meandering regime with an obstacle, has not previously being considered. Such interactions can be very complex (Olmos & Shizgal, 2008; Yermakova & Pertsov, 1986), and the determination of the conditions for which a meandering spiral wave attaches to an obstacle is an important endeavor. On the other hand, it has been considered that the presence of obstacles can be only of a stabilizing nature, which is not always the case. Therefore, the main objective of this work is to present a numerical study of the interaction of spiral waves with obstacles and to show the existence of different transitions due to the presence of obstacles.

By considering non-excitable and partially excitable obstacles we will show that obstacles cannot only stabilize the dynamics as shown in (Ikeda et al., 1997; Kim et al., 1999; Lim et al., 2006), but also, they can act as destabilizers. In both cases and by different mechanisms, the obstacle might act as a switch between two arrhythmic regimes, in which one is less dangerous than the other. In the case of non-excitable obstacles, it is shown that under certain conditions like the size of the obstacle, a more complex arrhythmia might appear.

To this end, this work will consist in the following sections. We start by presenting a general background about generation and propagation of action potentials (Section 2). In Section 3, we describe the model equations considered in the simulations. Then, in Section 4 the formation of a spiral wave is discussed. In the same section, we discuss the concepts of meandering and drift of spirals, which will be essential in explaining the results in this work. We follow this section by presenting the results obtained with partially excitable obstacles and non-excitable obstacles (Sections 5 and 6). We finish this work with Section 7 by presenting some conclusions, limitations and open questions in this topic.

2. Generation and propagation of an action potential

An important electrical property of atrial and ventricular cells is excitability. At rest, a ventricular cell has a transmembrane potential of about $u = -84mV$ (Beeler & Reuter, 1977), which is called the resting membrane potential (RMP). If a short time pulse of current is applied such that the new potential is below $-60mV$, the value of u will return to the RMP immediately. However, if the potential is raised above $u = -60mV$, the transmembrane potential will undergo a large excursion raising its value approximately to $28mV$, generating a peak, then a plateau and finally return to the RMP (Fig. 1). This phenomenon is called an action potential (AP) and cells with this property are called excitable cells. The value of u above which an AP is elicited, which in this case is $u \approx -60mV$, is called the threshold potential value u_{th}.

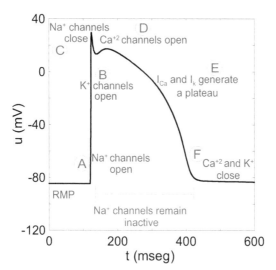

Fig. 1. Membrane potential u versus time during an AP. Representative mechanisms involved in the generation of an AP in a cardiac cell.

Changes in the membrane potential are due mainly to the passage of Na^+, K^+ and Ca^{++} ions via ion channels and other mechanisms through the cell membrane. The ion channels are membrane proteins which allow the passage across the membrane of specific type of ions between the interior and exterior of the cell. An essential part of the work by Hodgkin and Huxley (Hodgkin & Huxley, 1952) was to establish that the Na, K and Ca channels can be opened or closed, and that state depends on the membrane potential at a given time.

The general mechanism by which an AP is generated is as follows: Initially the cell is at rest i.e. the potential across the cell membrane is at the RMP value. When the current is applied such that the new potential is above u_{th}, Na channels open in a fast time scale and a flux of Na^+ inside the cell, follows (Fig. 1A). The Na current is responsible for the rapid change in u, which changes dramatically from $-60mV$ to $28mV$ in a phenomenon called depolarization. In Fig. 1B, K channels open in a slow time scale compared to the time scale of the Na channels opening, and K^+ flow outside the cell. In Fig. 1C, the Na channels close and the K^+ current lowers the membrane potential generating a peak in the AP. After that, Ca channels open in a slow time scale and a flow of Ca^{++} from outside to inside the cell occurs (Fig. 1D). During this stage, K and Ca currents move in the opposite direction, generating what is called a plateau (Fig. 1E). Finally, both channels close and the membrane potential returns to the RMP value (Fig. 1F).

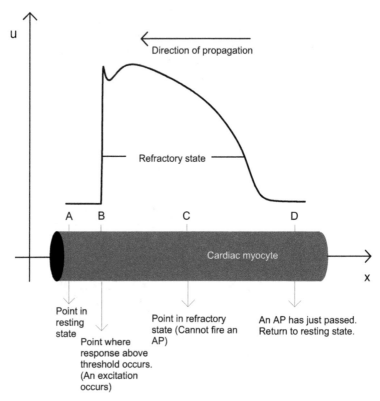

Fig. 2. Propagation of an AP. The propagation is taken over a hypothetical large myocyte.

Each location of the cell membrane, once it has a response above u_{th}, will experience an AP. The AP generated in a cell location, with the proper conditions (Kléber & Rudy, 2004), will propagate through the rest of the cell and through the cardiac tissue. The general mechanism by which an AP travels through cardiac muscle can be explained by considering a large single cell as shown in Fig. 2. In Fig. 2, it is considered that an AP is propagating only in the x direction and from right to left. At location A, the membrane potential is at the RMP value and it is ready to accept an AP. At point B, an AP has just been elicited. At point C, an AP is in process and at this location the cell is in refractory state and another AP cannot be generated. Durig this stage the Na channels, responsible for the depolarization of the cell, are closed and remain inactive for a time called the refractory period. Finally, at location D, an AP has just passed and at this location the membrane potential has almost returned to the RMP value.

Therefore, the propagation of the AP is as follows. At location B, where the AP has just been elicited, Na ions are entering to the cell. These ions generate a current in the x direction due to the concentration gradient in a neighborhood of point B. These ions move to location A, increasing its corresponding u value until it reaches u_{th}. Then, an AP is elicited at location A and the AP advances in space. Therefore, propagation of the AP follows.

3. The model equations

In order to make simulations we consider equations of the reaction-diffusion type given by

$$\frac{\partial u}{\partial t} = \nabla \cdot (D\nabla u) - \frac{1}{C_m}(I_{ion}) \tag{1}$$

where, u is the transmembrane potential, D is the conductivity tensor, C_m is the capacitance and I_{ion} is the sum of the different ionic currents. There are different forms in which I_{ion} can be chosen, depending on which cell type is considered. For example the Luo-Rudy (Luo & Rudy, 1994) or the Priebe-Beuckelmann (Priebe & Beuckelmann, 1998) models are considered for ventricular cells, whereas the Courtemanche (Courtemanche et al., 1998) and the Nygren (Nygren et al., 1998) models were developed for atrial cells. Other models are the Yanagihara model for the sinoatrial node (Yanagihara et al., 1980), and the DiFrancesco- Noble model for the Purkinje cells (DiFrancesco & Noble, 1985). A complete list of models can be found in (Fenton & Cherry, 2008).

In this work, we consider the ionic currents given by Fenton and Karma (Fenton & Karma, 1998). This set of equations is a minimal model and was designed to mimic the behavior of complex models with a minimum number of variables. The Fenton-Karma (FK) equations are of the reaction diffusion type. They are given by

$$
\begin{aligned}
\frac{\partial u}{\partial t} &= \nabla \cdot (D\nabla u) - \frac{1}{C_m}(I_{fi} + I_{so} + I_{si}) \\
\frac{\partial v}{\partial t} &= \frac{1}{\tau_v^-}\Theta(u_c - u)(1 - v) - \frac{1}{\tau_v^+}\Theta(u_c - u)v \\
\frac{\partial w}{\partial t} &= \frac{1}{\tau_w^-}\Theta(u_c - u)(1 - w) - \frac{1}{\tau_w^+}\Theta(u_c - u)w
\end{aligned}
\tag{2}
$$

where

$$
\begin{aligned}
I_{fi} &= -\frac{v}{\tau_d}\Theta(u - u_c)(1 - u)(u - u_c) \\
I_{so} &= \frac{u}{\tau_o}\Theta(u_c - u) + \frac{1}{\tau_r}\Theta(u - u_c) \\
I_{si} &= -\frac{w}{2\tau_{si}}(1 + \tanh[k(u - u_c^{si})]) \\
\tau_v^-(u) &= \Theta(u - u_v)\tau_{v1}^- + \Theta(u_v - u)\tau_{v2}^-
\end{aligned}
\tag{3}
$$

In this case, $u = u(x,t)$ measures the membrane potential at a location x and time t, whereas v and w are gate variables. I_{fi}, I_{so} and I_{si} denote fast inward, slow outward and slow inward currents, respectively. Also $D = 0.001$, $C_m = 1, \tau_d = 0.403, \tau_r = 50.0, \tau_{si} = 44.84, \tau_o = 8.3, \tau_v^+ = 3.33, \tau_{v1}^- = 1000.0, \tau_{v2}^- = 19.2, \tau_w^+ = 667.0, \tau_w^- = 11, u_c = 0.13, u_v = 0.055, u_c^{si} = 0.85$. $\Theta(x)$ is the Heaviside step function. Numerically, we consider $\Theta(x)$ as

$$\Theta(x) = \frac{1}{2}(1 + \tanh(50x))$$

Equations (2) are solved in a rectangular domain $\Omega = [-7,7] \times [-7,7]$ using finite differences with $N = 512$ points in each dimension. Advancing in time is done with Euler as in (Fenton & Karma, 1998) with $dt = 0.125$. At the domain boundary and at the boundary of non-excitable obstacles (Section 6), no-flux boundary conditions were imposed. Boundary conditions at obstacles were implemented as done in (Morton & Mayers, 2005).

4. Generation of a spiral wave

Spiral waves have been observed to occur in cardiac tissue (Ikeda et al., 1997; Isomura et al., 2008; Pertsov et al., 1993) and in computer models (Isomura et al., 2008; Olmos, 2010; Otani,

2000). There are different ways in which a spiral wave might be generated. For example, spiral waves arise when an unexcitable obstacle is stimulated with high frequency of AP (Panfilov & Kenner, 1993); they can also be generated by using the method of cross-field stimulation (Pertsov et al., 1993); and they might arise due to the appearance of ectopic beats (Otani, 2000). Ectopic beats can arise due to abnormal calcium cycling (Benson & Holden, 2005) or by overload of calcium inside the cell (Luo & Rudy, 1994).

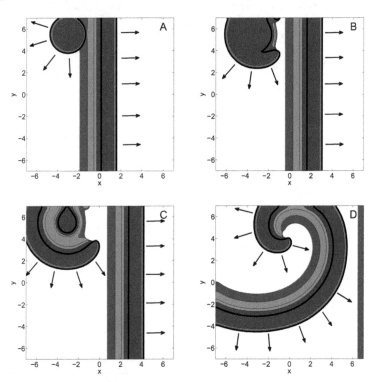

Fig. 3. Generation of a spiral wave due to ectopic activity. See text for details. The black bold line is the contour plot $u(x, y, t^*) = 0.1$. The different colored regions represent different levels of refractoriness of the medium. The region in white represents the medium completely recovered and an AP can be elicited. The region in red is a completely unexcitable region as an AP is occurring. The regions in orange and clear blue have a very low excitability level. The region in dark blue is more excitable and an AP might propagate in this region. The arrows point the direction of wave propagation. (x and y are in cm)

A particular and simple way in which the formation of a spiral wave can be explained, is shown in Fig. 3, where a solution of Eq. (2) is shown for four different integration times. In Fig. 3A, a pulse travels from left to right as shown by the direction of the arrows. After the pulse has passed, an ectopic firing appears at the back of the pulse. The ectopic firing starts propagating in all directions except at the back of the front where the region is still in refractory state (Fig. 3B). The abnormal firing generates a curved front with a free end that propagate downwards (Fig. 3C). The original AP moves to the right, disappears at the right boundary and the region that was initially in refractory state is now ready to accept another AP. Then, the free end can propagate on the recovered region generating a spiral wave (Fig. 3D). After a spiral wave has been generated, if its rotation frequency is faster than the stimulation frequency from the sinoatrial node, then the spiral wave becomes the new pacemaker of the heart (Lee, 1997).

4.1 Meandering and drift of a spiral wave

When a spiral wave evolves in excitable media in general, its dynamics are ruled by (i) the local conducting mechanisms, and; (ii) the heterogeneities of the medium. The former gives rise to a phenomenon called meandering, whereas the later to a phenomenon referred to as drift of a spiral wave.

One way to get a better understanding of meandering and drift of a spiral wave, is by studying the evolution of the position of its tip. The tip of a spiral wave can be defined in a variety of ways and a resume can be found in (Fenton et al., 2002). In this work it is considered the tip of the spiral wave as the point over the level curve $u = 0.5$ with zero normal velocity (Fenton et al., 2002).

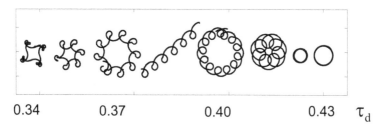

0.34   0.37   0.40   0.43 τ_d

Fig. 4. Tip trajectories of the spiral waves obtained with Eqns. (2), with $u_c = 0.13$ and varying the parameter τ_d from 0.34 to 0.43. An increase in the value τ_d implies a reduction in the excitability of the medium.

4.1.1 Meandering of a spiral wave

In Fig. 4, different tip trajectories of spiral waves corresponding to different values of τ_d are shown. The value τ_d controls the speed at which the depolarizing ions enter to the cell and is a measure of the excitability of the cell (Efimov et al., 1995; Fenton et al., 2002). An increase in the value τ_d implies a reduction in the excitability of the medium. When $\tau_d = 0.43$ the tip of the spiral wave traces a circumference. When the value of τ_d is reduced to 0.425 the radius of the circular trajectory is reduced. However, when the value of τ_d is reduced to about 0.415 the trajectory is no longer circular but a curve that resembles an epitrochoid (Fig. 5B). Decreasing the value of τ_d increases the radius R (Fig. 5B) of the epitrochoidal trajectory. For $\tau_d = 0.3965$ the value of R tends to infinity obtaining a trochoidal trajectory (Epitrochoid with $R = \infty$). For smaller values of τ_d the tip trajectory resembles an hypotrochoid of radius R (Fig. 5A). For values less than $\tau_d = 0.34$ deformations of hypotrochoidal trajectories are obtained (Fig. 4).

The phenomenon shown in Fig. 4, is called meandering of the tip trajectory or meandering. In order to understand the mechanisms behind meandering it is necessary to study the recovery regions when the spiral wave is propagating in the medium. In Fig. 6, it is shown the contour of the variable $u(x, y, t^*) = 0.1$ for a particular time t^* (Labeled bold line in Fig. 6B); Also, are shown different regions corresponding to the level of recovery of the medium, given by the variable v in Eqns. 2, plotted also for the time t^*. The region in black means that the region is

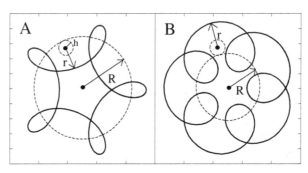

Fig. 5. (A) An hypotrochoid and; (B) an epitrochoid. From (Olmos, 2007)

completely unexcitable (v in this case is close to zero); As the region becomes clearer, the value of v gets closer to 1 and therefore the region is able to accept more easily another AP. The line in blue is the trajectory followed by the tip for a time interval around t^*.

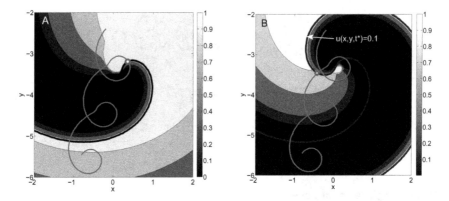

Fig. 6. Propagation of a spiral wave generated with Eqns. (2) with $\tau_d = 0.3965$. The line in blue represents the trajectory of the tip. The different coloured regions represents different levels of refractoriness given by the v variable. For v close to 0 (black), the region is in its maximum level of refractoriness and an AP cannot be elicited here. For $v \approx 1$ (white), the region is almost or totally recovered and an AP can be elicited in this region. (A) Formation of a petal; (B) Formation of an arc. The blue dot filled in white, is the location of the tip of the spiral.

In Figures 4 and 6, it is shown that the trajectory of the tip of the spiral wave has high and low curvature in an alternate and periodic fashion. The part with high curvature is referred to as a petal, whereas the part with low curvature, an arc. In Fig. 6A, the tip is tracing a petal, whereas in Fig. 6B, an arc.

In Fig. 6A, it is shown the spiral wave at the time where the tip is tracing a petal. In this case, the front that is close to the tip (blue dot filled in white) of the wave, propagates through a region that is almost completely recovered giving a maximum in the curvature of the trajectory. A different scenario occurs in Fig. 6B, where the tip is tracing an arc. Here, it is clear that the front close to the tip of the spiral propagates through a region that is not completely recovered. This causes the front to propagate in another direction, where the medium is more excitable. This deviation generates the low curvature part of the trajectory or the arc. This process occurs periodically and the trajectory shown in Fig. 6 is obtained.

In order to give an explanation about the occurrence of the different trajectories obtained in Fig. 4, we use the information of the previous paragraph and the facts that (i) $1/\tau_d$ is the speed at which the Na ions enter to the cell to depolarize it. For shorter τ_d the ions enter faster to the cell, and; (ii) from Eqns. (2), changing the value of τ_d does not affect the threshold value u_{th}. Consider the case shown in Fig. 6, where $\tau_d = 0.3965$, ie, when the tip trajectory is trochoidal. In Fig. 6A, a petal is being traced. When the value of τ_d is reduced then the flux of Na ions (In Eqns. (2), I_{fi} is carried by Na ions) is increased. Therefore, the larger amount per time unit of ions with a constant diffusion coefficient, makes that the spiral wave will trace a petal with larger curvature than in the case with $\tau_d = 0.3965$. In the same way, it will follow that the front of the spiral wave will reach its own tail before than the case with $\tau_d = 0.3965$. Therefore, it is obtained an hypotrochoidal trajectory like the one shown in Fig. 4 with $\tau_d = 0.37$. A similar argument follows for epitrochoidal trajectories.

4.1.2 Drift of a spiral wave

Drift of a spiral wave is a directed change of its location with time in response to perturbations (Biktashev, 2007). There are different ways in which drift might occur and an complete list can be found in (Biktashev, 2007). In this work we focus on two different ways in which drift occurs (Fig. 7). In Fig. 7A, it is shown the drift of a spiral wave due to the presence of inhomogeneities. Initially, we considered a spiral wave with $\tau_d = 0.43$. With this choice of τ_d, the tip of the spiral wave traces a circumference. After some integration time, we changed the value of τ_d to 0.39 for $y < 0$. The result of this change in the value of τ_d is shown in Fig. 7A. In the figure, it is observed that the tip trajectory no longer traces a circumference but a trajectory that resembles a spring. When the tip is far from the interphase $y = 0$, the trajectory traces the usual circumference. However, when the tip hits the region above $y = 0$, the curvature generated is higher than the curvature below $y = 0$ due to the decrease in τ_d. This causes a drift of the position of the center of the circumference. It follows that the trajectory moves along the line $y = 0$ where there is a difference in τ_d between the two phases.

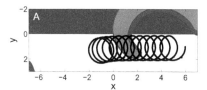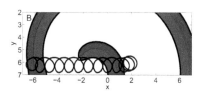

Fig. 7. Drift of a spiral wave due to (A) Inhomogeneities in the medium, and; (B) Interaction with a boundary. In (A) $\tau_d = 0.43$ for $y \geq 0$ and $\tau_d = 0.39$ for $y < 0$.

In Fig. 7B, it is shown the drift of a spiral wave due to the presence of a boundary. In this case, when a spiral wave with a circular tip trajectory gets close enough to a boundary, there is an increase in the curvature of the trajectory giving as a consequence drift of the center of the circular trajectory. Therefore, the trajectory drifts along the boundary. The physical mechanism by which the gain in curvature of the trajectory is observed, is apparently as follows: The impermeable boundary prevents the spread of the current produced by the spreading wavefront, which is equivalent to local rise in the excitability of the medium close to the boundary (Yermakova & Pertsov, 1986), and therefore an increase in the curvature of the trajectory (Subsection 4.1.1).

5. Partially excitable obstacles

Partially excitable obstacles are inhomogeneities in the tissue that originate from changes in single-cell properties such as the conductance of ion channels (Shajahan et al., 2009). Such inhomogeneities can arise from damaged or scar tissue (Starobin et al., 1996), when a lesion is created via ablation (Azene et al., 2001) or by regional hyperkalemia (Xie et al., 2001). These changes affect the propagation speed of the pulse (Kléber & Rudy, 2004), the action potential duration (Beeler & Reuter, 1977; Efimov et al., 1995; Shajahan et al., 2009) and prolongs recovery of excitability after the occurrence of an action potential (Xie et al., 2001).

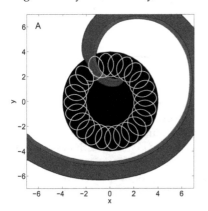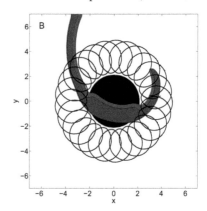

Fig. 8. Tip trajectories of spiral waves obtained with Equations (2) with a partially excitable circular obstacle (A) $\tau_d = 0.38$ outside the circular obstacle and $\tau_d = 0.43$ inside, $r = 4$; (B) $\tau_d = 0.43$ outside the obstacle and $\tau_d = 0.38$ inside, $r = \sqrt{4.5}$.

The stability of spiral waves depending on inhomogeneities in the medium has been studied by Shajahan (Shajahan et al., 2009) and Xie (Xie et al., 2001). In this work, we focus on partially excitable obstacles of circular shape. A pair of simulations are shown in Fig. 8. In Figure 8A, $\tau_d = 0.38$ outside the circular obstacle and $\tau_d = 0.43$ inside. The radius of the obstacle is $r = 4$. In the previous section, the tip of the spiral wave followed the boundary between the two regions. In Figure 8A, it is shown that the trajectory also follows such boundary, which corresponds to the boundary of the inhomogeneity. In this case, it is shown that the tip traces a curve that resembles an hypotrochoid. In the case where the value of τ_d is inverted, i.e. $\tau_d = 0.43$ outside the inhomogeneity and $\tau_d = 0.38$ inside, with a radius $r = \sqrt{4.5}$, we obtain the trajectory shown in Fig. 8B. Here, the trajectory obtained resembles an epitrochoid. This last result has been presented in (Biktashev, 2007) within a frame of drift due to inhomogeneities where inside the obstacle the refractory period is longer than outside.

Now, consider varying the radius of the obstacle. In Fig. 9 we present the results of considering the two cases presented in Fig. 8. In the top row, we show the case when the trajectory resembles a hypotrochoid. In order to obtain these trajectories, we took $\tau_d = 0.43$ inside the obstacle, such that inside the obstacle the trajectory is circular. Outside the obstacle τ_d was taken as 0.38, such that the trajectory outside is hypotrochoidal. The radius of the obstacle is increased from left to right. When the radius of the obstacle is less than the radius of the circumference traced by the tip trajectory, the trajectory is circular. As the radius of the obstacle is increased, the trajectory changes from circular to hypotrochoidal. Then, by considering an increase in the radius of the obstacle, the circular trajectory experiences a bifurcation as the one periodic rotation changes to a two period rotation. This result was reported by Mikhailov et al. (Mikhailov et al., 1994) where a circular domain with no flux boundary conditions was considered.

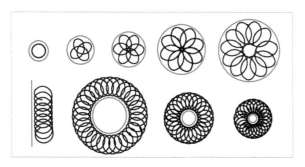

Fig. 9. Trajectories obtained with Eqns. (2) with a partially excitable circular obstacle and different radii. The red circle in each case, represents the boundary of the obstacle. Top row: $\tau_d = 0.38$ outside the circular obstacle and $\tau_d = 0.43$ inside. Circular and hypotrochoidal trajectories are obtained; Bottom row $\tau_d = 0.43$ outside the obstacle and $\tau_d = 0.38$. Epitrochoidal trajectories are obtained

In the bottom row of Fig. 9 is shown the case when the trajectory traces an epitrochoid. In this case, if we take a smaller radius, an epitrochoidal trajectory remains even by taking R tending to zero. Additionally to this result, it is also clear that by considering partially excitable obstacles it is possible to obtain the case of an epitrochoidal trajectory with $R = \infty$ and therefore a transition between the hypotrochoidal and epitrochoidal cases. Just like the case of meandering discussed in subsection 4.1.1.

The results presented in the top row of Figure 9, have a completely different meaning from those presented in (Mikhailov et al., 1994). As an example, consider the tip trajectory shown in Fig. 10, which corresponds to the upper left case shown in Fig. 9. Initially, the tip of the spiral wave is located outside of the obstacle. Because $\tau_d = 0.38$ outside the obstacle, an hypotrochoid is obtained. However, as soon as the trajectory hits the obstacle, the tip of the spiral wave gets trapped by the obstacle and the trajectory becomes circular (Fig. 10).

Therefore, in this section we have shown that heterogeneities in the conducting properties of the medium can give different results. (i) If inside the obstacle we take a value of τ_d^1 such that the tip trajectory is a circumference of radius r_1 and outside the obstacle the value of τ_d is less than $\tau_d^2 < \tau_d^1$, where τ_d^2 gives a circular trajectory with radius $r_2 < r_1$, then if the radius of the obstacle is $r \in [r_2, r_1]$ then a circular tip trajectory due to the interaction between the tip of the spiral wave and the obstacle is obtained. Clearly, this case includes the situation of having an epitrochoidal or hypotrochiodal trajectory outside the obstacle (with the values of τ_d given in Fig. 4). (ii) Under the same conditions as above but the radius r of the obstacle larger than r_1, then the trapped trajectory will trace a hypotrochoid. Observe that in this regime, we can obtain a transition from epitrochoidal (given by meandering) to hypotrochoidal trajectory

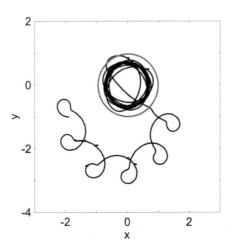

Fig. 10. $\tau_d = 0.38$ outside $\tau_d = 0.43$ inside the obstacle. The radius of the obstacle is $r = 1$. The simulation was done in the domain $\Omega = [-7,7] \times [-7,7]$, but a zoom of the region of interest is shown. x and y in cm.

(given by drift of the spiral wave). (iii) Finally, when the values of τ_d inside and outside the obstacle are reverted, what is obtained is an epitrochoidal trajectory.

It is important to observe that two periodic rotations, named epitrochoidal and hypotrochoidal trajectories, and transitions from circular to hypotrochoidal regimes, are also obtained through drift. Therefore, the presence of partially excitable obstacles in cardiac tissue may induce the existence of trajectories that mimic the meandering behavior.

6. Non-excitable obstacles

Obstacles in cardiac tissue have been modeled with regions where the zero flux condition is imposed (Azene et al., 2001; Isomura et al., 2008; Panfilov & Kenner, 1993; Shajahan et al., 2009; Starobin et al., 1996; Valderrábano et al., 2000). Arteries (Valderrábano et al., 2000) and the natural orifices in the atria, (Azene et al., 2001) are examples of this type of obstacles. Also, these obstacles can be artificially generated in experimental preparations by making cuts in the tissue (Cabo et al., 1996; Ikeda et al., 1997).

The interaction of spiral waves with non excitable obstacles has been considered by different authors (Azene et al., 2001; Ikeda et al., 1997; Isomura et al., 2008; Panfilov & Kenner, 1993; Shajahan et al., 2009; Starobin et al., 1996; Valderrábano et al., 2000). Of particular interest is the work by Ikeda (Ikeda et al., 1997), where it is observed that when a spiral wave attaches to an obstacle, a transition between two different classes of arrhythmias is observed.

In the present section we extend the results observed by Ikeda (Ikeda et al., 1997) and show that the presence of non excitable obstacles, just as the partially excitable ones, can stabilize or destabilize spiral wave dynamics. Initially, it is considered a spiral wave in the circular regime ($\tau_d = 0.426$), with a circular obstacle with radius $r = 1.7$ and center in the origin. In this regime, we placed the tip of the spiral wave near the obstacle. The result is shown in Fig. 11. In this situation, it is observed that the spiral rotates and at the same time starts moving around the obstacle. Due to the drift at an impermeable boundary plus the circular shape of the obstacle, it is observed that the tip of the spiral traces a curve very similar to an epitrochoid. Therefore, the presence of a circular obstacle, has changed the simple rotation of the spiral wave into a two periodic rotation. This phenomenon, was observed for obstacles of all sizes above mesh partition. The speed of the drift was a decreasing function of the radius.

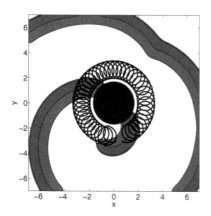

Fig. 11. Drift of a spiral wave around a circular obstacle. $\tau_d = 0.426$, radius $r = 1.7$.

In our second experiment, we considered a spiral wave in the epitrochoidal regime ($\tau_d = 0.405$). In the same way, we placed the spiral wave in such way that the tip of the spiral interacts with the obstacle. The results are shown in Fig. 12. In the figure, it is shown a spiral wave in the epitrochoidal regime interacting with the circular obstacle at different integration times. In Figs. 12A,B, it is shown that the spiral wave traces an epitrochoid. As soon as the spiral wave hits the boundary, the tip trajectory changes its direction due to the boundary effects (Olmos & Shizgal, 2008; Yermakova & Pertsov, 1986). In the figure, it is shown that the tip of the spiral wave hits the boundary four times. In the first three interactions, it is observed that the spiral bounces at the obstacle. However, in the fourth interaction it is observed that the spiral wave attaches to the obstacle (Fig. 12C). A major consequence obtained is that the two frequency rotation given by the epitrochoidal regime, changes after a transient, to a simple rotation given by the circular regime.

The change from the two rotation period to simple rotation was due to attachment of the spiral wave to the obstacle (Olmos, 2010). However, this experiment raises different questions. When the tip of the spiral hits the obstacle, why in some cases bouncing is observed and then attachment?, Does attachment always occur? Does attachment depend on the size of the radius of the obstacle?, How long it takes to a spiral to attach to the obstacle? To answer these questions is a very difficult task.

In order to show the complexity of this problem, we consider a previous analysis done in (Olmos & Shizgal, 2008). We interact the tip of spiral waves in the trochoidal regime ($R = \infty$ in Fig.5) with a flat boundary. With these settings we remove the effect of the curvature of the obstacle and the curvature of the epitrochoidal and hypotrochoidal regimes. We took initial conditions such that the trajectory had an incident angle θ_i with respect to the boundary (Fig. 13A).

When the tip of a spiral wave interacts with a boundary, there are two possible outcomes. The tip of the spiral wave bounces at the boundary as in Fig. 13A, or disappears at the boundary, in which case the spiral wave also disappears from the domain (Olmos & Shizgal, 2008). When

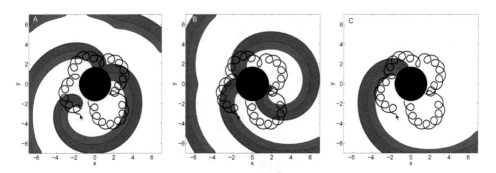

Fig. 12. Interaction of a spiral wave in the epirtrochoidal regime with a circular obstacle for different integration times. The arrow points at the place where the trajectory starts. (A) shows the trajectory of the spiral wave meandering; (B) the spiral wave hits the obstacle and bounces, and; (C) the spiral wave hits the obstacle and gets anchored. Note the difference in the frequency of excitation between (A)-(B) and (C).

considering obstacles, the effect of bouncing is the same for a boundary and for the obstacle. However, the effect of annihilation at a boundary becomes attachment of the spiral wave to the obstacle (Olmos, 2010). In Fig. 13B, we show the probability of annihilation of a spiral wave at the boundary as a function of the incident angle, following the procedure in (Olmos & Shizgal, 2008). From the figure, it is clear that for $\theta_i \in [0^o, 60^o] \bigcup [160^o, 180^o]$ the tip of the spiral wave bounces at the boundary. For $\theta_i \in (60^o, 160^o)$ in some cases, there was observed bouncing but also annihilation. As we increase the value of θ_i from 60° to 140°, there is an increase in the proportion of spiral waves that annihilate at the boundary. For $\theta_i = 140^o$ all the trajectories considered in the simulations disappeared at the boundary giving annihilation. From there, as the value of θ_i is increased up to $\theta_i = 160^o$, the proportion of spirals that bounced at the boundary increased again.

Based on the previous information, we run several examples in the epitrochoidal regime ($\tau_d = 0.405$) as the one shown in Fig. 12. We considered obstacles with three different radius, $r = 0.8$, $r = 1.1$ and $r = 1.7$. From there, we took all the cases where attachment of the spiral wave to the obstacle was obtained. It was observed from this numerical experiment that the angles at which attachment occurred, ranged from 10° to 100°. From this observation and from Fig. 13B, it is shown that for incident angles $\theta_i \in [10^o, 60^o]$, annihilation at the flat boundary is not possible, but attachment to the circular obstacle is possible.

The phenomenon of obtaining attachment for angles θ_i that in the flat boundary gave bouncing might be expected from the studies in (Leal-Soto, 2011; Olmos, 2010), where a spiral wave in the trochoidal regime interacted with the face of a square shaped obstacle. In these studies, it is shown that a spiral wave that would experience bouncing in a flat boundary, will experience attachment to the obstacle, as the interaction of the spiral wave takes place near a corner of the obstacle. Therefore, when we consider a circular obstacle, the interactions of the tip of the spiral wave with the obstacle can be thought as the interaction of the tip of a spiral with a smoothed corner of a square shaped obstacle. This explains why attachment is observed for angles less than $\theta_i = 60^o$ observed in the simulations.

Attachment to the circular obstacle was observed to happen with angles θ_i between 10° to 100°. This does not imply that attachment is not possible for θ_i outside this range of values. In fact, from the simulations, the interaction of the spiral wave with the obstacle rarely

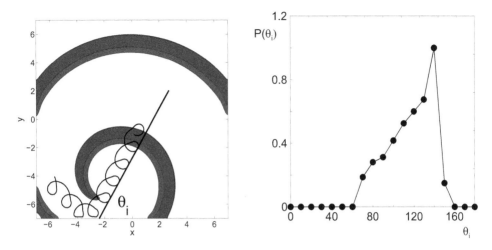

Fig. 13. (A) Interaction of a spiral wave in the trochoidal regime ($R = \infty$ in Fig. 5, $\tau_d = 0.3965$) with a boundary. θ_i is the angle of incidence. In the figure, the tip of the spiral wave bounces at the boundary. (B) Probability of annihilation of the spiral wave at the boundary for a particular angle of incidence θ_i.

occurs with angles greater than 100°. This basically happens because we are considering epitrochoidal trajectories. If we consider hypotrochoidal trajectories, then interactions will take place mostly with angles above 90°.

6.1 More complex dynamics

The interaction of a meandering spiral wave with an obstacle has different outcomes. In Fig. 14A, we show how complex dynamics can be. We took a spiral wave in the epitrochoidal regime such that the tip touches the obstacle and bounces at it. The dynamics of the tip trajectory are shown in Fig. 14A. From the figure it is clear that the trajectory hits the obstacle repeatedly following no visible pattern. As seen in the figure, there is no attachment of the spiral to the obstacle for large time integrations. Clearly, the activation of the tissue is completely irregular and might be considered as being in a fibrillatory regime.

When we consider an obstacle of a very small size, and an epitrochoidal trajectory, it is observed that the trajectory follows a more stable pattern (Fig. 14B). In this case, the trajectory gets close to the obstacle periodically and it can be said that it happens each time the trajectory traces an epitrochoid. As soon as the tip of the trajectory gets close to the obstacle, the boundary effects induce an increase in the curvature of the trajectory, producing drift of the spiral wave. It is important to note that the increase in the curvature is very small as the size of the obstacle is also very small. This small perturbation in the tip trajectory allows the trajectory to preserve the epitrochoidal trajectory as opposed in what is shown in Fig. 14A.

In this section, we have shown that obstacles might act as a switch between the one and two periodic rotations. Therefore, it follows that the presence of obstacles does not necessarily induce a more stable regime in the spiral wave. Moreover, if the spiral wave is in the epitrochoidal regime, the result might be (*i*) A transition to a simple rotation scheme; (*ii*)

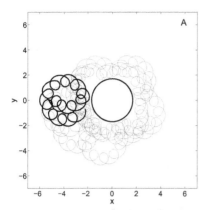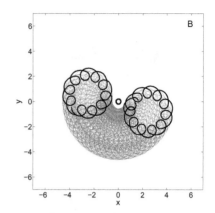

Fig. 14. Tip trajectories traced by a spiral wave solutions of Eqns. (2) when a circular obstacle is imposed. (A) The trajectory does not follow a regular pattern; (B) When the size of the obstacle is small enough a three periodic trajectory is obtained.

A transition to a more complex pattern, and; (*iii*) if the radius of the obstacle is sufficiently small, a transition to a three period rotation [1].

7. Conclusions, limitations and open questions

In this work, it was considered the interaction of spiral waves in the circular and meandering regime with partially and non excitable obstacles of circular shape. The aim was to understand the transitions that occur between three different regimes: the circular, the epitrochoidal and the hypotrochoidal. The presence of a spiral wave in the circular regime, provides a periodic stimulation of the tissue in a more stable fashion than the other two regimes, as only one excitation frequency is present. When a spiral wave attaches to an obstacle the arrhythmic regime is the same as is the tip of a spiral wave were tracing a circle.

When partially excitable obstacles were considered (Section 5), it was shown that the presence of such inhomogeneities induced the appearance of epitrochoidal and hypotrochoidal trajectories, commonly associated to meandering. This implies that epitrochoidal and hypotrochoidal trajectories might arise due to meandering or drift. It is important to point out that tip trajectories obtained with meandering, like linear trajectories (Fenton et al., 2002), were not obtained with drift. Nonetheless it is important to understand the nature of these trajectories to apply the proper procedure to remove them.

Transitions between different spiral wave regimes were obtained when an obstacle was placed in the medium (Sections 5 and 6). In Section 5, tip trajectories changed from epitrochoidal or hypotrochoidal to circular ones. Also, the reversed process might be obtained, i.e. circular trajectories can switch to epitrochoidal or hypotrochoidal trajectories. Finally, transitions from epitrochoidal to hypotrochoidal might also be obtained. On the other hand, in Section 6, it was shown that the presence of an obstacle, might act as a switch between two different arrhythmic regimes. (*i*) Simple rotating spirals changed to a two period meandering spiral wave; (*ii*) Two periodic meandering spiral waves changed to (*a*) simple rotating spiral; (*b*) Three periodic meandering spiral wave and; (*c*) More complex trajectory with no regular pattern associated.

---

[1] Strictly speaking, the trajectory is not three periodic, but there are three frequencies associated to the tip motion.

In general, it was shown that the presence of inhomogeneities in the medium not only stabilizes the spiral wave dynamics as shown in (Ikeda et al., 1997; Kim et al., 1999; Shajahan et al., 2007) but also might generate more complex dynamics, which implies that the presence of obstacles might induce a more dangerous arrhythmic regime than the one without the obstacle.

Drift of a spiral wave had been considered only for planar boundaries (Yermakova & Pertsov, 1986) and inside circular domains (Mikhailov et al., 1994). In this work, it was presented the drift of a spiral wave around a circular obstacle which was not previously reported. Up to now, there are still missing conditions for general shape obstacles that allow drift of the spiral wave around the obstacle, when the spiral tip traces a circle. A similar analysis for partially excitable obstacles is missing. i.e. which geometric properties must have an obstacle such that the tip trajectory of a spiral wave will follow its boundary?

The study of attachment of meandering spiral waves to non-excitable obstacles is a very difficult task, as there is not a clear a pattern that relates the radius of the obstacle and the radius of the epitrochoid. Also, it is still the question of studying which type of trajectory, epitrochoidal or hypotrochoidal, will attach more easily to an obstacle of a given size. In this work it was not considered the study of hypotrochoidal trajectories and non-excitable obstacles as the original study was to establish conditions to consider an obstacle as a switch between the circular and epitrochoidal regime.

8. Acknowledgements

The author would like to acknowledge ACARUS at the University of Sonora, for their facilities for the numerical computations. This work was supported by PROMEP.

9. References

Azene, E. M.; Trayanova, N. A. & Warman, E. (2001). Wave Front-obstacle interactions in cardiac tissue: a computational study. *Ann. Biomed. Eng.*, Vol. 29, No. 1, (January 2001) (35-46), 0090-6964

Beeler, G. W. & Reuter, H. (1977). Reconstruction of the action potential of ventricular myocardial fibres. *J. Physiol.*, Vol. 268, No. 1, (June 1977) (177-210) 0022-3751

Benson, A. P. & Holden, A. V. (2005). Calcium oscillations and ectopic beats in virtual ventricular myocytes and tissues: bifurcations, autorhythmicity and propagation, In: *Lecture Notes in Computer Science*, Frangi, F; Radeva P. I.; Santos A. & Hernandez, Springer, (895-897), Springer-Verlag Berlin, 3-540-26161-3, Berlin, Germany

Biktashev V. N. (2007). Drift of spiral waves. *Scholarpedia*, Vol. 2, No. 4, (2007) (1836), 1941-6016

Cabo, C.; Pertsov, A. M.; Davidenko, J. M.; Baxter, W. T.; Gray, R. A. & Jalife J. (1996). Vortex shedding as a precursor of turbulent electrical activity in cardiac muscle. *Biophys. J.*, Vol 70, No. 3, (March 1996) (1105-1111), 0006-3495

Comtois, P. & Vinet, A. (2005). Multistability of reentrant rhythms in an ionic model of a two-dimensional annulus of cardiac tissue. *Phys. Rev. E*, Vol. 72, No. 5, (November 2005) 051927(1-11), 1539-3755

Courtemanche, M.; Ramirez, R. J. & Nattel S. (1998). Ionic mechanisms underlying human atrial action potential properties: insights from a mathematical model. *Am. J. Physiol. and Heart Circ. Physiol.*, Vol. 275, No. 1, (July 1998) (H301-H321), 0363-6135

Davidenko, J. M.; Pertsov, A. V.; Salomonsz, R.; Baxter, W. & Jalife, J. (1992). Stationary and drifting spiral waves of excitation in isolated cardiac muscle. *Nature*, Vol. 355, No. 6358, (January 1992) (349-351), 0028-0836

DiFrancesco, D. & Noble, D. (1985). A model of cardiac electrical activity incorporating ionic pumps and concentration changes. *Phil. Trans. R. Soc. Lond.*, Vol. 307, No. 1133, (January 1985), (353-398), 0962-8436

Efimov, I. R.; Krinsky, V. I.; & Jalife, J. (1995). Dynamics of rotating vortices in the Beeler-Reuter model of cardiac tissue. *Chaos, Sol. and Frac.*, Vol. 5, No.3-4 (March-April 1995) (513-526), 0960-0779

Fenton, F. H. & Cherry, E. M. (2008). Models of cardiac cell. *Scholarpedia*, Vol. 3, No. 8, (2008) (1858), 1941-6016

Fenton, F. H. & Karma, A. (1998). Vortex dynamics in three-dimensional continuous myocardium with fiber rotation: Filament instability and fibrillation. *CHAOS*, Vol. 8, No. 1, (March 1998) (20-47), 1054-1500

Fenton, F. H.; Cherry, E.; Hastings, H. M. & Evans, S. J. (2002). Multiple mechanisms of spiral wave breakup in a model of cardiac electrical activity. *CHAOS*, Vol. 12, No. 3, (September 2002) (852-892), 1054-1500

Hodgkin, A. L. & Huxley, A. F. (1952). A quantitative description of membrane current and its application to conduction and excitation in nerve. *J. Physiol*, Vol. 117, (August 1952), (500-544), 0022-3751

Ikeda, T.; Yashima, M.; Uchida, T.; Hough, D.; Fishbein, M. C.; Mandel, W. J.; Chen, P. S. Karagueuzian, H. (1997). Attachment of meandering reentrant wave fronts to anatomic obstacles in the atrium - Role of the obstacle size. *Circ. Res.*, Vol. 81, No. 5, (November 1997) (753-764), 0009-7330

Isomura, A.; Hörning, M.; Agladze, K. & Yoshikawa, K. (2008). Eliminating spiral waves pinned to an anatomical obstacle in cardiac myocytes by high-frequency stimuli. *Phys. Rev. E.* Vol. 78, No. 6, (December 2008) 066216(1-6), 1539-3755

Kim, Y.; Xie, F.; Yashima, M.; Wu, T.; Valderrábano, M.; Lee, M.; Ohara, T.; Voroshilovsky, O.; Doshi, R. N.; Fishbein, M. C.; Qu, Z.; Garfinkel, A.; Weiss, J. N.; Karagueuzian, H. S. & Chen, P. (1999). Role of papillary muscle in the generation and maintenance of reentry during ventricular tachycardia and fibrillation in isolated swine right ventricle. *Circulation*, Vol. 100, No. 13, (September 1999), 1450-1459, 0009-7322

Kléber, A. G. & Rudy, Y. (2004). Basic Mechanisms of cardiac impulse propagation and associated arrhythmias. *Physiol. Rev.*, Vol. 84, No. 2, (April 2004) (431-488), 0031-9333

Leal-Soto, D. A. (2011). M. Sc. Thesis: Interacción de ondas en espiral y obstáculos en medios excitables con la ecuación de Fitzhugh-Nagumo (In Spanish). Universidad de Sonora, México.

Lee K.J. (1997) Wave Pattern Selection in an Excitable System. *Phys. Rev. Lett.* Vol. 79, No. 15, (October 1997) (2907-2910) 0031-9007

Lim, Z. Y.; Maskara, B.; Aguel, F.; Emokpae R. & Tung, L. (2006). Spiral wave attachment to millimeter-sized obstacles. *Circulation*, Vol 114, No. 20 (November 2006) (2113-2121), 0009-7322

Luo, C.-S. & Rudy, Y. (1994). A Dynamic Model of the Cardiac Ventricular Action Potential.I. Simulations of ionic currents and concentration changes. *Circ. Res.*, Vol. 74, No. 8, (June 1994) (1071-1096), 0009-7330

Luo, C.-S. & Rudy, Y. (1994). A Dynamic Model of the Cardiac Ventricular Action Potential.II. Afterdepolarizations, triggered activity, and potentiation. *Circ. Res.*, Vol. 74, No. 8, (June 1994) (1097-1113), 0009-7330

Mikhailov, A. S.; Davydov, V. A.; Zykov, V. S. (1994). Complex dynamics of spiral waves and motion of curves. *Physica D*, Vol 70, No. 1-2, (January 1994) (pages 1-39) 0167-2789

Morton K. W. & Mayers D. F. (2005). *Numerical Solution of Partial Differential Equations*, Cambridge University Press, 978-0-521-60793-0, Cambridge.

Nygren, A.; Fiset, C; Firek, L.; Clark, J. W.; Lindblad, D.S.; Clark, R. B.; Giles W. R. (1998). Mathematical Model of an Adult Human Atrial Cell: The Role of K^+ Currents in Repolarization *Circ. Res.*, Vol 82, No. 1, (January 1998) (63-81), 0009-7330

Olmos, D. (2007). Ph. D. Thesis: Pseudospectral solutions of reaction-diffusion equations that model excitable media: convergence of solutions and Applications. University of British Columbia, Canada.

Olmos, D. & Shizgal B. D. (2008). Annihilation and reflection of spiral waves at a boundary for the Beeler-Reuter model. *Phys. Rev. E*, Vol. 77, No. 3, (March 2008) (031918 1-14), 1539-3755

Olmos, D. (2010). Reflection and attachment of spirals at obstacles for the Fitzhugh-Nagumo and Beeler-Reuter models. *Phys. Rev. E*, Vol. 81, No. 4, (April 2010) 041924(1-9), 1539-3755

Otani, N. F. (2000). Mini Review: Computer Modeling in Cardiac Electrophysiology. *J. Comput. Phys.*, Vol. 161, No. 1, (June 2000) (21-34), 0021-9991

Panfilov, A. V. & Keener, J. P. (1993). Effects of high frequency stimulation on cardiac tissue with an inexcitable obstacle, *J. Theor. Biol*, Vol. 163, No. 4, (August 1993) (439-448), 0022-5193

Pertsov, A. M.; Davidenko, J. M.; Salomonsz, R.; Baxter, W. T. & Jalife, J. (1993). Spiral waves of excitation underlie reentrant activity in isolated cardiac muscle. *Circ. Res.*, Vol. 72, No. 3, (March 1993) 631-650, 0009-7330

Priebe, L. & Beuckelmann, D. J. (1998). Simulation Study of Cellular Electric Properties in Heart Failure. *Circ. Res.*, Vol. 82, No. 11 (June 1998) (1206-1223) 0009-7330

Priori, S. G.; Aliot, E.; Blømstrom-Lundqvist, C.; Bossaert, L.; Breithardt, G.; Brugada, P.; Camm, J. A.; Cappato, R.; Cobbe, S. M.; Di Mario, C.; Maron, B. J.; McKenna, W. J.; Pedersen, A. K.; Ravens U.; Schwartz, P. J.; Trusz-Gluza, M.; Vardas, P.; Wellens, H. J. J. & Zipes, D. P. (2002). Task Force on Sudden Cardiac Death, European Society of Cardiology. *Europace*, Vol. 4 (January 2002) (3-18), 1099-5129

Shajahan, T. K.; Sinha, S. & Pandit, R. (2007). Spiral-wave dynamics depend sensitively on inhomogeneities in mathematical models of ventricular tissue. *Phys. Rev. E*, Vol. 75, No. 1, (January 2007) 011929(1-8), 1539-3755

Shajahan, T. K.; Nayak, A. R. & Pandit, R. (2009) Spiral-Wave Turbulence and its Control in the Presence of Inhomogeneities in Four Mathematical Models of Cardiac Tissue. *Plos One*, Vol. 4, No. 3, (March 2009) (1-21), 1932-6203

Starobin, J. F.; Zilberter, Y. I.; Rusnak, E. M. & Starmer, C. F. (1996). Wavelet formation in excitable cardiac tissue: the role of wavefront-obstacle interactions in initiating high-frequency fibrillatory-like arrhythmias. *Biophys. J.*, Vol. 70, No. 2, (February 1996) (581-594), 0006-3495

Tang, A. S.; Ross, H.; Simpson, C. S.; Mitchell, L. B.; Dorian, P.; Goeree, R.; Hoffmaster, B.; Arnold M. & Talajic, M. (2005). Canadian cardiovascular society / Canadian heart rhythm society position paper on implantable cardioverter defibrillator use in Canada. *Can J. Cardiol*, Vol. 21, Suppl A, (May 2005) (11A-18A), 0828-282X

Ten Tusscher, K. H. W. J. & Panfilov, A. V. (2002). Reentry in heterogeneous cardiac tissue described by the Luo-Rudy ventricular action potential model. *Am J. Physiol. Heart Circ. Physiol.*, Vol. 284, No. 2, (February 2002) (H542-H548), 0363-6135

Valderrábano, M.; Kim, Y.-H.; Yashima, M.; Wu, T.-J.; Karagueuzian, H. S. & Chen, P.-S. (2000). Obstacle-induced transition from ventricular fibrillation to tachycardia in isolated swine right ventricles: Insights into the transition dynamics and implications for the critical mass. *J. Am. Col. Cardiol.*, Vol. 36, No. 6, (November 2000) (2000-2008), 0735-1097

Veenhuyzen, G. D.; Simpson, C. S. & Abdollah, H. (2004). Atrial Fibrillation. *CMAJ*, Vol. 171, No. 7, (September 2004) (755-760), 0820-3946

Xie, F.; Qu, Z.;Garfinkel A. & Weiss J. N. (2001). Effects of simulated ischemia on spiral wave stability. *Am. J. Heart Circ. Physiol.*, Vol. 280, No. 4, (April 2001) (H1667-H1673). 0363-6135

Yanagihara, K.; Noma, A. & Irisawa, H. (1980). Reconstruction of sino-atrial node pacemaker potential based on the voltage clamp experiments. *Jap. J. Physiology*, Vol. 30, No. 6, (1980) (841-857), 0021-521X

Yermakova, Y. A. & Pertsov, A. M. (1986). Interaction of rotating spiral waves with a boundary. *Biophysics*, Vol. 31, No. 5,(932-940) 0006-3509

Zaret, B. L.; Moser, M. & Cohen, L. S. (1992). *Yale University School of Medicine Heart Book*, Hearst books, 0-688-09719-7, New York.

Zipes, D. P. (2005). Epidemiology and mechanisms of sudden cardiac death. *Can J. Cardiol*, Vol. 21, Suppl A, (May 2005) (37A-40A), 0828-282X

4

Electrical Storm

Federico Guerra, Matilda Shkoza, Marco Flori and Alessandro Capucci

Cardiology Clinic, Marche Polytechnic University

Italy

1. Introduction

Electrical storm (ES) is usually defined as a clustering of destabilizing episodes of ventricular tachycardia or ventricular fibrillation in a short period of time, requiring multiple cardioversions or defibrillations. Many criteria have been proposed to define ES since the early 1990s, when the term was first introduced to indicate a state of electrical instability with several ventricular tachycardias (VT) or ventricular fibrillations (VF) over a few hours. At present an official and widespread definition of ES is not available. ES has been defined differently, from two or more to twenty or more episodes within 24 hours. Some definitions were based on number of hemodynamically unstabilizing episodes, others relied on number of shocks needed (or just delivered, whether appropriate or not), and some others on time between each single episode. More imaginative definitions include "VT recurring immediately after termination", "VT for an half of each of three days" and "VT resulting in more total ventricular ectopic beats than sinus beats in 24 hours" (Israel et al, 2007). Fortunately, nowadays most cardiologists define ES as recurrent VT or VF, at least 3 in a 24 hours period, as this is probably the most appropriate and solid definition. This definition does not include the presence of haemodynamic instability, since the intervention of modern implanted cardioverter-defibrillator (ICD) usually terminates the arrhythmia before its clinical and hemodynamical consequences.

Similarly to definitions, many names have been used as synonymous to ES, such as arrhythmic storm, recurrent short-term ventricular arrhythmia, VT clusters and electrical instability. In this chapter we will use the term ES, as the most used and widespread in clinical practice.

ES is more frequently seen as an acute complication of myocardial infarction, as a not-so-uncommon adverse event in ischemic and non ischemic dilated cardiomyopathy and in genetic arrhythmia syndromes, such as congenital long QT syndrome and Brugada syndrome. However, the highest incidence of ES is reported in heart failure patients with ICD. This incidence, which ranges from 4% to 60% according to different studies, is mainly due to two factors. First, ICD can detect the VT of VF underlying a clinical episode of dizziness, syncope or even aborted sudden cardiac death, thus making the diagnosis far easier. Second, and most important, it can effectively treat the first and second VT or VF, thus saving the patient from sudden cardiac death and making him able to withstand more arrhythmic episodes.

The current chapter will summarize the current epidemiology and diagnosis of electrical storm, as well as give some insight on current recommendation regarding pharmacological and non pharmacological treatment.

2. Epidemiology of electrical storm

2.1 Incidence of electrical storm and its different causative arrhythmias
In the last twenty years, several studies were carried out to determine the incidence of ES (table 1).

Author	Year	Definition	Population	%
Wood	1995	≥3 VT/VF ≤24 h	ICD (secondary prevention)	10
Kowey	1996	≥2 VT/VF ≤24 h	All ES patients	-
Villacastin	1996	≥2 shocks for VT	ICD (secondary prevention)	20
Fries	1997	>2 VT ≤ 1 h	ICD (secondary prevention)	60
Credner	1998	≥3 VT/VF ≤24 h	ICD (secondary prevention)	10
Nademanee	2000	≥20 VT/VF ≤24 h ≥4 VT/VF ≤1 h	All ES patients	-
Greene	2000	≥3 VT/VF ≤24 h	ICD (secondary prevention)	18
Bansch	2000	≥3 VT/VF ≤24 h	ICD (secondary prevention)	28
Exner	2001	≥3 VT/VF ≤24 h	ICD (secondary prevention)	20
Verma	2004	≥2 VT/VF ≤24 h	ICD (secondary prevention)	10
Arya	2005	≥3 VT/VF ≤24 h	ICD (30% primary prevention)	13
Brigadeau	2006	≥2 VT/VF ≤24 h	ICD (secondary prevention)	58
Honhloser	2006	≥3 VT/VF ≤24 h	ICD (secondary prevention)	23
Sesselberg	2007	≥3 VT/VF ≤24 h	ICD (primary prevention)	4
Nordbeck	2010	≥3 VT/VF ≤24 h	ICD (55% primary prevention)	7
Streinert	2011	≥3 VT/VF ≤24 h	ICD (81% primary prevention)	7

Table 1. Incidence of electrical storm according to different definitions and populations.

However, due to different definitions of ES and different populations, results vary widely. Most of the evidences come from ICD populations implanted after sustained ventricular arrhythmias, in which ES incidence ranges from 10 to 60 %. ICD recipients implanted for primary prevention, either with underlying ischemic or idiopathic dilated cardiomyopathy, have a lower incidence of ES (from 4 to 7%).

Little is known about incidence after acute myocardial injury, except that is more common in acute ST-elevation myocardial infarction (STEMI), when STEMI is associated with an important left ventricular dysfunction and when reperfusion therapy (either fibrinolysis or percutaneous angioplasty) is late or ineffective.

Similarly, exact incidence and prevalence of ES in genetic arrhythmic syndromes such as Brugada syndrome, familiar long QT syndrome, short-coupled variant of torsade de pointes and right ventricular arrhytmogenic cardiomyopathy is still unknown. Albeit they are all rare conditions, patients afflicted by genetic arrhythmic syndromes are tipically young and otherwise healthy subjects, therefore in immediate need for ES primary prevention.

More than 8 out of 10 arrhythmic episodes constituting ES are monomorphic VT (mVT), with polymorphic VT (pVT) and VF far behind in prevalence (Table 2).

Author	Year	mVT (%)	pVT+VF (%)
Credner	1998	71	29
Greene	2000	97	3
Bansch	2000	91	8
Exner	2001	86	14
Verma	2004	52	48
Brigadeau	2006	90	10
Honhloser	2006	91	9
Sesselberg	2007	78	22
Nordbeck	2010	85	15
Streinert	2011	73	27

Table 2. Prevalence of different ventricular arrhythmia types in ES.

Sustained monomorphic VT is usually related to structural heart disease. Monomorphic VT self-propagation is made possible by a reentry mechanism around a fixed anatomic barrier, which is often represented by a myocardial scar from a previous MI. The same ischemic cardiomyopathy, as it progresses, leads to fibrosis which in turn leads to conduction slowdowns, creating the perfect pathway for reentrant VT. In this particular setting an otherwise harmless trigger such as a premature ventricular contraction is necessary to start monomorphic VT. Monomorphic reentrant VT does not require active ischemia as a trigger, and is an uncommon cause of ES in acute myocardial infarction.

VF and pVT are due to different mechanisms, comprehending multiple activation of different ventricular foci (pVT) or chaotic activation of the whole endocardial ventricular surface (VF). These two arrhythmias are more common in acute myocardial infraction or when a long QT interval is present. Therefore QT interval should be assessed in all patients with ES due to pVT or VF as soon as sinus rhythm has been restored. Acquired causes of long QT, such as hypokalemia, hypocalcemia, hypomagnesemia, hypothyroidism and medication known to prolong QT interval, should be corrected as soon as possible. Inherited causes of long QT should be suspected whether an acquired cause cannot be found.

2.2 Short and long-term prognosis of electrical storm

Available data strongly suggest that patients who experience an ES have a poor outcome. Only a few trials were inconclusive regarding the role of ES as a mortality marker, and those usually had a wider definition of ES or a shorter follow-up. In secondary prevention populations such as the one of the AVID trial (Exner et al, 2001), patients with ES had a higher risk for non-sudden cardiac death (OR 2.4). In a substudy of the MADIT-II trial, which enrolled primary prevention patients, the risk of death was even higher (OR 7.4). Consistent findings suggest that the increase in mortality is mainly due to the worsening of ventricular dysfunction leading to end stage heart failure, with only a small proportion of sudden cardiac or other deaths (Gatzoulis et al, 2005). This hypothesis is also supported by the fact that risk of death after ES reaches its peak around 2-3 months after the acute event.

Another main clinical consequence of ES is hospitalization, which is required for a proper treatment in approximately 80% of patients (Bänsch et al, 2000). Hospitalization rates grow higher with each shock delivered, reaching 100% if 3 or more shocks are needed. Hospitalization is in turn associated with a poorer quality of life and higher costs.

Patients who experience an ES are more likely to have multiple ES over time. Recent data showed that recurrence of ES happens in more than half of all patients with ES, and is more common within the first year after the original ES episode (Streitner et al, 2011).

2.3 Pseudo-storm

Sometimes multiple recurrent ICD discharges are not associated with ES but are due to device malfunctioning. Pseudo-storm is defined as recurrent inappropriate ICD discharges over 24 hours. Far from being a minor complication, pseudo-storm is usually physical and psychological harmful and potentially lethal. The most common causes of inappropriate ICD shock include supraventricular tachycardia with high ventricular response and oversening of peaked T waves, myopotentials or electrical noise (Gradaus et al, 2003).

Recurrent ICD shocks can cause myocardial injury by direct electrocution cell injury and by activation of signaling pathways in the molecular cascade of HF, the most important of all being adrenergic neurohormonal system. Adrenergic iperactivity may then synergize with recurrent ventricular arrhythmias in exacerbating ventricular dysfunction and worsening heart failure. In a recent paper on a typical ICD population, Sweeney et al. demonstrated that electrical shocks were associated with an increased risk of death independently of underlying ventricular arrhythmia (Sweeney et al, 2010). Authors esteemed that for every delivered shock, whether appropriate or not, the risk of death increases by 20%. On the other hand, no increased risk was associated with anti-tachycardia pacing (ATP) therapies. Pseudo-storm does not only cause myocardial damage, but can deplete a full device battery within hours, potentially leaving the patient unprotected from life-threatening arrhythmic events. Although a very rare complication, fatal arrhythmias actively caused by pseudo-storm are possible. Messali and coworkers described a patient who, three months after an ICD replacement, received six consecutive shocks related to detection of noise interpreted as VF. Unfortunately, the sixth shock triggered a true VF, which was not treated due to the end of the therapeutic sequence, and which led to the patient's death (Messali et al, 2004).

Pseudo-storm should be treated by immediate intervention to suppress ICD shocks. Moreover, inappropriate discharges from ICD should be avoided at all cost by an optimal device programming. ATP therapy should be preferred over shock in the therapeutic sequence, due to its more favorable risk profile.

3. Clinical presentation of electrical storm

3.1 Electrical storm in acute myocardial infarction

Electrical storm, when present, is often the initial manifestation of ischemia and usually starts in the first 48 hours of an ST-elevation MI. In that case, pVT is almost always the ventricular arrhythmia underlying ES. Ischemia and adrenergic activation increase Purkinje cell automaticity, thus letting multiple spontaneous firing. Necrosis, altered myocite membrane potential, electrolytic imbalance and even reperfusion damage can all contribute to increase dispersion of refractory periods between epicardium and endocardium, thus facilitating the propagation of multiple reentry waves.

ES is a strong negative prognostic factor in acute myocardial infarction. In one study where ES was defined as ≥20 VT or VF episodes/day or ≥4 VT/VF episodes/hour, one-week incidence of non-sudden death was as high as 50%. The majority of patients who survived the acute phase, however, have a prognosis relatively comparable with other ES populations. Along with pharmacological therapy, swift and effective reperfusion is crucial to end arrhythmic episodes. Retrospective studies and registry data suggest the hypothesis that, with modern reperfusion therapy currently available, the incidence of ES could be associated with reperfusion time.

3.2 Electrical storm in heart failure

Heart failure is an important risk factor for ES. Most of the times, idiopathic dilated cardiomyopathy is the structural heart disease underlying heart failure in ES patients, followed in prevalence by ischemic cardiomyopathy (Gasparini et al, 2008). Hypertrophic cardiomyopathy and valvular cardiomyopathy, albeit uncommon, has been associated with heart failure worsening leading to ES (Credner et al, 1998).

Left ventricular ejection fraction (LVEF) is the most widespread and easy to obtain marker of systolic dysfunction and has been used to test the association between heart failure and ES. Several studies have found an altered LVEF as an independent risk factor for ES, along with older age, chronic renal failure, causative arrhythmia and electrolytic imbalances (Exner et al, 2001 and Brigadeau et al, 2006). On the other hand, Streitner and coworkers found that a LVEF lower than 30% was not predictive for the initial ES event, but brought a 2.2-fold increased risk for ES recurrence (Streitner et al, 2011).

Current evidence suggests that, more than the presence or absence of heart failure by itself, it is the progression of heart failure and structural cardiomyopathy the real factor in promoting ES and ES recurrence. Therefore, prevention of further systolic function deterioration after an initial ES is mandatory and must be achieved through optimization of medical and resynchronization therapy.

3.3 Electrical storm in patients with congenital pro-arrhythmic diseases

Genetic arrhythmic syndromes or inherited arrhythmic disorders comprise a group of syndromes with unique genetic abnormalities and presentations but with very similar clinical outcomes, the most terrifying of which are life-threatening arrhythmias and sudden cardiac death. Some of them, such as Brugada syndrome and long QT syndrome, affect structural normal hearts, whereas others, such as arrhythmogenic right ventricular cardiomyopathy and left ventricular non-compaction affect deeply the myocardial tissue, and are included in the cardiomyopathies classification. ES has been described in the Brugada syndrome, in the familiar long QT syndrome, in the short-coupled variant of torsade de pointes, in catecholaminergic polymorphic ventricular tachycardia, in arrhythmogenic right ventricular cardiomyopathy and in myocardial non-compaction. Overall, these syndromes are quite rare, being Brugada syndrome the most prevalent with 5 cases out of 10.000, and association with ES in even rarer. However, patients affected by these syndromes are typically young and otherwise completely healthy, making diagnosis and treatment of these conditions challenging.

4. Laboratory and electrical storm

Although electrolytic imbalances, such as hypokalemia, hyperkalemia and hypomagnesemia are a well known risk factors for ventricular arrhythmias and hence ES, many papers report that an evident trigger in a majority of patients cannot be identified by laboratory alone. Credner et al. underlined the presence of hypokalemia, along with acute coronary syndrome and worsening heart failure as potential triggers in 26% of the patients in his case-records (Credner et al, 1998). Similarly, Bänsch et al. found hypokalemia as a potential cause of ES in 20% of their cohort. According to the SHIELD trial, electrolytic imbalance was responsible for storm triggering in only 4% of patients (Hohnloser et al, 2006).

In 2006 for the first time Brigadeau et al. highlighted a possible role of creatinine in predicting ES, identifying a storm trigger in 36% of the whole cohort. Among most common triggers (such as acute coronary syndrome, high body temperature, hypokalemia or hyperkalemia, hyperthyroidism and acute heart failure) chronic renal failure, identified as a creatinine clearance lower than 60 ml/min, was independently associated with ES occurrence. Thus, this study concluded that the patients with a defibrillator who are likely to undergo electrical storm are those who have both low left ventricular ejection fraction and chronic renal failure (Brigadeau et al, 2006). In a recent MADIT II chronic kidney disease was associated with a 2.1–fold increase in risk for ES in both primary and secondary prevention patient (Sesselberg et al., 2007).

Thyroid disorders (both hypothyroidism and hyperthyroidism) have been suggested as a trigger for ES. However, at present there is scarce evidence of an important role of thyroid hormones in ventricular arrhythmias pathogenesis. In one case report ES was attributed to amiodarone-induced thyrotoxicosis (Marketou et al, 2001). The patient was unresponsive to medical therapy and the ES was successfully terminated by thyroidectomy.

In conclusion, in an ES setting laboratory could play an important role. Electrolytic abnormalities such as hypokalemia, hyperkalemia and hypomagnesemia should be promptly diagnosed and corrected, as potential triggers of arrhythmic events. High serum levels of BNP, creatinine and PCR are valid markers for respectively decompensated heart failure, chronic renal insufficiency and pro-inflammatory state, and should be assessed in every patients experiencing ES as useful stratification tools.

5. Electrical storm therapy

5.1 Pharmacological therapy
5.1.1 Amiodarone

Amiodarone is widely used in the treatment of ventricular arrhythmias. Intravenous amiodarone appears to be the most effective agent for ES, and may even suppress ventricular tachycardia that recurs despite chronic oral amiodarone therapy. In acute ES, a rapid intravenous amiodarone administration (300 mg or 5 mg/kg rapid push followed by repeated boluses at half the above doses for breakthrough episodes) blocks fast sodium channels in a use-dependent fashion (producing more channel blockade at faster heart rates), inhibits norepinephrine release, and blocks L-type calcium channels without prolonging ventricular refractoriness. On the other hand, prolonged ventricular refractory periods are seen in oral amiodarone therapy over periods ranging from days to weeks. Amiodarone has few negative inotropic effects and is safe in patients who have depressed systolic function. It is in fact the only anti-arrhythmic drug with solid safety evidences in patients with NYHA class III and IV or recently decompensated heart failure. Moreover, the incidence of torsades de pointes is low in such patients despite the potential significant prolongation of the QT interval. Amiodarone efficacy in terminating ES is approximately 60%. When compared with placebo in the ARREST trial, amiodarone improved survival to hospital admission in patients who had a cardiac arrest that involved VF or pulseless VT (Kudenchuk et al, 1999). Amiodarone can be effective even when other agents have been ineffective. Levine and colleagues examined 273 hospitalized patients who had electrical storm that was refractory to lidocaine, procainamide, and bretylium therapy (Levine et al, 1996). When amiodarone was given, 46% of the patients survived for 24 hours without another episode of VT, and another 12% improved after taking amiodarone plus lidocaine or procainamide. Side effects of short-term amiodarone intravenous use are rare. A combination of intravenous amiodarone and propranolol improves survival rates and should be the mainstay of therapy in acute management of ES.

Oral amiodarone is effective as adjunctive therapy to prevent recurrent ICD shocks. The OPTIC (Optimal Pharmacological Therapy in Implantable Cardioverter) study compared amiodarone (200 mg maintenance dose following 6 weeks of loading) plus β-blocker with sotalol (240 mg adjusted for renal function) or β-blocker alone (Connolly et al, 2006). Appropriate shocks were reduced by amiodarone compared with β-blocker therapy only by 70%, inappropriate shocks were reduced by 78%, appropriate shocks and ATP were reduced by 70%, and all-cause shocks excluding the first 21 days were reduced by 82%. The mean number of shocks per year was 4.32 in the beta-blocker only group, 0.93 in the sotalol group, and 0.51 in the amiodarone group. Although long-term amiodarone therapy is usually successful, substantial side effects include pulmonary fibrosis, hypothyroidism, liver toxicity, and corneal deposits. In addition, amiodarone may increase the energy required for successful defibrillation, so patients with ICDs should undergo repeated defibrillation threshold testing. Patients who have episodes of electrical storm despite amiodarone therapy may benefit from β-blockers adjunctive therapy or undergo RF ablation.

5.1.2 β-blockers

β-blockers play a key role in the management of electrical storm. Their effects were discovered in the 1970s, when they were studied as therapy for acute MI. First evidences regarding a possible role as anti-arrhythmic drugs come from canine models (Anderson et al, 1983). All β-blockers increased 6-fold the fibrillation threshold and made the animals less susceptible to fibrillation under ischemic and non-ischemic conditions. The improvement was greater with the use of more potent β-blockers and with those that antagonized both β1 and β2 receptors. Although several β-blockers decrease susceptibility to VF, most of the studies have focused on propranolol. Propranolol consistently decreases the incidences of fatal VF during acute MI and sudden cardiac death after MI (Tsagalou et al, 2005). In patients with congestive heart failure, propranolol decreases sympathetic outflow more than does metoprolol, perhaps because β2 receptors prevail in failing hearts (Newton et al, 1996). The lipophilic nature of propranolol enables active penetration of the central nervous system and the blockade of central and prejunctional receptors in addition to peripheral β receptors. Propranolol may effectively suppress an electrical storm even when metoprolol has failed (Tsagalou et al, 2005). Therefore, propranolol, given at a dose of 0.15 mg/kg intravenous bolus over 10 minutes followed by a 3-5 mg dose every 6 hours, is a first line therapy in emergency ES setting. Nademanee and coworkers investigated the efficacy of sympathetic blockade in electrical storm comparing propranolol, esmolol, and left stellate ganglionic blockade to combined lidocaine, procainamide, and bretylium therapy (Nademanee et al, 2000). All their patients have experienced a recent MI and more than 20 episodes of VT within 24 hours or more than 4 episodes per hour. Sympathetic blockade provided a marked survival advantage (78% versus 18% at one week, and 67% versus 5% at one year). Despite the high doses of propranolol, an increase in heart failure progression was not reported in this study, although it is known from previous studies that propranolol can exacerbate heart failure in patients with poor systolic function and use in these patients should be carefully monitored. The short acting intravenous esmolol may also be used but its dosing and titration are somewhat more complicated. Miwa et al. have demonstrated that landiolol, an ultra-short acting β1-selective blocker is useful as a life-saving drug for amiodarone-resistant ES (Miwa et al, 2010). Landiolol in ES is used intravenously with an initial dose of 2.5 μg/kg*min, which can be doubled every 10 minutes if first dose is ineffective, up to a maximum dose of 80 μg/kg*min. Landiolol has a shorter plasma half-life (4 minutes) than esmolol (9 minutes) or propanolol (2 hours) and higher β1 selectivity. These properties suggest that adverse respiratory effects, such as bronchial asma, are less likely to develop and to persist with landiolol, which make it more suitable for emergency medical care. When amiodarone was ineffective, landiolol inhibited ES in 33 patients (79%) at a mean dose of 7.5 μg/kg*min. All patients in whom landiolol was ineffective died of arrhythmia. Of the 33 patients in whom landiolol was effective, 25 survived and were discharged (60% of all patients). At present, landiolol is not available in most European countries and its safety profile in ES still needs to be assessed, making this drug a promising alternative to propranolol when amiodarone alone is ineffective.

5.1.3 Lidocaine

Intravenous sodium-channel blockers (lidocaine, procainamide) are minimally effective in suppressing shock-resistant VT/VF and ES (Credner et al, 1996 and Nademanee et al, 2000). Lidocaine binds to fast sodium channels in a use-dependent fashion. Binding increases under cellular conditions that are common in ischemic VT, such as reduced pH, faster stimulation rate and reduced membrane potential. However, lidocaine has relatively weak antiarrhythmic properties outside the ischemic setting: conversion rates from VT to sinus rhythm range from 8% to 30%. In one study enrolling patients with out-of-hospital, shock-resistant VT or VF, only 12% of those randomized to lidocaine survived to hospital admission, versus 23% who received amiodarone. On the basis of this and other findings, amiodarone has replaced lidocaine as first line therapy for refractory VT and VF. Actual recommendations suggest intravenous lidocaine only in the treatment of polymorphic VT associated with acute ischemia. If lidocaine is used, it should be administered as an intravenous bolus of 0.5 to 0.75 mg/kg that is repeated every 5 to 10 min as needed. A continuous intravenous infusion of 1 to 4 mg/min maintains therapeutic levels. The maximum total dose is 3 mg/kg over 1 hr.

5.1.4 Procainamide
Procainamide blocks fast sodium channels in a use-dependent fashion and is metabolized to N-acetylprocainamide, which in turn blocks potassium channels and accounts for much of the antiarrhythmic effect in vivo. When given as a loading dose of 100 mg over 5 min, procainamide is a reasonable choice for terminating monomorphic VT. In patients with depressed systolic function procainamide can cause hypotension or prolong QRS width by more than 50%, either of which would necessitate discontinuation of the drug. Procainamide prolongs the QT interval and therefore could cause torsade de pointes. Its use is contraindicated in patients with impaired renal function, because N-acetylprocainamide is excreted by the kidneys.

5.1.5 Azimilide
Azimilide is an experimental class III antiarrhythmic drug that blocks calcium channels and prolongs the energy potential and refractory periods. The recently published SHIELD trial showed that azimilide is effective and helps to reduce the number of ICD discharges, though not mortality (Stefan et al, 2006). A secondary analysis of the SHIELD data found that during a prospective one-year follow up azimilide significantly reduced the incidence of ES in comparison with placebo. Azimilide could become an alternative for the treatment of ES whenever it becomes commercially available.

5.1.6 Polypharmacological approach
Optimization of β-blocker therapy is the first important step, particularly when the electrical storm is triggered by ischemia or increased sympathetic tone. The next step is initiating anti-arrhythmic therapy if patient still experiences ES. In the absence of contraindications (such as QT lengthening or polymorphic ventricular tachycardia), amiodarone is generally the antiarrhythmic drug of choice and has been validated in numerous clinical trials (Kowey et al, 1995 and Wood et al, 1995). Most of the time, optimized β-blocker therapy plus intravenous amiodarone will control the electrical storm within 24 to 48 hours. This appears to be the most effective therapy for electrical storm. If the intravenous combination of amiodarone and β-blockers proves inefficacious, the addition of lidocaine is a reasonable option. Although controlled data are not available, combination of anti-arrhythmic drug allows lower and better tolerated doses of individual drugs, and offers the potential of synergistic effects.

5.1.7 Sedation
The physical and emotional stress that patients experience in association with electrical storm and multiple electrical cardioversions increases adrenergic tone and often perpetuates

arrhythmias. All patients who have electrical storm should be sedated. Sedation or general anesthesia are needed in resistant cases where repeated shocks or anti-tachicardia transthoracic pacing are needed. Short-acting anesthetics such as propofol, benzodiazepines, and some agents of general anesthesia have been associated with the conversion and suppression of VT (Burjorjee & Milne, 2002). Left stellate ganglion blockade and thoracic epidural anesthesia have also suppressed electrical storms that were refractory to multiple antiarrhythmic agents and β blockade (Nademanee et al, 2000). These therapeutic approaches directly target nerve fibers that innervate the myocardium, and a reduced adrenergic tone is most likely responsible for the reported efficacy. Is currently unknown whether sedative and anesthetic agents may have direct antiarrhythmic effects.

5.2 Implantable defibrillators: First-line therapy and first-line diagnostic?

ES is quite common in ICD recipients. In different studies the incidence of ES in patients with an ICD ranges from 10 to 60% when ICDs are implanted for secondary prevention (Arya A et al, 2005) and 4% to 7% when ICDs are implanted for primary prevention (Sesselberg et al, 2007). A higher incidence of ES in ICD patients is related to an higher cardiovascular mortality and morbidity among ICD recipients. As previously said the presence of ICD allows the physician to recognize more arrhythmias and the patient to survive the arrhythmia and hence manifest more episodes.

Occurrence of ES after ICD implant has changed over time. A paper from the late 1990s reported the peak of incidence of ES between 4 and 5 months after implant (Credner et al, 1998). On the other hand recent evidences pushed the onset of ES to 26 months after implant (Streitner et al, 2011). Total number of episodes varied over time too: as much as 55 mean episodes per patient have been reported (Greene et al, 2000), whereas more recent papers describe far less VT/VF per single patient (Streitner et al, 2011). Both these findings could be explained by changes in antiarrhythmic therapy and ICD technology occurred in this last decade which in turn led to fewer total arrhythmic episodes and improved overall prognosis.

There is a multitude of etiologies of ES in ICD patients: hypokalemia or other electrolytic imbalance, drugs (diuretics, b-adrenergic drugs, alcohol), ischemia, medication noncompliance and less common causes such as fever or stress (Huang et al, 2005 and Israel et al, 2007). The most common cause of ES in ICD patients is exacerbation of heart failure, as underlying ischemic or idiopathic dilated cardiomyopathy could progress despite medical therapy and arrhythmic prevention. Nevertheless, most ES have no clear etiology and even an exhaustive search for acute cause may prove fruitless.

Clinical presentation can vary dramatically depending on arrhythmias typology (monomorphic VT, polymorphic VT or VF) and patient's characteristics (EF, NYHA class, comorbidities). The presence of syncope associated with arrhythmia depends both on hemodynamic factors and on ICD settings (mostly shock charging time). The most important acute consequence related to ES is hospitalization that is required in more than 80% of patients, particularly when shocks are delivered (Bansch et al, 2000). ICD patients presenting ES have higher morbidity and mortality, hence determination of predictors is needed to identify high risk patients.

Data on risk factors of ES are far from comprehensive or conclusive but most studies consider low EF and secondary prevention as major risk factors for developing ES in ICD recipients. High NT-proBNP and hs-CRP, history of atrial fibrillation before implant or single/dual chamber pacing over CRT are also described as predisposing to ES (Streitner et al, 2011).

ICD patients who experienced a first ES are also more likely to experience one or more ES recurrence. Recurrence rate is as high as 80% within 12 months after the first episode, according to Steinert, who described LVEF < 30%, age > 65 years, chronic obstructive pulmonary disease and lack of ACE inhibitors therapy as independent predictors of ES recurrence (Steinert et al, 2011).

Most authors report poor prognosis associated whit ES with a risk of death increased from 1.9 to 17.8 fold. Death rate is usually low during hospitalization and acute episode but increases afterward, particularly during the first year after ES.

Lately, new tools have become available to detect and manage ES in ICD patients. All major ICD companies now offer some sort of home or remote monitoring along with their devices. Home monitoring offers the physician reports for arrhythmic events, device battery and parameters status in real-time. Asymptomatic or lightly symptomatic ES could be then promptly recognized and the patient immediately called in for a check-up without the need to wait for the next programmed ambulatory visit. Figure 1 shows how an ES looks like on auto-generated home monitoring report: the patient experienced 37 arrhythmic episodes in less than 24 hours, 36 VT terminated with a shock after ATP sequence was ineffective and 1 VF episode terminated with ATP.

Figure 2 shows how EGM can be seen and interpreted via remote monitoring. In this EGM VT has been correctly detected and treated by ICD shock.

5.3 Is cardiac resynchronization therapy useful in preventing electrical storm?

Cardiac resynchronization therapy (CRT) is a well established therapy for treatment of moderate to severe heart failure. Several studies assessed benefits from biventricular pacing resulting in prevention of left ventricular remodeling and improvement of hemodynamic, ejection fraction, NYHA class, quality of life, morbidity and mortality (Cleeland et al, 2005). Effects of CRT on ventricular arrhythmias are less well established. Some evidence suggests that pacing itself might cause arrhythmias and some authors reported an increase in incidence of atrial fibrillations, ventricular arrhythmias or even electrical storms after biventricular pacing (Kantharia et al, 2006). However, currently available large-scale trials showed no significant proarrhythmic effects of CRT. On the other hand, there is no strong evidence of a direct antiarrhythmic effect of CRT over single or dual chamber pacing either. Nordbeck et al. compared incidence of ES in 168 CRT and 561 ICD patients. They found significant lower incidence of ES in CRT group (0.6% versus 7%), suggesting that, beside the well known hemodynamic improvements, cardiac resynchronization therapy may reduce the arrhythmia burden in heart failure patients (Nordbeck et al, 2010). An Italian group found a higher incidence of ES (11.3% vs 5.3%) in patients non responder to CRT therapy, defined as minor improvement in NYHA class and ejection fraction (Gasparini et al, 2008). These data support the hypothesis that CRT may have an indirect antiarrhythmic effect, due to factors which are still unclear. Nordbeck suggests that the reduction of arrhythmic burden could be due to improvement of cardiac output and ejection fraction from CRT, as ejection fraction is a known risk factor for ventricular arrhythmias. Another hypothesis by Kowal found some evidences in clinical cases reporting a specific role of cardiac pacing site in development or suppression of VT. He hypothesized that the mechanism of arrhythmia suppression under biventricular pacing could be ascribed to preexcitation of the area of slow conduction responsible for the reentrant arrhythmia (Kowal et al, 2004).

Nevertheless, electrophysiologic effects of CRT are still poorly understood. Biventricular pacing remains a major therapeutic tool in the treatment of heart failure but additional data are required to assess its efficacy as antiarrhythmic therapy.

To:		
Report	Patient ID: **S** **P**	
from 28-Jul-2011	Device / Device SN:	Patient device SN:
11:45	**Lumax 300 HF-T / 60462319**	46817123

Recordings

Recordings - Episode list:

No.	Detection time	Type	Details	Predetection PP/RR	Pretermination PP/RR
84	29-Apr-2011 10:41:41	VT1	ATP: 3; Shocks delivered: 1	772 / 390	835 / 668
83	29-Apr-2011 10:37:42	VT1	ATP: 3; Shocks delivered: 1	772 / 387	816 / 719
82	29-Apr-2011 10:14:07	VT1	ATP: 3; Shocks delivered: 1	773 / 387	845 / 763
81	29-Apr-2011 10:06:14	VT1	ATP: 3; Shocks delivered: 1	770 / 387	922 / 998
80	29-Apr-2011 10:01:45	VT1	ATP: 3; Shocks delivered: 1	787 / 394	795 / 785
79	29-Apr-2011 09:51:22	VT1	ATP: 3; Shocks delivered: 1	787 / 393	801 / 823
78	29-Apr-2011 09:49:28	VF	ATP: 1; ATP One Shot: YES; Shocks aborted: 1	> 1998 / 271	599 / 553
77	29-Apr-2011 09:47:14	VT1	ATP: 3; Shocks delivered: 1	889 / 390	663 / 646
76	29-Apr-2011 09:41:47	VT1	ATP: 3; Shocks delivered: 1	784 / 383	695 / 880
75	29-Apr-2011 09:34:03	VT1	ATP: 3; Shocks delivered: 1	662 / 383	1409 / 917
74	29-Apr-2011 09:20:11	VT1	ATP: 3; Shocks delivered: 1	853 / 379	437 / 654
73	29-Apr-2011 09:04:47	VT1	ATP: 3; Shocks delivered: 1	582 / 387	1049 / 797
72	29-Apr-2011 08:50:27	VT1	ATP: 3; Shocks delivered: 1	786 / 393	> 1998 / 922
71	29-Apr-2011 08:27:16	VT1	ATP: 3; Shocks delivered: 1	672 / 390	555 / 898
70	29-Apr-2011 08:23:31	VT1	ATP: 3; Shocks delivered: 1	638 / 392	1244 / 915
69	29-Apr-2011 08:10:59	VT1	ATP: 3; Shocks delivered: 1	685 / 395	601 / 554
68	29-Apr-2011 06:46:20	VT1	ATP: 3; Shocks delivered: 1	751 / 374	931 / 804
67	29-Apr-2011 06:00:11	VT1	ATP: 3; Shocks delivered: 1	1008 / 405	1225 / 976
66	29-Apr-2011 05:30:13	VT1	ATP: 3; Shocks delivered: 1	784 / 390	566 / 851
65	29-Apr-2011 05:19:23	VT1	ATP: 3; Shocks delivered: 1	690 / 384	727 / 856
63	29-Apr-2011 04:52:44	VT1	ATP: 3; Shocks delivered: 1	766 / 383	1310 / 842
62	28-Apr-2011 23:59:30	VT1	ATP: 3; Shocks delivered: 1	588 / 386	584 / 598
61	28-Apr-2011 22:08:25	VT1	ATP: 3; Shocks delivered: 1	525 / 387	> 1998 / 747
60	28-Apr-2011 20:56:48	VT1	ATP: 3; Shocks delivered: 1	872 / 387	> 1998 / 868
59	28-Apr-2011 19:44:17	VT1	ATP: 3; Shocks delivered: 1	649 / 396	754 / 703
58	28-Apr-2011 19:16:43	VT1	ATP: 3; Shocks delivered: 1	677 / 387	655 / 740
57	28-Apr-2011 19:10:38	VT1	ATP: 3; Shocks delivered: 1	758 / 397	475 / 896
56	28-Apr-2011 19:06:48	VT1	ATP: 3; Shocks delivered: 1	671 / 382	610 / 536
55	28-Apr-2011 19:03:33	VT1	ATP: 3; Shocks delivered: 1	801 / 392	670 / 804
	28-Apr-2011 17:11:56	Follow-up			
54	28-Apr-2011 16:53:24	VT1	ATP: 3; Shocks delivered: 1	873 / 389	508 / 728
53	28-Apr-2011 16:43:14	VT1	ATP: 3; Shocks delivered: 1	1101 / 390	827 / 680
52	28-Apr-2011 16:31:38	VT1	ATP: 3; Shocks delivered: 1	1267 / 390	> 1998 / 878
51	28-Apr-2011 16:15:21	VT1	ATP: 3; Shocks delivered: 1	> 1998 / 385	> 1998 / 783
50	28-Apr-2011 15:49:35	VT1	ATP: 3; Shocks delivered: 1	> 1998 / 394	774 / 768
49	28-Apr-2011 15:34:34	VT1	ATP: 3; Shocks delivered: 1	885 / 396	538 / 760

Fig. 1. 78 year-old patient with dilated idiopathic cardiomyopathy. In this report the patient experienced 37 arrhythmic episodes in less than 24 hours. Physicians can check the report directly online in real time, allowing fast diagnosis of ES and, hence, immediate treatment of ES.

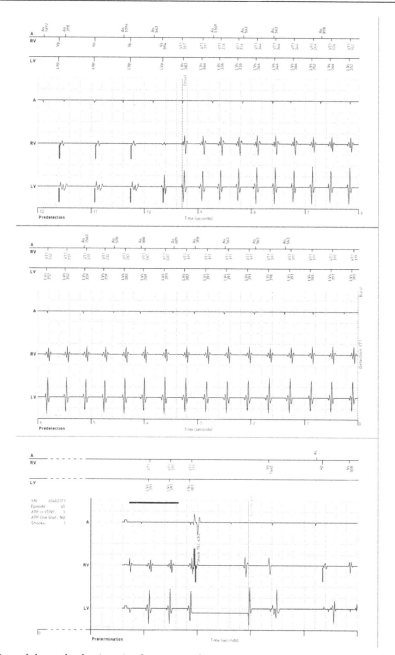

Fig. 2. One of the arrhythmic episodes reported in Fig.1. In this EGM a ventricular tachycardia in VT zone starts abruptly following a premature ventricular contraction. Atrioventicular dissociation is easily visible. ATP was ineffective whereas 15J delivered shock successfully terminated VT.

5.4 Specific therapy in congenital pro-arrhythmic diseases

Although electrical storm associated with Brugada syndrome is exceptional, it is a major and life threatening event that requires rapid and effective treatment. In most cases presented to date, infusion of isoproterenol (as a 1-2 µg bolus injection followed by continuous infusion at 0.15 µg/min, or at a rate of about 0.003 µg/kg/min tritated to result in a 20% increase in heart rate), was used to terminate electrical storm. Other cases reported intravenous orciprenaline infusion or quinidine as effective in terminating ES. Direct β adrenergic stimulation by isoproterenol and orciprenaline increases the L-type calcium current, which restores the epicardial action potential dome, normalizes ST segment elevations and suppresses ventricular arrhythmias. It should be emphasized that orciprenaline or quinidine use as last resort approach in ES is limited to cases of confirmed Brugada syndrome, while in the majority of ES associated with ischemic or dilated cardiomyopathy, orciprenaline or quinidine application may result in fatal outcome.

In the congenital long QT syndrome, high dose β-blockers can suppress the occurrence of ES and frequent ICD discharges. In refractory cases, left cardiac sympathetic denervation results in marked reduction in ES incidence.

In the ES associated with the short-coupled variant of torsade de pointes ventricular tachycardia, verapamil or the combination of verapamil and mexiletine is somewhat effective. Intravenous magnesium and overdrive pacing are the treatment of choice for drug-induced torsade de pointes.

Arrhythmogenic right ventricular cardiomyopathy and myocardial non-compaction deeply modify heart structure, and ES associated with these conditions is usually resistant to medical therapy. Heart transplantation represents nowadays the only viable option for terminating recurrent, haemodynamically destabilizing arrhythmias in these patients.

5.5 Last resource therapies. Radio-frequency ablation and heart transplantation
5.5.1 Radio-frequency ablation

Although radiofrequency catheter ablation (CA) has an established role in the treatment of recurrent VT, only recently it has been suggested as a method of choice in management of ES, especially when pharmacological and ICD therapies fail. The best candidates for CA are those ventricular arrhythmias in which the initiating beat or premature ventricular contractions morphologically identical to the initiating beat can be localized with electroanatomical mapping. In patients affected with ischemic cardiomyopathy the typical site of the initiating beat is around the border zone of the scar tissue. The procedure can be performed under light anesthesia or deep sedation, according to the hemodynamic state of the patient. If the VT is not incessant, a stimulation protocol from right and left ventricle and up to three extrastimuli is usually applied to induce clinical VT and determine its characteristics. Mapping and ablation is usually performed by an irrigated-tip catheter introduced into the right ventricle or left ventricle by direct femoral vein approach or retrograde transaortic or transseptal approach, respectively. Electroanatomical mapping is nowadays the standard of care, being safe and effective.

The largest series of patients undergoing CA for refractory ES has been described by Carbucicchio and coworkers. Solid electrophysiological evidence of the effective treatment of the presenting VT was achieved in 89% of patients, whereas a transient effect of CA causing short-term stabilization but ineffective in long-term ES prevention was observed in the remaining 11% of patients (Carbucicchio et al, 2008). In this latter group, CA acted only as a temporary bailout, with no impact on ES recurrence. In a recent Czech study RF ablation proved effective in suppression of ES in 84% of cases; however, repeated procedures were necessary in 1 out of 4 patients (Kozeluhova et al, 2011). Severely depressed left ventricular ejection fraction, highly-dilated left ventricle, renal insufficiency, and ES recurrence after previous ablation procedure were independently associated with adverse outcome within the first 6 months after the procedure. Is it still unclear whether inducibility testing of the VT at the end of the study is predictive of mortality and arrhythmic recurrences, as currently available data are controversial.

Successful CA of refractory ES in the absence of a detectable trigger has also been described. Schreieck and colleagues reported a case series of 5 ischemic patients with unmappable recurrent VTs, in which CA was attempted targeting delayed local potentials guided by voltage mapping and pace mapping (Schreieck et al, 2004). These isolated delayed potentials are found exclusively in areas of dense scar, making this kind of technique ineffective in idiopathic dilated cardiomyopathy.

On a side note, patients with pseudo-storm due to inappropriate ICD shocks induced by atrial tachyarrhythmias can benefit from CA of atrial flutter, atrial fibrillation or even AV node ablation.

5.5.2 Heart transplantation

Patients with no significant comorbidities except for recurrent ES who experienced no improvements from pharmacological, device-related and surgical treatment should be considered for cardiac transplantation. Patients with refractory ES associated with a genetic arrhythmia syndromes may also be reasonable candidates for heart transplantation as these patients are typically young, otherwise healthy individuals with good quality of life and prognosis.

In haemodynamically instable patients, intraaortic balloon pump and cardiac assist devices should be used as bridge-to-transplant, as potentially lifesaving.

6. References

Anderson JL, Rodier HE, Green LS. (1983) Comparative effects of beta-adrenergic blocking drugs on experimental ventricular fibrillation threshold. *American Journal of Cardiology*, 51, 1196-1202.

Arya A, Haghjoo M, Dehghani MR, et al. (2005) Prevalence and predictors of electrical storm in patients with implantable cardioverter-defibrillator. *American Journal of Cardiology*, 97, 389–392.

Bansch D, Bocker D, Brunn J. (2000) Clusters of ventricular tachycardias signify impaired survival in patients with idiopathic dilated cardiomyopaty and implantable cardioverter defibrillators. *Journal of the American College of Cardiology*, 36, 566-573.

Brigadeau F, Kouakam C, Klug D, et al. (2006) Clinical predictors and prognostic significance of electrical storm in patients with implantable cardioverter defibrillators. *European Heart Journal*, 27, 700–707.

Burjorjee JE, Milne B. (2002) Propofol for electrical storm; a case report of cardioversion and suppression of ventricular tachycardia by propofol. *Canadian Journal of Anesthesia*, 49, 973-977.

Carbucicchio C, Santamaria M, Trevisi N, et al. (2008) Catheter ablation for the treatment of electrical storm in patients with implantable cardioverter-defibrillators: short- and long-term outcomes in a prospective single-center study. *Circulation*, 29, 117, 462-469.

Cleeland JGF, Daubert JC, Erdman E, et al. (2005) The effect of cardiac resynchronization on morbidity and mortality in heart failure. *New England Journal of Medicine*, 352, 1539-1549.

Connolly SJ, Dorian P, Roberts RS, et al. (2006) Comparison of beta-blockers, amiodarone plus beta-blockers, or sotalol for prevention of shocks from implantable cardioverter defibrillators: the OPTIC Study: a randomized trial. *Journal of the American Medical Association*, 295, 165-171.

Credner SC, Klingenheben T, Mauss O, et al. (1998) Electrical storm in patients with transvenous implantable cardioverter-defibrillators: incidence, management and prognostic implications. *Journal of the American College of Cardiology*, 32, 1909-1915.

Exner DV, Pinski SL, Wyse DG, et al. (2001) Electrical storm presages nonsudden death: the antiarrhythmics versus implantable defibrillators (AVID) trial. *Circulation*, 103, 2066-2071.

Gasparini M, Lunati M, Landolina M et al. (2008) Electrical storm in patients with biventricular implantable cardioverter defibrillator: Incidence, predictors and prognostic implications. *American Heart Journal*, 156, 847-854.

Gatzoulis KA, Andrikopoulos G, Apostolopoulos T, et al. (2005) Electrical storm is an independent predictor of adverse longterm outcome in the era of implantable defibrillator therapy. *Europace*, 7, 184-192.

Gradaus R, Block M, Brachmann J, et al. (2003) Mortality, morbidity, and complications in 3,344 patients with implantable cardioverter defibrillators: results from the German ICD registry EURID. *Pacing and Clinical Electrophysiology*, 26, 1511-1518.

Greene M, Newman D, Geist M, et al. (2000) Is electrical storm in ICD patients the sign of a dying heart? Outcome of patients with clusters of ventricular tachyarrhythmias. *Europace*, 2, 263-269.

Huang DT, Traub D. (2008) Recurrent ventricular arrhythmia storms in the age of implantable cardioverter defibrillator therapy: a comprehensive review. *Progress in Cardiovascular Diseases*, 51, :229-236.

Hohnloser SH, Al-Khalidi HR, Pratt CM, et al. (2006) Electrical storm in patients with an implantable defibrillator: incidence, features, and preventive therapy: insights from a randomized trial. *European Heart Journal*, 27, 3027-3032.

Israel CW, Barold SS. (2007) Electrical storm in patient with implanted defibrillator: a matter of definition. *Annals of Noninvasive Electrocardiology*, 12, 375-82.

Kantharia BK, Patel JA, Nagra BS, et al. (2006) Electrical storm of monomorphic ventricular tachycardia after a cardiac resynchronization therapy defibrillator upgrade. *Europace*, 8, 625-628.

Kowal RC, Wasmund SL, Smith ML, et al. (2004) Biventricular pacing reduces the induction of monomorphic ventricular tachycardia: a potential mechanism for arrhythmia suppression. *Heart Rhythm*, 1:295-300.

Kowey PR, Levine JH, Herre JM, et al. (1995) Randomized, double-blind comparison of intravenous amiodarone and bretylium in the treatment of patients with recurrent, hemodynamically destabilizing ventricular tachycardia or fibrillation. The

Intravenous Amiodarone Multicenter Investigators Group. *Circulation*, 92, 3255-3263.

Kozeluhova M, Peichl P, Cihak R, et al. (2011) Catheter ablation of electrical storm in patients with structural heart disease. *Europace*, 13, 109-13.

Kudenchuk PJ, Cobb LA, Copass MK, et al. (1999) Amiodarone for resuscitation after out-of-hospital cardiac arrest due to ventricular fibrillation. *New England Journal of Medicine*, 341, 871-878.

Levine JH, Massumi A, Scheinman MM, et al. (1996) Intravenous amiodarone for recurrent sustained hypotensive ventricular tachyarrhythmias. Intravenous Amiodarone Multicenter Trial Group. *Journal of the American College of Cardiology*, 27, 67-75.

Marketou ME, Simantirakis EN, Manios EG, et al. (2001) Electrical storm due to amiodarone induced thyrotoxicosis in a young adult with dilated cardiomyopathy: thyroidectomy as the treatment of choice. *Pacing and Clinical Electrophysiology*, 24, 1827-1828.

Messali A, Thomas O, Chauvin M, et al. (2004) Death due to an implantable cardioverter defibrillator. *Journal of Cardiovascular Electrophysiology*, 15, 953-956.

Miwa Y, Ikeda T, Mera H, et al. (2010) Effects of landiolol, an ultra-short-acting beta1-selective blocker, on electrical storm refractory to class III antiarrhythmic drugs. *Circulation Journal*, 74, 856-863.

Newton GE, Parker JD. (1996) Acute effects of beta 1-selective and nonselective beta-adrenergic receptor blockade on cardiac sympathetic activity in congestive heart failure. *Circulation*, 94, 353-358.

Nordbeck P, Seidl B, Fey B et al. (2010) Effect of cardiac resynchronization therapy on the incidence of electrical storm. *International Journal of Cardiology*, 143, 330-336.

Schreieck J, Zrenner B, Deisenhofer I, et al. (2004) Rescue ablation of electrical storm in patients with ischemic cardiomyopathy: a potential-guided ablation approach by modifying substrate of intractable, unmappable ventricular tachycardias. *Heart Rhythm*, 2, 10-14.

Sesselberg HW, Moss AJ, McNitt S, et al. (2007) Ventricular arrhythmia storms in postinfarction patients with implantable defibrillators for primary prevention indications: a MADIT-II substudy. *Heart Rhythm*, 4, 1395–1402.

Stefan H, Hussein R, Craig M, et al. (2006) Electrical storm in patients with an implantable defibrillator:incidence, features, and preventive therapy: insights from a randomized trial. *European Heart Journal*, 27, 3027-3032.

Streitner F, Kuschyk J, Veltmann C et al. (2009) Role of proinflammatory markers and NT-proBNP in patients with and implanted cardioverter defibrillator and an electrical storm. *Cytokine*, 47, 166-172.

Streitner F, Kuschyk J, Veltmann C, et al. (2011) Predictors of electrical storm recurrences in patients with implantable cardioverter-defibrillators. *Europace*, 13, 668-674.

Sweeney MO, Sherfesee L, DeGroot PJ, et al. (2010) Differences in effects of electrical therapy type for ventricular arrhythmias on mortality in implantable cardioverter-defibrillator patients. *Heart Rhythm*, 7, 353-360.

Tsagalou EP, Kanakakis J, Rokas S, et al. (2005) Suppression by propranolol and amiodarone of an electrical storm refractory to metoprolol and amiodarone. *American Journal of Cardiology*, 99, 341-342.

Wood MA, Simpson PM, Stambler BS, et al. (1995) Long-term temporal patterns of ventricular tachyarrhythmias. *Circulation*, 91, 2371-2377.

5

Bradycardia Secondary to Cervical Spinal Cord Injury

Farid Sadaka and Christopher Veremakis
St John's Mercy Medical Center, St Louis University
USA

1. Introduction

Acute spinal cord injury (SCI) is most commonly traumatic in origin but may also result from degenerative spine disease, ischemia, demyelination, inflammation, or rapidly expanding neoplastic, hemorrhagic, or pyogenic masses (Ghezzi et al, 2001). In the United States, traumatic SCI with or without bony injury has an annual incidence of 28 to 55 per million, with an average of 10,000 new cases a year and a prevalence of 200,000 (Sekhon & Fehlings, 2001). The average age at the time of injury is 32 years and the male/female ratio is 4:1. More than half (55%) of traumatic SCI involves the cervical cord. The most common causes of SCI are traffic accidents (motor vehicle, bicycle, pedestrian) (40%– 50%), assault (10%–25%), falls (20%), work-related injuries (10%–25%), and sports/recreation-related injuries (10%–25%) (Cheung et al, 2002; Surkhin et al, 2000). In traumatic cervical SCI, 3-month mortality is 20% to 21%. The independent predictors of mortality are level of cord injury, Glasgow Coma Scale, respiratory failure, and age. Principal causes of death are respiratory disorders, cardiovascular disorders, pulmonary embolism, infections, and suicide (Claxton et al, 1998; DeVivo et al, 1999, Yeo et al, 1998). Cardiovascular disorders are responsible for 40.5% of deaths, being the most common cause of mortality in patients with SCI (Garshick et al, 2005).

2. Cardiovascular instability

Cardiovascular instability is a frequent complication of SCI, especially when the upper thoracic or cervical cord is involved (Figure 1). Peripheral sympathetic denervation results in arteriolar dilation and pooling of blood in the venous compartment, while interruption of cardiac sympathetic innervation (T1– T4) promotes bradycardia (Figure 2) and reduces myocardial contractility. The autonomic nervous system modulates cardiac electrophysiology, and, consequently, autonomic dysfunction can lead to ventricular arrhythmias. Concomitantly, parasympathetic input to the heart (from the vagus nerve, cranial nerve [CN] X) remains intact and may frequently result in bradycardia, especially with cervical SCI. Less commonly, cardiac arrest has been documented. Bradycardia is often precipitated by tracheal stimulation (for example, during suctioning) and hypoxia (Mathias et al, 1976; Piepmeier et al, 1985). Reflex bradycardia and cardiac arrest occur due to a vago–vagal reflex. Under normal circumstances, this reflex is opposed by sympathetic activity. As a compensatory response to hypoxia, a pulmonary–vagal reflex occurs, designed to increase respiratory rate and pulmonary inflation. However, in patients with SCI, compensatory sympathetic activity is eliminated, leaving parasympathetic activity unopposed, leading to severe bradycardia and potentially cardiac arrest. Studies of cardiovascular abnormalities after SCI show that as many as 100% of patients with motor complete cervical injuries (American Spinal Injury Association [ASIA] grades A and B) develop bradycardia, 68% are hypotensive, 35% require pressors, and 16% have primary cardiac arrest. Of persons with motor incomplete cervical injuries (ASIA grades C and D), 35-71% develop bradycardia, but few have hypotension or require pressors. Among patients with thoracolumbar injuries, 13-35% have bradycardia (Lehmann et al, 1987; Wirth et al, 2007). Bradycardia is more frequently encountered in the acute phase, and is more severe in the first 2–6 weeks after trauma (Krassioukov et al, 2007; McKinley et al, 2006). Cardiovascular dysfunctions improve in time. The reasons are not well understood, but synaptic reorganization or hyperresponsiveness of alpha receptors may play a role (Gondim et al, 2004).

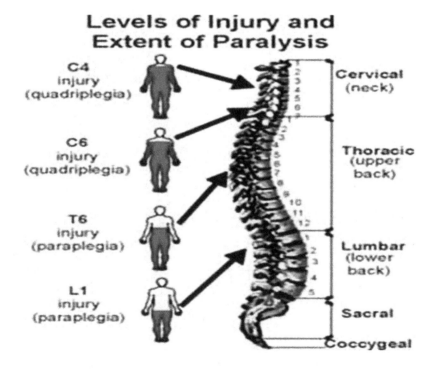

Fig. 1. Spinal cord and level of injury.

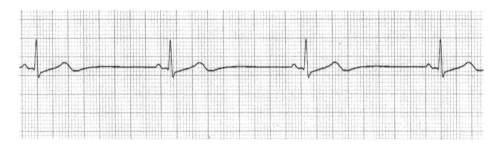

Fig. 2. Sinus Bradycardia during cervical SCI.

Cardiovascular control in acute and chronic SCI has been investigated by measuring the response to a variety of cardiovascular markers (blood pressure, heart rate, and plasma levels of norepinephrine and epinephrine) before ,during and after application of noxious stimuli below the level of the lesion. In acute SCI, noxious stimuli (eg. bladder stimulation) caused minimal changes in heart rate and plasma norepinephrine and epinephrine levels. In chronic SCI, noxious stimuli induced bradycardia and elevation in plasma norepinephrine but not in epinephrine levels. Resting plasma norepinephrine and epinephrine levels in both the acute and chronic SCI were lower than in normal subjects (Mathias et al, 1979).

The tilt test has been used to evaluate and delineate alterations in sympathetic cardiovascular compensation, which reflect the degree of autonomic dysfunction. Autonomic and cardiovascular responses to tilt test are blunted in persons with quadriplegia or paraplegia (Welch et al, 2005). Such tests could be used to noninvasively assess autonomic dysfunction in persons with SCI, determine the degree of sympathetic disruption, and assess the risk of developing cardiac arrhythmias, especially bradycardia. However, there are very few studies on these bedside tests upon which to solidly base conclusions and recommendations.

3. Treatment

3.1 Pharmacotherapy

Although bradycardia after cervical SCI usually resolves within 6 to 8 weeks after injury, it may progress to complete heart block and cardiac arrest. As such, the acute management and maintenance of cardiovascular stability in these patients may range from a practical clinical chore to a potentially lifesaving responsibility. There is limited data available regarding the optimal and best treatment available for symptomatic bradycardia in this patient population (Table 1). All data on therapeutic management of bradycardia secondary to cervical spinal cord injury is based on case reports, case series and observational studies.

Atropine, an anticholinergic agent, is generally recommended as the first-line agent for bradycardia after cervical spinal cord injury. Atropine improves conduction through the atrioventricular (AV) node by reducing vagal tone through muscarinic receptor blockade. The dose ranges from 0.4 to 0.6 mg, administered intravenously every 4 hours for short-term therapy (Abd & Braun, 1989; Pansoori & Leesar, 2004; Piepmeier et al, 1985; Sadaka et al,

2010; Sakamoto et al, 2007; Schulz-Stubner, 2005; Weant et al, 2007; Whitman et al, 2008; Winslow et al, 1986). Atropine should be kept readily available at the bedside at all times with this patient population, as acute episodes of bradycardia and hypotension may occur suddenly and without warning in the immediate few hours and days following injury.

Modality	Route of administration	Mechanism of action
Atropine	IV	reduces vagal tone by muscarinic receptor blockade
Dopamine	IV infusion	Beta$_1$ receptors on the heart
Epinephrine	IV infusion	Beta$_1$ receptors on the heart
Aminophylline	IV	inhibition of PDE enzyme thus increasing c-AMP with subsequent rise in catecholamines
Theophylline	Enteral or parenteral	inhibition of PDE enzyme thus increasing c-AMP with subsequent rise in catecholamines
Propantheline	Enteral	postganglionic parasympathetic acetylcholine receptor blocker
Permanent Pacemeker	invasive	

Table 1. Therapeutic modalities for bradycardia secondary to cervical SCI.

Another frequently utilized category of intravenous medications includes sympathomimetic agents such as Dopamine or Epinephrine which increase heart rate through action on Beta$_1$ receptors in the heart. Continuous infusions of dopamine at a rate of 2 to 10 mcg/kg/min or epinephrine at a rate of 0.01 to 0.1 mcg/kg/min has been used in the acute setting (Abd & Braun, 1989; Piepmeier et al, 1985; Sadaka et al, 2010; Winslow et al, 1986). Complications include tachyarrythmias, angina pain, palpitations, vasoconstriction, nausea, vomiting and headache.

When intermittent boluses of atropine or continuous infusions of sympathomimetic drugs have failed to prevent recurrent symptomatic bradycardia, or reverse high or complete heart block , permanent pacemaker placement has often been used as the next therapeutic alternative (Franga et al, 2006; Ruiz-Arango et al, 2006). Cardiac pacemaker implantation is advocated for patients with high cervical spinal cord injuries with persistent bradycardia not responding to medical management (Giloff et al,1991). However, specific criteria for placement of a pacemaker are not well defined. The reported number of SCI patients requiring a pacemaker varies from 9 to 17% (Abd & Braun, 1989; Lehmann et al, 1987). Complications of permanent pacemakers include infection, lead malfunction, death during attempted insertion, and death associated with failure to capture.

The methylxanthine agents, including aminophylline and theophylline, have been used effectively for the management of refractory symptomatic bradycardia when other agents have failed (Pansoori & Leesar, 2004; Sadaka et al, 2010; Sakamoto et al, 2007; Schulz-Stubner, 2005; Weant et al, 2007; Whitman et al, 2008). In addition, there are recent reports of methylxanthines used specifically as a successful first line treatment for bradycardia associated with cervical spinal cord injury. None of the patients in the case series needed a pacemaker placement and none of the patients developed drug related side effects (Sadaka et al, 2010). The proposed mechanism for the chronotropic effect of these drugs is via inhibition of phosphodiesterase (PDE) enzyme thus increasing the cyclic adenosine monophosphate with subsequent rise in catecholamines. A clear benefit of these agents is that they may be administered on a fixed schedule as an enteral preparation. An oral (or intravenous) loading dose between 200 and 300 mg was administered in most cases with maintenance doses starting at 100 mg three times daily and continued for up to 12 weeks. Drug serum levels were variable and differed widely among patients. The effective dose of theophylline resulted in serum levels that were below the therapeutic range defined in the literature (10-20 mcg/ml), and ofcourse below the toxic range (>25 mcg/ml). Since no therapeutic index for symptomatic bradycardia has been established, the methylxanthine dose was titrated according to clinical response. The main side effects of these agents are nausea, vomiting, tremor, headache, and seizures. However, No adverse effects were noted in any of the reports. Nonetheless until more experience is gained with this modality, careful attention should be made to monitor drug levels and avoid toxicity. Methylxanthine has also been associated with diaphragmatic strengthening in animal models, another potential beneficial effect to consider in spinal cord injury patients (Whitman et al, 2008).

In patients requiring long-term therapy, there are case reports of successful treatment with propantheline 7.5 to 30 mg every 4 to 6 hours (Abd & Braun, 1989; Winslow et al, 1986). Propantheline competitively blocks the action of acetylcholine at postganglionic parasympathetic receptors. The main side effect reported from chronic propantheline therapy is a reduction in gastrointestinal motility due to its anticholinergic effects.

3.2 Anticipation, prevention & positioning

Bradycardia and potential for cardiac arrest should be anticipated in any patient with spinal cord injury. Bedside care providers should be alerted to the fact that life threatening events occur more frequently with high spinal cord lesions. Personnel should anticipate and document triggers for serious bradycardic episodes. Hyperoxygenation and ambu "bagging" may be helpful prior to tracheal suctioning. Prophylactic atropine administration before tracheal suction, laryngoscopy, or oral intubation has been shown to minimize severity of events (Frankel et al, 1974; Mathias ,1976;Welphy et al, 1975). Theophylline may also be started at the first indication of bradycardia. Particular attention should be paid to other potential exacerbating factors, including rapid changes in positioning, prolonged recumbency, drug adverse effects, underlying infection, and hypovolemia.

Before moving the patient out of supine position, abdominal binder, thigh-high stockings, and elastic bandages to the lower extremities can be applied. These measures decrease venous pooling in the lower extremities and splanchnic vasculature. The patient can be moved slowly, from a supine position to a relatively upright position. A tilt table can be used to slowly bring the patient to the upright position.

3.3 Rehabilitation measures

Active arm exercises can be used to maintain blood pressure while the patient is on the tilt table (Mckinley et al, 2006). Bilaterally functional electric stimulation to lower-limb muscles, quadriceps, hamstrings, tibialis anterior and gastrocnemius during tilting improves orthostatic tolerance in patients with cervical SCI. Functional electric muscle stimulation during tilting maneuver, significantly increases heart rate (Chao et al, 2005).

4. Conclusion

Spinal cord injury is a very common and devastating disease process that can occur as a consequence of motor vehicle collisions, falls or other traumatic injuries. Cardiac disorders are common consequences following SCI. Cardiovascular disturbances are the leading causes of morbidity and mortality in both acute and chronic phases of SCI. Disruption of descendent pathways from superior centers to spinal sympathetic neurons, originating into the intermediolateral nuclei of T1- L2 spinal cord segments results in a reduced overall sympathetic activity and unopposed parasympathetic activity. As a result, the most common cardiac dysrrhythmia is bradycardia. There are a few well established therapeutic modalities (Table 1) for the treatment of bradycardia associated with cervical SCI. All therapeutic options are based on anecdotal reports and small retrospective reviews. Atropine should be kept readily available at the bedside at all times. Based on recent evidence with methylxanthines, we recommend further studies to establish the role of these agents as a first line therapy in this specific patient population. Optimal dose and duration of therapy need to be established. Theophylline's use via entral route as a first line therapy for spinal cord injury-related bradycardia can help avoid the long term use of inotropic and chronotropic infusions and their associated risks and complications, as well as prevent and/or decrease the use of cardiac pacemaker placement and its associated procedural risks and complications. We further recommend the study of xanthine derivates as prophylactic treatment for the first 2-6 weeks of the injury based on the frequency of bradycardia in patients with cervical SCI which is reported to be 100%. Currently, there are no established guidelines regarding permanent pacemaker placement in this patient population. Permanent pacemaker should still be considered in patients with refractory or recurrent bradycardia more than two weeks after the injury. In addition, the incidence of bradycardia after cervical SCI may be decreased by proper prophylactic measures, cardiac exercises and appropriate rehabilitation.

5. References

Abd AG & Braun NM. Management of life-threatening bradycardia in spinal cord injury. Chest.; 95(3):701-702.

Chao CY & Cheing GL. The effects of lower-extremity functional electric stimulation on the orthostatic responses of people with tetraplegia. Arch Phys Med Rehabil. 2005; 86(7):1427-33.

Cheung AT, Weiss SJ, McGarvey ML, Stecker MM, Hogan MS, Escherich A, & Bavaria JE. Interventions for reversing delayed-onset postoperative paraplegia after thoracic aortic reconstruction. Ann Thorac Surg. 2002; 74:413–9.

Claxton AR, Wong DT, Chung F, et al. Predictors of hospital mortality and mechanical ventilation in patients with cervical spinal cord injury. Can J Anaesth. 1998; 45:144–9.

DeVivo MJ, Krause JS, & Lammertse DP. Recent trends in mortality and causes of death among persons with spinal cord injury. Arch Phys Med Rehabil. 1999; 80:1411–9.

Franga DL, Hawkins ML, Medeiros RS, & Adewumi D. Recurrent asystole resulting from high cervical spinal cord injuries. Am Surg. 2006 ; 72(6):525-9.

Frankel HL, Mathias CJ, & Spalding JM. Mechanisms of reflex cardiac arrest in tetraplegic patients. Lancet. 1975; 2(7946):1183-5.

Garshick E, Kelly A, Cohen SA, Garrison A, Tun CG, Gagnon D, & Brown R. A prospective assessment of mortality in chronic spinal cord injury . Spinal Cord. 2005;43[7]:408–416.

Ghezzi A, Baldini SM, & Zaffaroni M. Differential diagnosis of acute myelopathies. Neurol Sci. 2001; 22(suppl 2):60–4.

Giloff IS, Ward SL, & Hohn AR. Cardiac pacemaker in high spinal cord injury. Arch Phys Med Rehab 1991; 72(8):601-3.

Gondim FA, Lopes AC Jr, Oliveira GR, Rodrigues CL, Leal PR, Santos AA, & Rola FH. Cardiovascular control after spinal cord injury. Curr Vasc Pharmacol. 2004; 2(1):71–79.

Krassioukov AV, Karlsson AK, Wecht JM, Wuermser LA, Mathias CJ, & Marino RJ. Assessment of autonomic dysfunction following spinal cord injury: rationale for additions to international standards for neurological assessment . JRRD. 2007; 44(1):103–112.

Lehmann KG, Lane JG, Piepmeier JM, & Batsford WP.Cardiovascular abnormalities accompanying acute spinal cord injury in humans: incidence, time course and severity. J Am Coll Cardiol. Jul 1987; 10(1):46-52.

Mathias CJ. Bradycardia and cardiac arrest during tracheal suction—mechanisms in tetraplegic patients. Eur J Intensive Care Med. 1976; 2(4):147-56.

Mathias CJ, Christensen NJ, Frankel HL, & Spalding JM. Cardiovascular control in recently injured tetraplegics in spinal shock. Q J Med. 1979; 48(100):273–287.

McKinley W, Garstang SV, Wieting JM, Talavera F, Foye PM, Allen KL, & Campagnolo DI. Cardiovascular concerns in spinal cord injury. Cord Injury: eMedicine Specialties/Physical Medicine and Rehabilitation/Spinal; 2006.

Pasnoori VR & Leesar MA. Use of aminophylline in the treatment of severe symptomatic bradycardia resistant to atropine. Cardiol Rev. 2004; 12(2):65-68.

Piepmeier JM, Lehmann KB, & Lane JG. Cardiovascular instability following acute cervical spinal cord trauma. Cent Nerv Syst Trauma. 1985; 2(3):153-60.

Ruiz-Arango AF, Robinson VJ, & Sharma GK. Characteristics of patients with cervical spinal injury requiring permanent pacemaker implantation. Cardiol Rev. 2006; 14(4):e8-e11.

Sadaka F, Naydenov SK, & Ponzillo JJ. Theophylline for bradycardia secondary to cervical spinal cord injury. Neurocrit Care. 2010 Dec;13(3):389-92.

Sakamoto T, Sadanaga T, & Okazaki T. Sequential use of aminophylline and theophylline for the treatment of atropine-resistant bradycardia after spinal cord injury: a case report. J Cardiol. 2007; 49(2):91-96.

Schulz-Stubner S. The use of small-dose theophylline for the treatment of bradycardia in patients with spinal cord injury. Anesth Analg. 2005; 101(6):1809-1811.

Sekhon LHS & Fehlings MG. Epidemiology, demographics, and pathophysiology of acute spinal cord injury. Spine. 2001;26(suppl 24):2–12.

Surkin J, Gilbert BJ, Harkey HL 3rd, Sniezek J, & Currier M. Spinal cord injury in Mississippi: findings and evaluation, 1992–1994. Spine. 2000; 25: 716–21.

Weant KA, Kilpatrick M, & Jaikumar S. Aminophylline for the treatment of symptomatic bradycardia and asystole secondary to cervical spine injury. Neurocrit Care. 2007; 7(3):250-252.

Welch JM, Radulovic M, Weir JP, Lesser J, Spungen AM, & Bauman WA. Partial angiotensin-converting enzyme inhibition during acute orthostatic stress in persons with tetraplegia. . J Spinal Cord Med. 2005; 28(2):103–105.

Welphy NC, Mathias CJ, & Frankel HL. Circulatory reflexes in tetraplegics during artificial ventilation and general anaesthesia. Paraplegia. 1975; 13(3):172-82.

Whitman CB, Schroeder WS, Ploch PJ, & Raghavendran K. Efficacy of aminophylline for treatment of recurrent symptomatic bradycardia after spinal cord injury. Pharmacotherapy. 2008; 28(1):131-135.

Winslow EB, Lesch M, Talano JV, & Meyer PR Jr. Spinal cord injuries associated with cardiopulmonary complications. Spine. 1986; 11(8):809-812.

Wirth B, van Hedel HJ, Kometer B, Dietz V, & Curt A. Changes in activity after a complete spinal cord injury as measured by the Spinal Cord Independence Measure II (SCIM II). Neurorehabil Neural Repair. Aug 30 2007.

Yeo JD, Walsh J, Rutkowski S, Soden R, Craven M, 7 Middleton J .Mortality following spinal cord injury. Spinal Cord. 1998; 36:329–36.

Part 2

Electrophysiology Study of the Heart: Mapping Procedure

6

Novel Technologies for Mapping and Ablation of Complex Arrhythmias

Shahnaz Jamil-Copley, Louisa Malcolme-Lawes and Prapa Kanagaratnam
Imperial College Healthcare NHS Trust, St Mary's Hospital, London,
National Heart and Lung Institute, Imperial College London,
UK

1. Introduction

1.1 The burden of complex arrhythmias

Atrial fibrillation (AF) is the most common cardiac arrhythmia, affecting about 9% of the population over 70 years of age (Feinberg, Blackshear et al. 1995). It is characterised by an irregular pulse, leading to symptoms of shortness of breath, dizziness, palpitations, chest pain, lethargy and an increased risk of stroke (Kannel, Abbott et al. 1982). Current widely accepted indications for catheter ablation of AF are significant symptoms uncontrolled by anti-arrhythmic medications, however more recent European Guidelines have suggested catheter ablation may be used as a first line treatment for symptomatic paroxysmal AF in patients with no or minimal heart disease. Randomised trials from 2003 - 2010 have shown a range of success rates for catheter ablation of AF from 56 - 89% (freedom from AF off anti-arrhythmic drugs) compared to the use of AADs alone ranging from 4 - 43% (Camm, Kirchhof et al. ; Kannel, Abbott et al. 1982).

Atrial tachycardia (AT) is relatively rare, accounting for 5-15% of all supraventricular tachycardias (SVTs). It can be encountered in patients with a structurally normal heart or those with underlying structural or scar-related heart disease. In patients with structurally normal hearts, atrial tachycardia is associated with a low mortality rate. However spontaneous resolution of symptomatic episodes is uncommon. Prolonged episodes (typically months or years) of continuous atrial tachycardia can be problematic leading to irreversible changes of the atria, including negative remodeling with atrial enlargement and myopathy causing symptomatic congestive cardiac failure. In addition, prolonged episodes can make reversion and maintenance of normal sinus rhythm more difficult. In recent years, the significance of AT in the initiation and perpetuation of atrial fibrillation has become apparent. Paradoxically AT occurs in up to 50% of patients undergoing extensive ablation for persistent AF.

Sustained ventricular tachycardia (VT) is a significant cause of morbidity and sudden death especially in patients with underlying structural heart disease. Coronary heart disease is the most common cause of clinically documented VT occurring in 76–82% of the patients (CASCADE Study 1993; Kuch et al 2000; AVID Study 1997; CIDS Study 2000). Although implantable cardioverter defibrillators (ICD) prevent sudden cardiac death and antiarrhythmic drugs reduce the frequency of VT episodes, drug side-effects and repeated device therapies can have a major impact on quality of life (Moss et al 2004, Poole et al 2008, Schron et al 2002). Recurrent VT develops in 40-60% of patients receiving an ICD for ischaemic cardiomyopathy after an episode of spontaneous sustained VT however the first ICD therapy appears to be the most important predictor of subsequent therapy in this population and is likely to occur within the first two years of implant (Koa-Wing M et al 2007). VT ablation has been shown to reduce therapies from ICDs, but in its current state, is technically challenging and time consuming with procedural times up to 8 hours (Cao et al 1996).

1.2 The challenges of complex arrhythmias
1.2.1 Atrial Fibrillation
Several models have been proposed to explain the continuous irregular atrial activation of clinical AF. It is widely accepted that the initiation of AF is from an atrial ectopic 'trigger' originating from the pulmonary veins (Haissaguerre, Jais et al. 1998). The 'trigger' can continue to act as 'a focal driver' maintaining AF or can establish a self-sustaining spiral wave (or rotor) in a localised region of the myocardium leading to fibrillatory activation in the remaining atria (Haissaguerre, Jais et al. 1998; Jalife, Berenfeld et al. 2002; Sahadevan, Ryu et al. 2004).

Pulmonary vein isolation to remove the 'trigger' has been shown to be effective in paroxysmal AF (Haissaguerre, Jais et al. 1998) (Pappone, Santinelli et al. 2004). However, triggers outside the pulmonary veins have also been identified in the superior vena cava and coronary sinus and these have been more challenging to identify and treat. Linear ablation has been performed in both paroxysmal and persistent AF along the principles of the Cox Maze surgical procedures, but these have not achieved the same success as the surgical approach (Cox, Boineau et al. 1995; Cox, Schuessler et al. 1996; Hsu, Jais et al. 2004). Linear ablation at the roof of the left atrium (Hocini, Jais et al. 2005) and the mitral isthmus between the left lower pulmonary vein and annulus has been shown to improve outcomes when there is proven conduction block of these lines (Jais, Hocini et al. 2004; Willems, Klemm et al. 2006). However, conduction block is difficult to achieve due to lack of catheter stability and failure to achieve transmurality.

More recently, catheter-based substrate modification has targeted regions of highly fractionated electrograms that others suggest as drivers for persistent AF (Lellouche, Buch et al. 2007). Nadamanee et al achieved an 81% success rate for ablation after up to 4 procedures targeting only areas of complex fractionated atrial electrograms (CFAE) (Nademanee, Schwab et al. 2008). However several other groups have failed to reproduce these success rates with CFAE ablation alone (Estner, Hessling et al. 2008). Speculation as to the mechanistic basis for CFAE has implicated regions of autonomic innervations termed the ganglionated plexi, as these were noted to be co-located with regions of CFAE in animal studies. Alternatively, they may originate from regions of atrial scarring or fibrosis, and are thought to represent a combination of wavefronts approaching the recording electrode from multiple directions. Integration of delayed-enhancment MRI imaging, particularly containing information relating to scar, may provide greater insight on the origin of CFAE. This is discussed in more detail later in this chapter.

Wide area circumferential ablation with pulmonary vein isolation, designed to encircle the PVs at a distance from the ostia, is a widely accepted technique for AF ablation and appears to achieve greater success rates than segmental PVI. (Marrouche, Martin et al. 2003; Pappone, Rosanio et al. 2003; Ouyang, Bansch et al. 2004) The most widely practiced approach is to use a 3D-navigation system to recreate a virtual left atrium and move around the chamber delivering lesions around the pulmonary veins and marking lesion points on the virtual anatomy.(Pappone, Oreto et al. 1999) The 3D geometry aids the operator in manipulating catheters around the complex anatomy of the left atrium which can vary significantly from patient to patient. This can prove particularly challenging with only 2D fluoroscopy for navigation.

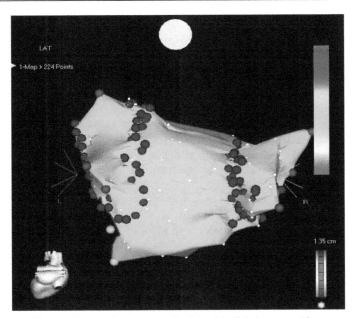

Example of virtual left atrium and points marked (red balls) during wide area circumferential ablation

Despite these novel approaches, published success rates for single procedure AF ablation range remain around 50% to 88% (Lim, Matsuo et al. 2007; Matsuo, Lim et al. 2007; Natale, Raviele et al. 2007; O'Neill, Jais et al. 2007; Marchlinski 2008) which are still not comparable to the >95% success rates expected from ablations for other arrhythmias.

1.2.2 Atrial Tachycardia

Endocardial activation allows categorisation of ATs into focal and macro-rentrant. However in the era of persistant AF ablation the presence of "micro-reentry" circuits particularly within regions of previous complex fractionated atrial electrograms (CFAE) ablation scar must be acknowledged. It is therefore imperative to clarify the mechanism of the underlying AT during electrophysiological procedures to guide ablation therapy. Currently established techniques for guiding ablation in complex atrial tachycardias include activation and/or entrainment mapping. Routinely the tachycardia is displayed as an activation map on a recreated atrial geometry from endocardial location points collected using 3-D mapping technology. However, activation mapping is limited by a point-by-point acquisition process which is not always systematic, is often time-consuming and can miss small areas crucial to the circuit. Detailed mapping often requires >150-200 points with each circuit potentially involving multiple loops and figure-of-8 circuits. In order to identify the critical isthmus maintaining the tachycardia a trained operator is required to set an accurate "window of interest" and collect activation data, which requires significant processing to ensure all collected points have been correctly annotated to the chosen reference. In addition conventionally established entrainment manoeuvres are often used to confirm the diagnosis represented by activation mapping however these can have limitations if there is a variation in the tachycardia cycle length particularly in scarred atria with multiple regions of block and slow conduction.

The most commonly recognised mechanisms seen post-AF ablation are macro re-entrant roof-dependant and mitral isthmus dependant tachycardias however with increasing linear and CFAE ablation lesions, micro-reentrant circuits must also be appreciated. In these situations diagnostic yield from mapping and entrainment can test the most skilled electrophysiologist and although acute success rates have been reported ranging from 88-100%, recurrences are disappointing with rates ranging from 0-47% over a mean follow-up of 2 to 16 months (Gerstenfeld 2004; Chugh 2005; Deisenhofer 2006; Mesas 2004; Haïssaguerre 2005).

Several other circuits capable of sustaining re-entrant tachycardias are seen following cardiac surgery, particularly congenital heart disease.

These are typically a challenge to map and ablate due to the unpredictable location and extent of the underlying iatrogenic scar exposing the limitations of the aforementioned diagnostic techniques.

1.2.3 Ventricular Tachycardia

The biggest challenge in VT ablation remains scar-related VT including ischaemic and dilated cardiomyopathy. The substrate for post-infarct VT is produced by channels of slow conduction within the scar border (the diastolic pathway), created by anatomical and functional lines of block. Identification and ablation of these diastolic pathways is required for successful VT ablation (Koa-Wing, Ho SY et al 2007; Stevenson, Khan et al 1993). Conventional techniques to identify the diastolic pathway consist of performing activation mapping followed by entrainment manoeuvres to locate areas within the scar that participate in the re-entrant circuit (Stevenson, Khan et al 1993; Huang & Wood 2006; Bogun, Good et al 2006), but non-inducibility, difficulty capturing scarred myocardium during entrainment, multiple different morphologies of VT, haemodynamic instability and circuit components deep to the sub-endocardium make this approach unreliable and prolonged with disappointingly high recurrence rates.

These limitations have led to a change in practice from targeting specific circuits to substrate modification of the scar by linear ablation in an attempt to transect potential diastolic pathways and render the VT non-inducible (Marchlinski, Callans et al 2000). Although acute ablation success rates at elimination of the "clinical" tachycardia have improved from 71-74% (Morady et al 1993, Gonska et al 1994, Kim et al 1994) in the mid-1990s to 90% in the 2000s (Sacher et al 2008) long-term outcomes remain unsatisfactory. This is despite the introduction of cardiac mapping systems, irrigated tip catheters and substrate based ablation strategies. Up to 31% of patients with an acutely successful ablation outcome of the "clinical" VT have arrhythmia recurrence. Ablation to non-inducibility of any VT has been reported with success rates approaching 65% but with recurrence rates of 29% during a median follow-up of 1 month (Sacher et al. 2008). The potential causes of recurrence or failure at the index procedure include inadequate mapping techniques of, often small, isthmi in a complex anatomic substrate and failure to achieve transmurality of lesions in those with circuits traversing the subendocardium and epicardium. Although epicardial circuits can be targeted percutaneously, this is not possible in up to 85% of patients with previous cardiac surgery (Sacher F, Roberts-Thomson K, et al. 2010).

2. Mapping

The development of intra-cardiac mapping was based on the use of individual contact catheters. Despite being able to record information from different sites using multipolar catheters, complex arrhythmias and complex substrates pose significant challenges using these techniques. 3-D electrophysiological mapping systems were developed to aid the localisation of the source of focal tachycardias and the critical isthmi of re-entrant circuits (Stevenson, Delacretaz et al 1998; Marchlinski, Callans et al 1998; Earley, Showkathali et al 2006; Schilling, Peters et al 1999; Shah, Jais et al 1997) Conventionally, these systems display electrical data from mapping catheters as either local activation time (isochronal) or local voltage (isopotential) maps. These methods indicate the parameter being displayed using a colour-scale on a 3D representation of the cardiac chamber of interest.

The current versions of these mapping systems are not only significantly more accurate but they offer many more features to facilitate mapping of complex arrhythmias; voltage mapping, propagation maps, rapid mapping using multipolar catheters and mapping of fractionated electrograms and the input of anatomical data from pre-operative CT or MRI scans of the heart or rotational angiograms. The latest feature allowing 4-dimensional mapping, 'ripple-mapping', will also be discussed in this chapter.

The use of mapping systems has not been shown to reduce the duration of the procedure or the efficacy of the procedure(Sporton, Earley et al. 2004), however, it has been shown to significantly reduce the fluoroscopy time, thereby reducing the exposure of patients and lab staff to harmful radiation.(Scaglione, Biasco et al.)

2.1 Current mapping systems

Current electroanatomic mapping systems build a 3-dimensional geometry of a cardiac chamber by recording sequential positional co-ordinates from the catheter tip in contact with the myocardium and combining this information with concomitantly acquired electrogram data. Low voltage areas and scar can be easily identified to develop a picture of the underlying substrate for arrhythmogensis. Electrogram timings with respect to a stable reference catheter, enables an activation map to be created, which is colour coded to differentiate between 'early' and 'late' signals.

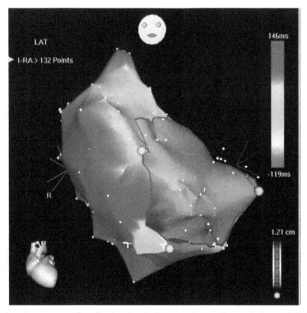

Colour coded activation map of a clockwise isthmus dependent right atrial flutter.

Alternatively, this can be displayed as a propagation map, which demonstrates activation of the excitatory wavefront as it advances across the chamber geometry. Maps can be rotated and viewed in multiple orientations at the same time so that the wavefront can be followed throughout the cardiac cycle. Electroanatomic mapping systems are primarily used for mapping stable tachycardias, however they can also facilitate substrate mapping during sinus rhythm, which is particularly useful when mapping VTs which cause significant haemodynamic compromise. Additionally, these systems facilitate encirclement of cardiac structures, the best example of which is the encirclement of pulmonary veins as part of the treatment for ablation of atrial fibrillation (AF). Areas targeted may lie between important scar boundaries (e.g. linear ablation lesions to transect the diastolic pathway in VT circuits) or between inert structures (e.g. linear ablation between the mitral valve annulus and the left inferior pulmonary vein in mitral isthmus-dependent atrial tachycardia).

2.2 Integration with robotic navigation

New Cohesion™ 3D visualisation module available with the Hansen Robotic Navigation system allows integration of the electroanatomic mapping system NavX or Velocity (St Jude Medical™) This facilitates navigation of the robotic catheter by producing an intuitive driving plane according to the orientation of the virtual geometry within the mapping system. This removes the requirement for the operator to re-orientate him or herself when using the virtual geometry of the left atrium to guide navigation. This has been tested in clinical studies and shown to reduce fluoroscopy times for robotic navigation and ablation of AF.(Steven, Servatius et al. 2009)

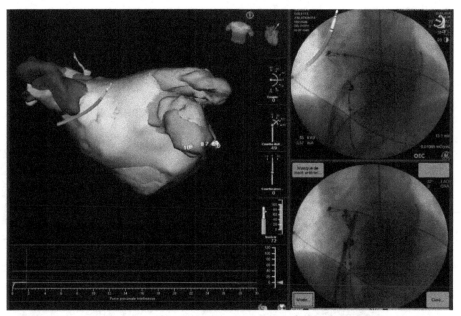

Example of Cohesion, Hansen Robotic navigation system fully integrated with NavX mapping system to provide intuitive driving in the orientation of the virtual LA geometry

2.3 Integration with MRI / CT imaging

The CARTO™ and NavX™ systems can both integrate digital computed tomography (CT) or magnetic resonance imaging (MRI) images of the heart into a mapping study, allowing navigation of "virtual" catheters within a high resolution model of the patient's anatomy.

CT / MRI studies can either be imported and segmented via the image processing platforms available in both mapping systems, or can be segmented offline by an experienced operator for direct import to the mapping system at the time of the procedure. Registration of the segmented chamber to the patient orientation is performed using fluoroscopy. Fixed anatomical landmarks close to the chamber of interest are acquired and subsequently registered with their corresponding sites on the CT/MRI image. The identified landmarks are then "merged" together to complete the registration process so that the catheter tip can be navigated within the detailed anatomical shell created on CT / MRI.

Electroanatomical mapping with CT/MRI image integration is particularly useful in patients with unusual or complex anatomy such as those with congenital heart disease and previous cardiac surgery. Detailed chamber anatomy is also helpful in pulmonary vein isolation procedures, by delineating the location, size and orientation of the pulmonary vein ostia. However, CT / MRI integration does not improve acute procedural efficacy or long term success rates.(Kistler, Rajappan et al. 2008)

2.4 Imaging of myocardial scar and integration with mapping systems

Delayed-enhanced Magnetic Resonance Imaging (DE-MRI) has been used for almost a decade to identify regions of ventricular scar. An increase in extracellular space within myocardial scar allows for an accumulation and prolonged wash-out time of the contrast agent, gadolinium.(Saraste, Nekolla et al. 2008). Information regarding ventricular or atrial scar can be obtained from voltage readings using intra-cardiac catheters. However, the integration of DE-MRI data may eliminate the need for acquisition of a detailed voltage map, and prevent inaccurate readings due to poor catheter contact.

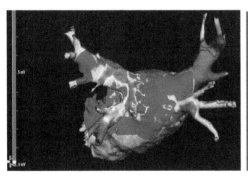 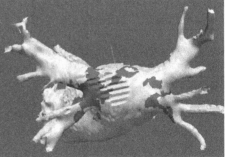

Example of similarity between endocardially collected voltage map and regions of LA scar identified by DE-MRI

2.4.1 Ventricular scar in ischaemic VT

DE-MRI enables detection, characterization and accurate quantification of acute and chronic myocardial infarction (Simonetti et al; McNamara et al 2001). Quantification of infarct size on DE-MRI has been validated against true infarct size as verified by histochemical staining in animal models (Kim RJ et al 1999). Heterogeneous tissue surrounding areas with dense LGE are hypothesized to be the imaging equivalent of slow conduction zones in patients with ischemic cardiomyopathy (Yan AT, Shayne AJ et al. 2006; Roes SD, Borleffs CJ et al 2009) although this is not a consistent finding. Until higher resolution images are possible we must accept the reality that the currently visualized "infarct core" and "heterogeneous tissue" is a mixture of true infarct core, true heterogeneous tissue, and artifacts, particularly those produced by volume averaging of infarct core with healthy tissue.

Utilising the technique described by Yan et al, Perez-David et al. demonstrated the connection between heterogeneous tissue on CMR and slow conduction zones identified by endocardial mapping. Furthermore, they confirmed that sites identified as critical VT isthmi by electrophysiological manoeuvres often reside in heterogeneous tissue identified by CMR.

2.4.2 Atrial scar in AF and AT

More recently, as scanners and scanning quality have improved, attention has turned to visualising atrial myocardium, in particular looking for regions of pre-existing fibrosis and iatrogenic scar following catheter ablation procedures.(Kim, Hillenbrand et al. 2000; Kim, Wu et al. 2000) Several recent studies have shown that high-spatial-resolution delayed enhancement MR (DE-MRI) imaging allows identification of scar induced by RF ablation in the left atrium(Peters, Wylie et al. 2007; McGann, Kholmovski et al. 2008; Badger, Adjei-Poku et al. 2009). Badger et al showed, however, that chronic atrial scar may not be formed and visible on MRI until up to 3 months following the ablation procedure. (Badger, Oakes et al. 2009) Integration of data from DE-MRI regarding location of scarred regions may benefit procedures such as repeat AF ablations and post-ablation atrial tachycardias. In particular, it may help identify the location of gaps within lines which are providing the substrate for ongoing AF / AT.

Methods for improved patient selection and non-invasive evaluation of the LA wall to assess the extent permanent tissue injury created by ablation, may be an important tool in improving ablation technique and increasing procedural success. Oakes et al demonstrated that the presence of left atrial fibrosis prior to ablation can also be detected using DE-MRI and that patients with higher levels of fibrosis had lower procedural success rates.(Oakes, Badger et al. 2009) On this basis they hypothesised that a further possible use of DE-MRI may be that of patient selection for atrial fibrillation ablation.

2.5 Novel mapping systems: CARTO Ripple

Despite the aforementioned advantages of current mapping systems there remain shortfalls and limitations to their use. The conversion of the raw electrical data to 'clean' activation maps requires operator expertise with the potential introduction of errors by incorrect assignment of local activation times or voltage thresholds. Furthermore interpolation of data within unmapped regions can lead to the display of false information. The introduction of integrated multielectrode mapping catheters should reduce this error by allowing creation of dense maps. This integration should also improve the rapidity with which maps are created with a likely increase in diagnostic yield (Patel et al 2008). Additionally, colour-spectrum isochronal maps are often converted to propagation maps that display moving activation wave fronts that are interpreted more intuitively but are mathematically extrapolated from the points collected and can give the operator a false sense of the resolution of the map. Isopotential maps created by grouping far-field reconstructed electrograms (Ensite Array) that are above a pre-specified activation threshold voltage to create activation wave fronts are prone to errors due to the subjective variation introduced by voltage threshold adjustments. In addition the hardware is limited by far-field reconstruction of low voltage electrograms.

Intracardiac electrograms provide unique site-specific data about local electrical activation and in-vitro studies have demonstrated that underlying anatomical substrate can be deduced from the electrogram morphology (Spach MS, Miller WT et al 1979). Electrograms are categorised by largely binary descriptors; simple or complex, early or late, high or low amplitude. Potentially crucial information contained within electrograms is lost to interpretation with current 3D mapping systems. CARTO does not assign any characteristics to potentials (diastolic or late systolic) within ventricular scar and is unable to appropriately display valuable data contained within complex fractionated electrograms often representing regions of slow conduction which may play a pivotal role in scar related artial arrhythmias. As the system can only assign a single value for the local activation time, isochronal and activation maps can be flawed if complex fractionated electrogams are annotated incorrectly.

ENSITE can collect simultaneous global activation data but is prone to far-field noise making low-amplitude fractionated signals difficult to differentiate from noise or repolarisation.

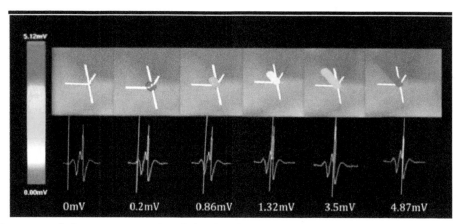

The top panel shows increasing Ripple bar height in correlation to the increasing magnitude of the electrogram voltage in the annotation window (shown in the lower window).

The bar height and colour are clearly visible. These can be correlated to the conventional reference colour bar from CARTO seen to the left of the panel with low voltage represented by red and high voltage represented by purple

The conventional 2D method for displaying electrograms is deflection from a baseline according to a voltage scale. The overall sequence of directions and rates of change and amplitudes of deflections define the electrogram "morphology". A new visualisation algorithm, Ripple Mapping, has allowed the reproduction of this 2D process on a 3D hull using a bar moving out from the cardiac surface conveying location, timing and electrogram morphology simultaneously (Linton, Koa-Wing. 2009). Multiple points collected in a small area will display bars, which change according to the local voltage change and in a temporally accurate sequence producing a 'ripple' effect which conveys the direction of wave propagation without any operator annotation. The program avoids interpolation and as it does not use a single local activation time, all the components of the electrogram are preserved and displayed. Therefore a sequence of small potentials and complex electrograms can be temporally related to adjacent electrograms. This method has the benefit of using high quality contact electrograms capable of demonstrating low amplitude signals with accurate 3D localisation, enabling the assessment of electrogram morphology within scar.

During the proof-of-concept study this novel method of cardiac mapping showed low-amplitude continuous activity in four of five tachycardias at the site of successful ablation, consistent with a re-entrant mechanism. Cardiac Ripple Mapping has been integrated onto an off-line CARTO ™ platform, which is currently undergoing validation and clinical evaluation.

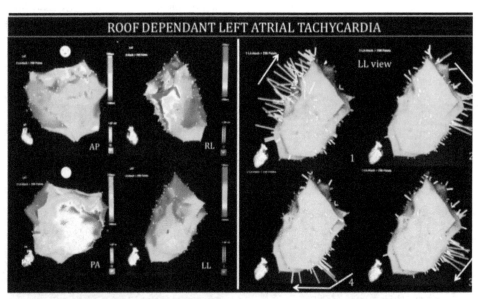

Left panel: Displays a left atrial CARTO-XP local activation time (LAT) map of a patient with left atrial tachycardia following circumferential pulmonary vein isolation for paroxysmal atrial fibrillation. Analysis of the LAT map suggests the possibility of a focal tachycardia origination from the posterior wall near the right pulmonary veins.
Right panel: The same atrial tachycardia as seen on the corresponding unaltered Ripple map (left lateral view) shows a roof dependant atrial tachycardia which was confimed by conventional entrainment manoeuvres.

3. Ablation of complex arrhythmias

The achievement of transmurality of ablation lesions for permanent VT abolition and pulmonary vein isolation is one of the ongoing challenges of ventricular tachycardia and atrial fibrillation ablation (Haissaguerre, Shah et al. 2000; Pappone, Santinelli et al.

2004);(Kosmidou, Inada et al. 2011 ; Willems, Steven et al. 2010). The Hansen™ robotic system was designed to improve catheter tip stability, lesion quality and clinical outcomes.

3.1 The Hansen robotic navigation system

The Hansen Sensei electromechanical robotic navigation system is capable of remotely steering a guide catheter to enable precise positioning and manipulation of any type of electrophysiological catheter within the heart for mapping and ablation. The Sensei system has been described in detail previously.(Saliba, Cummings et al. 2006; Kanagaratnam, Koa-Wing et al. 2008) In brief, the system comprises three linked components: the physician's workstation (Sensei™ robotic control system), remote catheter manipulator (RCM) and steerable guide catheter (Artisan™ Sheath). The steerable guide catheter comprises an outer (14F) and inner (10.5F) steerable sheath through which any 8.5F or less ablation catheter can be placed. The outer guide can be inserted, deinserted and can bend up to 90 degrees, whereas the inner guide is controlled by the 3D joystick and can be directed anywhere within the toroidal workspace. The Artisan sheath maintains the catheter position by the tensile strength of four pullwires so that the shape adopted by the sheath is uniquely suited to the point of interest to which the catheter is being positioned.(Kanagaratnam, Koa-Wing et al. 2008) This is in contrast to the manual approach, where the operator has to dynamically apply torque and flexion to prevent the catheter displacing from the point of interest. The Sensei™ robotic control system also incorporates a pressure sensor (Intellisense™), which calculates the contact force at the tip of the catheter using the differential resistance when continuously dithering the catheter in and out of the Artisan sheath. This tissue contact pressure enhances the validation of tissue contact and also provides for the ability to identify a pressure curve for optimal lesion production. (Kanagaratnam, Koa-Wing et al. 2008)

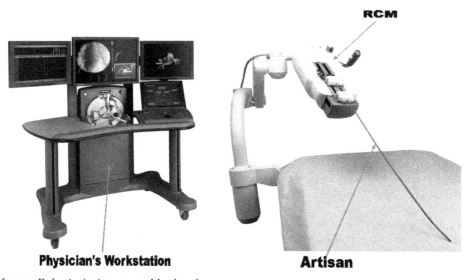

Physician's Workstation   **Artisan**

Hansen Robotic Artisan steerable sheath.

The Sensei system is currently compatible with all 8.5F or less mapping and irrigated ablation catheters. The physicians work station comprises 3 screens which can display any selected data including fluoroscopy, intracardiac echocardiography, electroanatomic mapping systems (Carto Biosense Webster, NavX St Jude Medical, Rotational Angiography imaging Philips ElectroNav etc.), and electrogram display systems (Bard Lab System Pro etc.) The free standing physician's work station and remote catheter manipulation system mounted on the patient table can be moved between laboratories and do not require any floor reinforcement such as that required for magnetic remote navigation systems.

The intended benefit of robotic catheter manipulation is that the catheter position is maintained once the physician has released the 3D joystick providing increased stability throughout the duration of RF delivery. In addition, the Intellisense system can confirm catheter contact during ablation.

3.1.1 Atrial and ventricular ablation

Several studies have been performed in animals to investigate whether the theoretical benefits of robotic ablation are translated into improved measurable parameters of lesion quality. In a study comparing robotic (Sensei) and manual ablation in 7 pig atria, robotic ablation reduced local electrogram amplitude to a greater degree than manual ablation (49+/- 2.6% vs 29 +/- 4.5% signal reduction after one minute p=0.0002) The incidence of >50% signal reduction was also greater for robotic (37%) than manual (21%) (p=0.0001).(Koa-Wing, Kojodjojo et al. 2009) Koa-Wing et al also noted that macroscopically the robotic lesions were more consistently transmural compared to the manual lesions, with no evidence of charring or perforation with either modality. In other in-vitro studies, 45W at 20-30g for 40secs, 83% of lesions were transmural, however 33% of lesions were associated with char formation. Using 30W and 20-30g pressure 0% were associated with char formation, however only 16% were associated with transmural lesion formation. (Di Biase, Natale et al. 2009),

Previous human studies comparing robotic and manual ablation have been non-randomised and have shown no significant difference in clinical outcomes. The primary aim of these studies was to prove safety and feasibility, however it is important to try to understand the potential reasons why these studies did not deliver the anticipated benefits of increased catheter precision and stability. (Willems, Steven et al 2010; Di Biase, Wang et al. 2009) The two studies both quoted using the same settings for both robotic and manual ablation (45W for 20secs and 20-25W for 60s) lesions. Interestingly, both reports comment on how robotic ablation required shorter radiofrequency duration. Therefore, in both series it appears that operators adjusted power according to anatomical location and local signal attenuation. Therefore, if the same target was being used for both manual and robotic arms, it is unsurprising that the clinical outcomes were similar.

The ability to titrate force and improve tissue contact are important attributes required during ablation in the ventricle which can be over a centimetre thick. Furthermore greater transmurality of delivered lesions should negate the need to gain epicardial access in this patient population who have often previously undergone cardiac surgery, making percutaneous access less practical. The reduction in operator radiation exposure during these long procedures is of added value. There are no large scale trials of robotic VT ablation however acute feasibility is suggested by occasional single case reports (Duncan, Johns et al 2010; Koa-Wing, Linton et al. 2009) Larger scale studies should help clarify the role of this technology in ablation of complex arrhythmias.

4. Conclusion

With the rapidly progressing field of catheter ablation, advances in mapping and ablation technologies will lead to improved therapeutic outcomes in complex cardiac arrhythmias. Innovative methods of assessing, displaying and integrating the underlying substrate of complex scar with electrophysiological data will further streamline our current practice in these challenging cases.

5. References

Anonymous (1997): A comparison of antiarrhythmic-drug therapy with implantable defibrillators in patients resuscitated from near fatal ventricular arrhythmias. The antiarrhythmics versus implantable defibrillators (AVID) Investigators. *N Engl J Med,* 337:1576- 1583.

Badger, T. J., R. S. Oakes, et al. (2009). "Temporal left atrial lesion formation after ablation of atrial fibrillation." *Heart Rhythm* 6(2): 161-8.

Badger, T. J., Y. A. Adjei-Poku, et al. (2009). "MRI in cardiac electrophysiology: the emerging role of delayed-enhancement MRI in atrial fibrillation ablation." *Future Cardiol* 5(1): 63-70.

Bogun F., Good E., Reich S., Elmouchi D., Igic P., Lemola K., Tschopp D., Jongnarangsin K., Oral H., Chugh A., Pelosi F. & Morady F. (2006) Isolated potentials during sinus rhythm and pace-mapping within scars as guides for ablation of post-infarction ventricular tachycardia. *J Am Coll.Cardiol,* 47: 2013-2019.

Calkins, H., J. Brugada, et al. (2007). "HRS/EHRA/ECAS expert Consensus Statement on catheter and surgical ablation of atrial fibrillation: recommendations for personnel, policy, procedures and follow-up. A report of the Heart Rhythm Society (HRS) Task Force on catheter and surgical ablation of atrial fibrillation." *Heart Rhythm* 4(6): 816-61.

Camm, A. J., P. Kirchhof, et al. "Guidelines for the management of atrial fibrillation: the Task Force for the Management of Atrial Fibrillation of the European Society of Cardiology (ESC)." *Europace* 12(10): 1360-420.

Cao, K. & Gonska, B. D. (1996). Catheter ablation of incessant ventricular tachycardia: acute and long-term results. *Eur Heart J.* 17:756-763.

Cappato, R., H. Calkins, et al. (2005). "Worldwide survey on the methods, efficacy, and safety of catheter ablation for human atrial fibrillation." *Circulation* 111(9): 1100-5.

Chugh A, Oral H, Lemola K, Hall B, Cheung P, Good E, Tamirisa K, Han J, Bogun F, Pelosi F, Morady F. Prevalence, mechanisms, and clinical significance of macroreentrant atrial tachycardia during and following left atrial ablation for atrial fibrillation. *Heart Rhythm.* 2005;2:464–471.

Connolly SJ, Gent M, Roberts RS, Dorian P, Roy D, Sheldon RS, Mitchell LB, Green MS, Klein GJ, O'Brien B (2000): Canadian implantable defibrillator study (CIDS): A randomized trial of the implantable cardioverter defibrillator against amiodarone. *Circulation,* 101:1297-1302.

Coumel, P. (1994). "Paroxysmal atrial fibrillation: a disorder of autonomic tone?" *Eur Heart J* 15 Suppl A: 9-16.

Coumel, P. (1996). "Autonomic influences in atrial tachyarrhythmias." *J Cardiovasc Electrophysiol* 7(10): 999-1007.

Cox, J. L., J. P. Boineau, et al. (1995). "Modification of the maze procedure for atrial flutter and atrial fibrillation. I. Rationale and surgical results." *J Thorac Cardiovasc Surg* 110(2): 473-84.

Cox, J. L., R. B. Schuessler, et al. (1996). "An 8 1/2-year clinical experience with surgery for atrial fibrillation." *Ann Surg* 224(3): 267-73; discussion 273-5.

Deisenhofer I, Estner H, Zrenner B, Schreieck J, Weyerbrock S, Hessling G, Scharf K, Karch MR, Schmitt C. Left atrial tachycardia after circumferential pulmonary vein ablation for atrial fibrillation: incidence, electrophysiological characteristics, and results of radiofrequency ablation. *Europace*. 2006;8:573–582.

Deisenhofer, I., H. Estner, et al. (2009). "Does electrogram guided substrate ablation add to the success of pulmonary vein isolation in patients with paroxysmal atrial fibrillation? A prospective, randomized study." *J Cardiovasc Electrophysiol* 20(5): 514-21.

Di Biase, L., A. Natale, et al. (2009). "Relationship between catheter forces, lesion characteristics, "popping," and char formation: experience with robotic navigation system." *J Cardiovasc Electrophysiol* 20(4): 436-40.

Di Biase, L., Y. Wang, et al. (2009). "Ablation of atrial fibrillation utilizing robotic catheter navigation in comparison to manual navigation and ablation: single-center experience." *J Cardiovasc Electrophysiol* 20(12): 1328-35.

Duncan, E., N. Johns, et al. (2010) "Robotic Catheter Navigation within the Left Ventricle." *Pacing Clin Electrophysiol.*

Earley MJ, Showkathali R, Alzetani M, et al. (2006) Radiofrequency ablation os arrhythmias guided by non-fluoroscopic catheter location: a prospective randomized trial. *Eur heart J* 27:1223-1229.

Estner, H. L., G. Hessling, et al. (2008). "Electrogram-guided substrate ablation with or without pulmonary vein isolation in patients with persistent atrial fibrillation." *Europace* 10(11): 1281-7.

Feinberg, W. M., J. L. Blackshear, et al. (1995). "Prevalence, age distribution, and gender of patients with atrial fibrillation. Analysis and implications." *Arch Intern Med* 155(5): 469-73.

Gerstenfeld EP, Callans DJ, Dixit S, Russo AM, Nayak H, Lin D, Pulliam W, Siddique S, Marchlinski FE. Mechanisms of organized left atrial tachycardias occurring after pulmonary vein isolation. *Circulation*. 2004; 110:1351–1357.

Gerstenfeld, E. P., S. Dixit, et al. (2002). "Utility of exit block for identifying electrical isolation of the pulmonary veins." *J Cardiovasc Electrophysiol* 13(10): 971-9.

Gonska D-B, Cao K, Schaumann A, Dorszewski A, von zur Muhlen F, Kreuzer H. (1994) Catheter ablation of ventricular tachycardia in 136 patients with coronary artery disease: results and long-term follow-up. *J Am Coll Cardiol.*;24:1506–1514.

Haines, D. E., D. D. Watson, et al. (1990). "Electrode radius predicts lesion radius during radiofrequency energy heating. Validation of a proposed thermodynamic model." *Circ Res* 67(1): 124-9.

Haïssaguerre M, Hocini M, Sanders P, Sacher F, Rotter M, Takahashi Y, Rostock T, Hsu LF, Bordachar P, Reuter S, Roudaut R, Clémenty J, Jaïs P. Catheter ablation of long-lasting persistent atrial fibrillation: clinical outcome and mechanisms of subsequent arrhythmias. *J Cardiovasc Electrophysiol*. 2005;16:1138 –1147.

Haissaguerre, M., D. C. Shah, et al. (2000). "Electrophysiological breakthroughs from the left atrium to the pulmonary veins." *Circulation* 102(20): 2463-5.

Haissaguerre, M., P. Jais, et al. (1998). "Spontaneous initiation of atrial fibrillation by ectopic beats originating in the pulmonary veins." *N Engl J Med* 339(10): 659-66.

Hocini, M., P. Jais, et al. (2005). "Techniques, evaluation, and consequences of linear block at the left atrial roof in paroxysmal atrial fibrillation: a prospective randomized study." *Circulation* 112(24): 3688-96.

Hsu, L. F., P. Jais, et al. (2004). "Catheter ablation for atrial fibrillation in congestive heart failure." *N Engl J Med* 351(23): 2373-83.

Huang SS, Wood MA. *Catheter Ablation of Cardiac Arrhythmias*. 1st Ed. 2006.

Jais, P., M. Hocini, et al. (2004). "Technique and results of linear ablation at the mitral isthmus." *Circulation* 110(19): 2996-3002.

Jalife, J., O. Berenfeld, et al. (2002). "Mother rotors and fibrillatory conduction: a mechanism of atrial fibrillation." *Cardiovasc Res* 54(2): 204-16.

Kanagaratnam, P., M. Koa-Wing, et al. (2008). "Experience of robotic catheter ablation in humans using a novel remotely steerable catheter sheath." *J Interv Card Electrophysiol* 21(1): 19-26.

Kannel, W. B., R. D. Abbott, et al. (1982). "Epidemiologic features of chronic atrial fibrillation: the Framingham study." *N Engl J Med* 306(17): 1018-22.

Kim, R. J., E. Wu, et al. (2000). "The use of contrast-enhanced magnetic resonance imaging to identify reversible myocardial dysfunction." *N Engl J Med* 343(20): 1445-53.

Kim, R. J., H. B. Hillenbrand, et al. (2000). "Evaluation of myocardial viability by MRI." *Herz* 25(4): 417-30.

Kistler, P. M., K. Rajappan, et al. (2008). "The impact of image integration on catheter ablation of atrial fibrillation using electroanatomic mapping: a prospective randomized study." *Eur Heart J* 29(24): 3029-36.

Koa-Wing, M., N. W. Linton, et al. (2009). "Robotic catheter ablation of ventricular tachycardia in a patient with congenital heart disease and Rastelli repair." *J Cardiovasc Electrophysiol* 20(10): 1163-6.

Koa-Wing, M., P. Kojodjojo, et al. (2009). "Robotically assisted ablation produces more rapid and greater signal attenuation than manual ablation." *J Cardiovasc Electrophysiol* 20(12): 1398-404.

Kosmidou, I., K. Inada, et al. (2011) "Role of repeat procedures for catheter ablation of postinfarction ventricular tachycardia." *Heart Rhythm* 8(10): 1516-22.

Kuck KH, Cappato R, et al. (2000). Randomized comparison of antiarrhythmic drug therapy with implantable defibrillators in patients resuscitated from cardiac arrest: The cardiac arrest study Hamburg (CASH). Circulation 102:748-754.

Lellouche, N., E. Buch, et al. (2007). "Functional characterization of atrial electrograms in sinus rhythm delineates sites of parasympathetic innervation in patients with paroxysmal atrial fibrillation." *J Am Coll Cardiol* 50(14): 1324-31.

Lim, K. T., S. Matsuo, et al. (2007). "Catheter ablation of persistent and permanent atrial fibrillation: Bordeaux experience." *Expert Rev Cardiovasc Ther* 5(4): 655-62.

Marchlinski FE, Callans DJ, Gottlieb CD, Zado E. (2000) Linear ablation lesions for control of unmappable ventricular tachycardia in patients with ischemic and nonischemic cardiomyopathy. *Circulation*. 101: 1288–1296

Marchlinski, F. E. (2008). "Atrial fibrillation catheter ablation: learning by burning continues." *J Am Coll Cardiol* 51(10): 1011-3.

Marrouche, N. F., D. O. Martin, et al. (2003). "Phased-array intracardiac echocardiography monitoring during pulmonary vein isolation in patients with atrial fibrillation: impact on outcome and complications." *Circulation* 107(21): 2710-6.

Matsuo, S., K. T. Lim, et al. (2007). "Ablation of chronic atrial fibrillation." *Heart Rhythm* 4(11): 1461-3.

McGann, C. J., E. G. Kholmovski, et al. (2008). "New magnetic resonance imaging-based method for defining the extent of left atrial wall injury after the ablation of atrial fibrillation." *J Am Coll Cardiol* 52(15): 1263-71.

Mesas CE, Pappone C, Lang CC, Gugliotta F, Tomita T, Vicedomini G, Sala S, Paglino G, Gulletta S, Ferro A, Santinelli V. Left atrial tachycardia after circumferential pulmonary vein ablation for atrial fibrillation: electroanatomic characterization and treatment. *J Am Coll Cardiol*. 2004;44:1071–1079.

Moss, A. J. *et al.* (2004). Long-term clinical course of patients after termination of ventricular tachyarrhythmia by an implanted defibrillator. *Circulation* 110: 3760–3765.

Nademanee, K., M. C. Schwab, et al. (2008). "Clinical outcomes of catheter substrate ablation for high-risk patients with atrial fibrillation." *J Am Coll Cardiol* 51(8): 843-9.

Natale, A., A. Raviele, et al. (2007). "Venice Chart international consensus document on atrial fibrillation ablation." *J Cardiovasc Electrophysiol* 18(5): 560-80.

Oakes, R. S., T. J. Badger, et al. (2009). "Detection and quantification of left atrial structural remodeling with delayed-enhancement magnetic resonance imaging in patients with atrial fibrillation." *Circulation* 119(13): 1758-67.

O'Neill, M. D., P. Jais, et al. (2007). "Catheter ablation for atrial fibrillation." *Circulation* 116(13): 1515-23.

Ouyang, F., D. Bansch, et al. (2004). "Complete isolation of left atrium surrounding the pulmonary veins: new insights from the double-Lasso technique in paroxysmal atrial fibrillation." *Circulation* 110(15): 2090-6.

Pappone, C., G. Oreto, et al. (1999). "Catheter ablation of paroxysmal atrial fibrillation using a 3D mapping system." *Circulation* 100(11): 1203-8.

Pappone, C., S. Rosanio, et al. (2003). "Mortality, morbidity, and quality of life after circumferential pulmonary vein ablation for atrial fibrillation: outcomes from a controlled nonrandomized long-term study." *J Am Coll Cardiol* 42(2): 185-97.

Pappone, C., V. Santinelli, et al. (2004). "Pulmonary vein denervation enhances long-term benefit after circumferential ablation for paroxysmal atrial fibrillation." *Circulation* 109(3): 327-34.

Patel A, d'Avila A, Neuzil P, Kim S, Mela T, Singh J, Ruskin J, ReddyV. Atrial Tachycardia After Ablation of Persistent Atrial Fibrillation : Identification of the Critical Isthmus

With a Combination of Multielectrode Activation Mapping and Targeted Entrainment Mapping. *Circ Arrhythm Electrophysiol* 2008;1;14-22.

Perez-David E, Arenal Á, Rubio-Guivernau JL, et al. (2011) Noninvasive identification of ventricular tachycardia-related conducting channels using contrast-enhanced magnetic resonance imaging in patients with chronic myocardial infarction: comparison of signal intensity scar mapping and endocardial voltage mapping. *J Am Coll Cardiol*, 57:184 –94.

Peters, D. C., J. V. Wylie, et al. (2007). "Detection of pulmonary vein and left atrial scar after catheter ablation with three-dimensional navigator-gated delayed enhancement MR imaging: initial experience." *Radiology* 243(3): 690-5.

Poole, J. E. *et al.* (2008). Prognostic importance of defibrillator shocks in patients with heart failure. *N. Engl. J. Med* 359: 1009–1017

Roes SD, Borleffs CJ, van der Geest RJ, et al. (2009) Infarct tissue hetero- geneity assessed with contrast-enhanced MRI predicts spontaneous ventricular arrhythmia in patients with ischemic cardiomyopathy and implantable cardioverter-defibrillator. *Circ Cardiovasc Imaging*, 2:183–90.

Sacher F, Roberts-Thomson K, Maury P et al. (2010) Epicardial ventricular tachycardia ablation. *J Am Coll Cardiol*, 55:2366-2372.

Sacher F, Tedrow UB, et al. (2008). Ventricular tachycardia ablation: evolution of patients and procedures over 8 years. *Circ Arrhythmia Electrophysiol*. 1: 153–16

Sahadevan, J., K. Ryu, et al. (2004). "Epicardial mapping of chronic atrial fibrillation in patients: preliminary observations." *Circulation* 110(21): 3293-9.

Saliba, W., J. E. Cummings, et al. (2006). "Novel robotic catheter remote control system: feasibility and safety of transseptal puncture and endocardial catheter navigation." *J Cardiovasc Electrophysiol* 17(10): 1102-5.

Sanders, P., P. Jais, et al. (2004). "Electrophysiologic and clinical consequences of linear catheter ablation to transect the anterior left atrium in patients with atrial fibrillation." *Heart Rhythm* 1(2): 176-84.

Saraste, A., S. Nekolla, et al. (2008). "Contrast-enhanced magnetic resonance imaging in the assessment of myocardial infarction and viability." *J Nucl Cardiol* 15(1): 105-17.

Scaglione, M., L. Biasco, et al. "Visualization of multiple catheters with electroanatomical mapping reduces X-ray exposure during atrial fibrillation ablation." *Europace* 13(7): 955-62.

Schilling RJ, Peters N, Davies W. (1999) Mapping and ablation of ventricular tachycardia with the aid of a non-contact mapping system. *Heart*, 81:570-575.

Schron, E. B. *et al.* (2002) Quality of life in the antiarrhythmics versus implantable defibrillators trial: impact of therapy and influence of adverse symptoms and defibrillator shocks. *Circulation* 105: 589–594.

Shah DC, Jais P, Haissaguerre M, et al. (1997) Three-dimensional mapping of the common atrial flutter in the right atrium. *Circulation*, 96:3904-3912.

Simonetti OP, Kim RJ, Fieno DS, et al. (2001) An improved MR imaging technique for the visualization of myocardial infarction. *Radiology*, 218:215–23.

Spach MS, Miller WT, Miller-Jones E, Warren RB, Barr RC (1979): Extracellular potentials related to intracellular action potentials during impulse conduction in anisotropic canine cardiac muscle. *Circ Res.* 45:188-204

Sporton, S. C., M. J. Earley, et al. (2004). "Electroanatomic versus fluoroscopic mapping for catheter ablation procedures: a prospective randomized study." *J Cardiovasc Electrophysiol* 15(3): 310-5.

Steven, D., H. Servatius, et al. (2009). "Reduced Fluoroscopy During Atrial Fibrillation Ablation: Benefits of Robotic Guided Navigation." *J Cardiovasc Electrophysiol.*

Stevenson W.G., Khan H., Sager P., Saxon L.A., Middlekauff H.R., Natterson P.D. & Wiener I. (1993) Identification of re-entry circuit sites during catheter mapping and radiofrequency ablation of ventricular tachycardia late after myocardial infarction. *Circulation*, 88: 1647-1670.

Stevenson WG, Delacretaz E, Friedman PL, Ellison KE. (1998) Identification and ablation of macroreentrant ventricular tachycardia with the CARTO electroanatomic mapping system. *Pacing Clin Electrophysiol*, 21:1448-1456.

Valles, E., R. Fan, et al. (2008). "Localization of atrial fibrillation triggers in patients undergoing pulmonary vein isolation: importance of the carina region." *J Am Coll Cardiol* 52(17): 1413-20.

Willems, S., D. Steven, et al. (2010) "Persistence of Pulmonary Vein Isolation After Robotic Remote-Navigated Ablation for Atrial Fibrillation and its Relation to Clinical Outcome." *JCardiovasc Electrophysiol*

Willems, S., H. Klemm, et al. (2006). "Substrate modification combined with pulmonary vein isolation improves outcome of catheter ablation in patients with persistent atrial fibrillation: a prospective randomized comparison." *Eur Heart J* 27(23): 2871-8.

Yokoyama, K., H. Nakagawa, et al. (2006). "Comparison of electrode cooling between internal and open irrigation in radiofrequency ablation lesion depth and incidence of thrombus and steam pop." *Circulation* 113(1): 11-9.

7

The Future of Cardiac Mapping

Pascal Fallavollita

Chair for Computer Aided Medical Procedures & Augmented Reality,
Technische Universität München,
Germany

1. Introduction

Severe disorders of the heart rhythm that can lead to sudden cardiac death (SCD) are often treated by radio-frequency (RF) catheter ablation. Using fluoroscopy as an imaging guide, the procedure consists of inserting a catheter inside the heart, near the area from which originates the abnormal cardiac electrical activity, then delivering RF currents through the catheter tip to ablate the arrhythmogenic area. Fluoroscopy is a conventional mapping technique that has been extremely useful in understanding and managing simpler arrhythmias. While the fluoroscopic procedure is still used in over 90% of ablations, its limitation in providing a reliable 3D geometry is evident when working upon complex cases like ventricular tachycardia (VT) or atrial fibrillation (AF) ablation. In turn, this results in impaired efficacy and length of the procedure lasting for several hours. Even though operator experience has decreased procedure times, radiation hazards still remain a major issue for the patient.

Recent 3D systems which integrate electrophysiological signals with anatomy to provide (3D+ t) geometry are extremely useful in situations where radiation needs to be limited as much as possible, and to increase the efficiency and shorten the duration of RF catheter ablation. During intracardiac mapping, it is not unusual to find sites at which the operator feels ablation is likely to succeed. Three-dimensional systems not only allow the surgeon to mark precise ablation points but also facilitate fixing reference points if the ablation process has to be repeated (Rajnish, 2009).

This chapter will summarize the most recent developments in catheter navigation and three-dimensional electroanatomic mapping. Conventional fluoroscopy techniques will be described followed by the CARTO and Ensite non-fluoroscopic mapping systems. Advances in ultrasound imaging for cardiac ablation guidance, and futuristic remote navigation technologies such as the Stereotaxis Magnetic Navigation system and the Hansen Sensei Robotic Catheter system will conclude the read.

2. Conventional catheter mapping

Every clinical electrophysiology (EP) laboratory is equipped with an X-ray system designed to provide fluoroscopic imaging of the heart. For many years this was the only form of procedural imaging available. A common characteristic of all X-ray images is that the soft tissue of the myocardium cannot be visualized (Figure 1), nevertheless, the walls of the left atrium can be indirectly assessed by bolus injection of contrast, which can be augmented by manoeuvres that minimize atrial emptying such as adenosine or rapid ventricular pacing. However, the major disadvantage of using X-ray fluoroscopy as the sole imaging modality is that all images obtained are two-dimensional representations of three-dimensional structures (D'Silva & Wright, 2011).

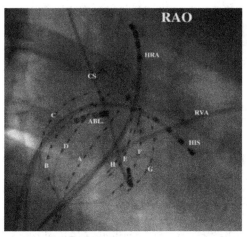

Fig. 1. A conventional fluoroscopy image showing a multielectrode basket array and other standard catheters inside the right atrium. Letters A to H identify basket splines and ABL indicates ablation catheter.
Image taken from Schmitt et al., 1999. (doi: 10.1161/01.CIR.99.18.2414).

2.1 Rotational angiography

Recently, three-dimensional rotational angiography (3DRA) has been introduced as an intraoperative modality for 3D imaging during cardiac ablation. In 3DRA, the C-arm typically performs a 200° rotation around the patient (Figure 2). Its cone-shaped radiation beam projects on a large flat-panel detector placed on the other end of the C-arm. A large number of two-dimensional projections are acquired over the course of the rotation. Reconstruction algorithms construct these into 3D images by volume or surface rendering. With adequate contrast agent administration and cardiac motion reduction (Figure 3), the image quality delivered by 3DRA has been shown to be comparable to or even exceeding classical cardiac computerized tomography (Wielandts et al., 2010). Three-dimensional rotational angiography images are more likely to represent the true anatomy than a remotely acquired image, such as CT or MRI, because of factors such as the patient's breathing and heart motion. This technique also reduces the financial and administrative burden of scheduling adjunctive and expensive imaging studies. In the case of patient movement, the geometry needs to be fully re-acquired; this can be promptly managed, but the consistent iodinated contrast agent load and radiation dose typically preclude the use of rotational angiography more than twice in a study (Casella et al., 2010).

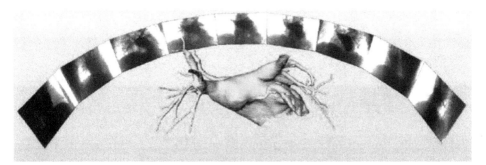

Fig. 2. A three-dimensional imaging sequence consists of 248 frames, imaged over a 200° rotation of the C-arm fluoroscope. Using advanced algorithms, a subsequent 3D volume reconstruction of the atrium is generated.
Image taken from Wielandts et al., 2010.

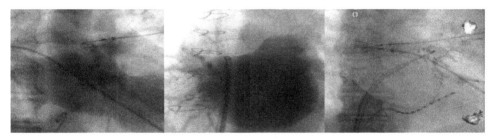

Fig. 3. Direct injection into the left atrium following segmentation of the resulting dataset. The subsequent 3D anatomical shell can then be superimposed on the live fluoroscopy. Image taken from D'Silva & Wright, 2011.

3. Electroanatomic mapping: CARTO

CARTO (*Biosense-Webster Inc, Diamond Bar, CA*) consists of a mapping catheter with miniaturized coils at the tip, a magnetic field generator located underneath the patient, a unit which analyses the current generated by the coils in the catheter-tip and a post-processing graphical display unit. The location pad fixed beneath the patient table has three coils that generate low magnetic fields (Figure 4). The emitted fields possess well-known temporal and spatial distinguishing characteristics that encode the mapping space around the patient's chest. The location is mapped in three-dimensions with reference to a fixed point. Each of the sensor locations is determined by its distance from the location pad. Three dimensional reconstruction is performed by calculating the distance between the two sensors. In case the patient moves, the distance of each sensor from the location pad is changed; however, the distance between the sensors is retained. The three distances determine the location, orientation and rotation of the catheter (Rajnish, 2009). Accuracy of the catheter tip location has been estimated to be within 0.54 ± 0.05mm (LaPage & Saul, 2011).

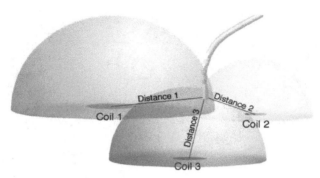

Fig. 4. Three electromagnetic fields originating from location pad coils. Spatial location of the catheter tip is accurately found by the electromagnetic fields, by determining the distance of the sensor on the catheter tip from each coil. This information is instantly computed to generate a real-time position of the catheter tip. Image courtesy of Biosense Webster.

The CARTO system is termed a point-by-point technology; multiple positions of the magnetic tip catheter are required inside the heart chamber to create a complete three-dimensional depiction of the chamber of interest (Figure 5). The activation time is referenced against an ECG lead or an intracardiac catheter (Rajnish, 2009).

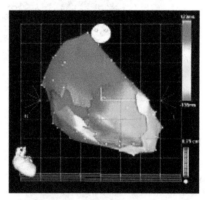

Fig. 5. Three dimensional anatomical reconstruction with superposition of activation times using the point-by-point CARTO technology. Earliest activation times are depicted in red. Image courtesy of Biosense Webster.

3.1 CARTO 3™

(Kabra & Singh, 2010) have recently reviewed the CARTO 3™ technology and some of the highlights of the system follow. First, the CARTO 3™ System is the third generation technology from Biosense Webster. Multiple catheter tips and curves can now be visualized on the electroanatomic map when compared to the traditional CARTO mapping system (Figure 6). In addition, CARTO 3™ uses a magnetic technology that calibrates the current-based technology, thereby minimizing distortions at the periphery of the electrical field. Mapping is performed in two steps. Initially, the magnetic mapping permits precise localization of the catheter with the sensor. As the catheter with the sensor moves around a chamber, multiple locations are created and stored by the system. The system then integrates the current based points with their respective magnetic locations, resulting in a calibrated current based field that permits accurate visualization of catheters and their locations (Kabra & Singh, 2010). Each electrode emits a unique frequency allowing each to be clearly distinguished, especially when in close proximity to one another. Both the catheters with and without the magnetic sensors can be visualized without spatial distortions. Lastly, CARTO 3™ has 'Fast Anatomical Mapping' (FAM) feature that permits rapid creation of anatomical maps. Unlike point-by-point electroanatomical mapping, volume data can be collected with FAM. Catheters such as the multi-polar Lasso can further enhance the collection of points and increase the mapping speed (Kabra & Singh, 2010).

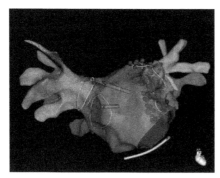

Fig. 6. The CARTO 3™ system with individually reconstructed catheters without spatial distortions. Image courtesy of Biosense Webster.

3.2 CARTOMerge
The major development for electroanatomic mapping in recent years has been the fusion of imaging technologies – MRI/CT – and electroanatomic mapping systems (Figure 7). The process of incorporating CT or MRI images into the electroanatomic mapping system involves 3D/3D registration of the catheter obtained geometry with the CT image. Typically, specific landmarks in the chamber are localized with the catheter and these points are then used to orient the CT/MRI image properly. (Rossillo et al, 2009) compared this method with a focused registration process during which they obtained multiple mapping points at each pulmonary vein using intracardiac echo guidance. They concluded that the focused registration process was a superior technique.

3.3 Advantages/disadvantages
The strengths of the CARTO technology are: (i) accurate heart chamber reconstruction, (ii) creation of linear ablations, (iii) color-coded activation maps, (iv) scar and ablation tagging capabilities. The weaknesses include: (i) incompatibility with other mapping catheters, (ii) limited utility in non-sustained arrhythmias, and (iii) orthogonal appearing volumes.

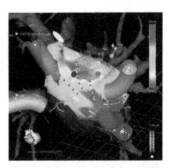

Fig. 7. The CARTOMerge technology allows the electroanatomic map of the left atrium using CARTO to be integrated with the CT/MRI images using CARTOMerge module. The circles depict the corresponding points on the two maps. Image taken from Thornton et al., 2008. (doi: doi:10.1093/europace/eun080)

3.4 Clinical study

In a recently published randomized study of 3DRA versus CARTO during atrial fibrillation ablation, the radiation exposure, procedural times and clinical outcomes at 10 months were similar in the groups investigated (Knecht et al, 2010). However the use of contrast makes it a less appealing option for patients with heart failure or renal failure. In addition, 3DRA was sensitive to patient movements during the study period. However further refinements are needed before it can be widely adopted. These include incorporation of respiratory and cardiac motion compensation and the ability to display electrogram data on the 3D (Kabra & Singh, 2010).

4. Electroanatomic mapping: ENSITE

The ENSITE system (*Endocardial Solutions, St. Jude Medical, Inc., St. Paul, MN, USA*) has two different techniques for mapping: the contact mapping system, wherein points assimilate anatomic and physiologic information in reference to five location patches applied to the skin at different places, and the non-contact mapping by a balloon array.

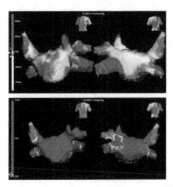

Fig. 8. Electroanatomical map acquired by the NavX system. (*Top*) Activation map of the left atrium during sinus rhythm, AP and PA views. (*Bottom*) Simultaneously-acquired voltage map of the left atrium. Image taken from Bhakta & Miller, 2008.

The contact mapping system, NavX™, is capable of displaying 3D positions of many catheters. This is achieved by applying a 5.6 kHz current through orthogonally-located skin patches on the patient. The recorded voltage and impedance at each catheter's electrodes generated from this current allows their distance from each skin patch to be triangulated with the help of a reference electrode. This determines their positions in space and the three-dimensional images of each catheter can then be displayed (Figure 8). Chamber geometry can be determined thereafter by moving a mapping catheter along the endocardial surface (Bhakta & Miller, 2008).

The non-contact mapping proceeds by using a multi electrode array (MEA). The array is comprised of 64 braided surgical-steel wires with a polyimide coating. The unipolar electrodes are created by removing a small area of insulation for each wire. The MEA is introduced into the body, like any other catheter through the femoral veins, and is inflated to 7.5 ml after positioning it at the centre of the chamber of interest (Figure 9).

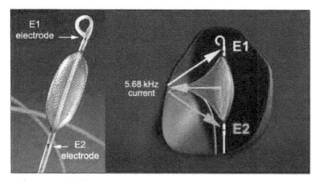

Fig. 9. Multielectrode array balloon catheter and in its deployed state. Image courtesy of Endocardial Solutions.

The balloon electrodes make galvanic contact with the blood and sense the electrical potentials induced upon them by the electrical fields generated by myocardial activity. Two ring electrodes (E1 and E2) used to build the geometry of the chamber are located on the catheter shaft about 1 cm proximal and distal to the MEA (Rajnish, 2009). A third ring electrode meant to serve as a reference for unipolar signals is located on the catheter shaft about 16 cm proximal to the MEA. The ENSITE array and a conventional catheter are placed in the heart in the same chamber. The Patient Interface Unit (PIU) sends a 5.6 kHz signal through the conventional catheter electrode, E1 and E2 alternately receive and return the signal to the PIU (Rajnish, 2009). Each of the 64 electrodes on the ENSITE array electrode senses the strength of the 5.6 kHz signal until the respective array electrode locations in three-dimensional are measured (Figure 10).

The latest version of the system, the ENSITE Velocity, has been reviewed by (Eitel et al., 2010). (Casella et al., 2009) evaluated the accuracy of the GeoMap – a new feature of Ensite Velocity that allows multipoint simultaneous geometry acquisition and activation mapping. They performed a typical point-by-point map and then a GeoMap of the right ventricle in 13 patients and compared them with MRI data from those patients. The GeoMap acquired more points in less time. The two mapping techniques disagreed in only 3% of regions and the GeoMap was more accurate at identifying low voltage correlated with areas of motion abnormality on MRI. (Schneider et al., 2010) provided one of the few recent pediatric-focused studies on noncontact mapping. They used the array in 20 patients with idiopathic ventricular tachycardia from the right ventricular outflow tract, left ventricle, or aortic root and achieved acute success in 17 of 18 patients for whom ablation was attempted with only three recurrences (LaPage & Saul, 2011). Previous versions of Ensite have been accurate within 0.7 ± 1.5mm.

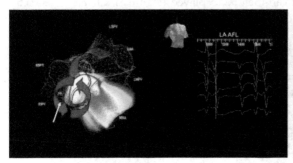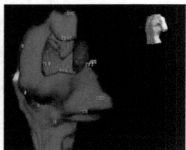

Fig. 10. Electroanatomic maps acquired by using a MEA. (*Left*) Activation map of macro-re-entrant LA flutter. The arrows depict wave front propagation within the flutter circuit. (*Right*) Anatomical reconstruction of the RA. Image taken from Bhakta & Miller, 2008.

4.1 Advantages/disadvantages
The strengths of the ENSITE technology are: (i) accurate heart chamber reconstruction, (ii) ability to use with any other catheter, (iii) respiratory and cardiac motion compensation, (iv) multiple catheter location display, and (v) useful in treating poorly sustained arrhythmias. The weaknesses include: (i) inaccurate anatomical reconstructions, (ii) limited utility in non-sustained arrhythmias, and (iii) difficult balloon deployment.

4.2 Clinical study
Recently, two clinical studies were performed to assess the impact of the NavX mapping system when compared to conventional fluoroscopy ablation.
The first study (Kwong et al, 2011) sought to assess the impact on paediatric catheter ablation fluoroscopy times. The authors retrospectively analysed the procedural data during a 7-year period (2002 – 2008), which spanned the transition between the standard fluoroscopic mapping and adoption of routine NavX™ mapping for catheter ablation of atrioventricular nodal re-entrant tachycardia (AVNRT) and right-/left-sided accessory pathways (RAP/LAP). Overall, success rates were similar between the two mapping systems (95.7% for conventional vs. 95.9% for NavX™). Secondly, NavX™ mapping significantly reduced the ablation fluoro time (15.9 + 14.3 min vs. 11.0 + 8.9 for NavX™) with a trend towards a decrease in total fluoro time (26.4 + 15.6 min vs. 23.8 +11.1 for NavX™). Lastly, the total procedure time was not significantly different between the two methods (210.1 + 66 vs. 222.8 + 61 min for NavX™, P ¼ 0.7). (Kwong et al, 2011) concluded that the NavX™ mapping reduced ablation fluoro times during paediatric catheter ablation, particularly in accessory pathways.
The second study (Liu et al., 2011) was to probe the feasibility and safety of non-fluoroscopic radiofrequency catheter ablation of atrioventricular nodal re-entrant tachycardia guided by Ensite NavX system. Non-fluoroscopic radiofrequency catheter ablation navigated by NavX system was performed in 18 cases (mean age 52.8 + 16.1 years, range 24 – 77 years) of

atrioventricular nodal re-entrant tachycardia with normal cardiac anatomy. Using NavX, right atrial and coronary sinus geometries were reconstructed. Diagnostic electrophysiological study and radiofrequency catheter ablation were performed in all patients without use of fluoroscopy. Each site with His bundle potential were mapped and marked in the 3D geometry before ablation. The real-time position of ablation catheter was confirmed by the relative position between CS catheter and ablation catheter, which were monitored simultaneously in the Ensite NavX system. The authors show the success rate of procedure was 100%. The fluoroscopic duration of each case was zero. The average procedure duration was 97.5 + 19.8 min (55 – 125 min, the coronary sinus access was obtained in 13.4 + 7.3 min (8 – 30 min). (Liu et al., 2011) conclude that the preliminary study suggests that non-fluoroscopic catheter navigation for radiofrequency catheter ablation of atrioventricular nodal re-entrant tachycardia is safe and feasible.

5. Remote navigation systems

Is robotic guidance for cardiac ablation procedures the future? We attempt to answer this question in this section. Remote navigation systems or robotic cardiac catheter ablation was essentially developed to eliminate potential errors in catheter manipulation. Also, the use of robots could systematically decrease clinician fatigue and fluoroscopy exposure. Some electrophysiologists agree that areas between mitral valves and pulmonary veins are typically difficult to reach and position correctly the mapping catheter. Robotics can thus provide more accuracy in these cases. Currently there are two robotic systems -the Niobe Stereotaxis Magnetic Navigation System (*Stereotaxis, Inc., St Louis, Missouri, USA*) and the Hansen Sensei Robotic Catheter System (*Hansen Medical, Mountain View, California, USA*) depicted in Figure 11 and Figure 12. Both systems allow the physician to perform the mapping and ablation procedure while sitting in a control room remote from the patient [LaPage & Saul, 2011].

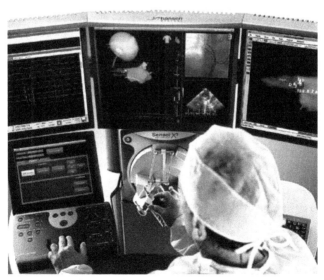

Fig. 11. The Hansen Sensei Robotic catheter system. Image taken from Hansen Medical.

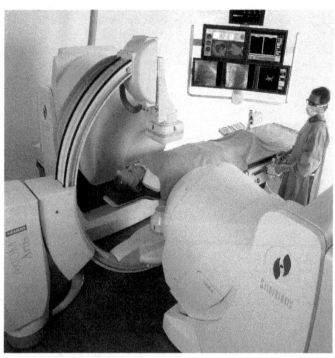

Fig. 12. Stereotaxis' Remote Magnetic Navigation System. Image taken from Stereotaxis.com.

The Stereotaxis system has been around for nearly a decade. Multiple studies have been published regarding its utility and several excellent review papers on the technology have been published (Xu et al., 2009; Wu et al., 2010 ; Thornton et al., 2010). The catheter has a magnet near the distal tip that can be oriented in any position using the fields produced by two magnets positioned bilaterally to the patient (LaPage & Saul, 2011). As an example application of Stereotaxis, (Azizian & Patel, 2011) used a magnetic tracking device to track the distal part of the ablation catheter in real time and a master-slave robot-assisted system is developed for actuation of a steerable catheter. The Sensei system facilitates catheter navigation through two coaxial sheaths steered with a pull wire mechanism controlled through a joystick remote control. The system is relatively novel and no pediatric applicable studies have been published. (Schmidt et al., 2009) achieved a high success rate using it for atrial fibrillation ablation and found the system equally compatible with both the CARTO and ENSITE systems. (LaPage & Saul, 2011) Both of these technologies have been integrated with electroanatomic mapping systems to store catheter location information for semi-automated re-navigation to regions of interest. These systems translate the operator's manipulation of a handle into precise movements of the catheter, thus allowing barely accessible regions of the heart to be reached, to create detailed electroanatomic mappings and precise ablation lesions (Casella et al., 2010).

5.1 Advantages/disadvantages
The strengths of the Sensei Hansen technology are: (i) can be used with any electroanatomic mapping system described previously, (ii) no fidelity devices or distortion effects, and (iii)

catheter stability. The limitations include: (i) sheath diameter and lengths and (ii) no catheter restriction.

The strengths of the Niobe Stereotaxis technology include: (i) low risk of perforation in anatomy, (ii) numerous experiments and trials published, (iii) semiautomatic mapping, and (iv)no fidelity devices or distortion effects. The limitations include: (i) restricted to expensive magnetic catheters, (ii) non real-time movement, and (iii) patients that have implanted devices.

5.2 Clinical study

(Chong et al., 2011a) performed two clinical studies using the Niobe Stereotaxis system. The first study aimed at determining the effectiveness and safety of single magnetic-guided catheter in the ablation of outflow tract tachycardias. At the outset of the clinical study, patients with symptomatic outflow tract tachycardia on surface ECG and without structural heart disease were recruited. Electrophysiology study and ablation were performed with the use of a single Navistar RMT Thermocool 8F ablation catheter. Both activation and pace mapping of ventricular tachycardia were performed. Three dimensional localization, using CARTO, was performed during activation mapping. As comparison, the patients were compared with a cohort of similar patients undergoing conventional catheter ablation via fluoroscopy. The results demonstrated that ablation was successful in all patients. Secondly, there was no difference in median procedure time between Niobe Stereotaxis (153 min) and conventional fluoroscopy (136 min) ablation groups. Nevertheless, the median fluoroscopy time was significantly reduced in the Niobe Stereotaxis group (8 vs. 29 min). (Chong et al., 2011a) concluded that the ablation of outflow tract ventricular tachycardia with a single magnetic-guided catheter is feasible, safe, and reduces fluoroscopy time.

In their second study, (Chong et al., 2011b) aimed at outlining their experiences in the ablation of incessant ventricular tachycardia with the use of the remote Niobe Stereotaxis magnetic-guided catheter system. In the course of the 1-year study, three patients with incessant ventricular tachycardia were recruited. All underwent ablation with Navistar RMT Thermocool 8F catheter guided via the Niobe Stereotaxis system and three dimensional localization using CARTO. Upon completion of procedure two of the patients' ventricular tachycardia could no longer be induced after successful ablation, and after a 12 month period, there was no recurrence. The third patient had ventricular ectopics and non-sustained ventricular tachycardia (NSVT) noted from two further sites these were ablated as well and there were no significant complications. Total fluoroscopy time was 17.4, 18.2, and 15.2 min, respectively, whereas the total procedure time was 3, 2, and 5 h, respectively. (Chong et al., 2011b) concluded that magnetic-guided catheter ablation is effective in the ablation of patients with incessant haemodynamically stable ventricular tachycardia.

(Zvereva et al., 2011) performed a prospective study to compare the incidence of oesophageal lesions using either the remote navigation system from Hansen Sensei to a manual approach for pulmonary vein isolation using a radiofrequency catheter. A total of 33 patients were recruited, 14 of which underwent manual approach. The oesophageal probe was placed and integrated with NavX™. When temperature rose to .39 FXC, ablation was immediately stopped until temperature decreased. Lastly, endoscopy was performed within 24 h after pulmonary vein isolation. Results demonstrated that in 2 of 19 patients with Hansen Sensei treatment had an oesophageal lesion found compared to only lesion found for 1 of 14 patients using the manual approach. Altogether, patients were comparable with respect to arterial hypertension, incidence of paroxysmal and persistent atrial fibrillation, or left atrial diameter. The oesophageal lesions showed brisk healing after re-endoscopy within 2 weeks in all patients. (Zvereva et al., 2011) concluded that the incidence of oesophageal lesions in patients using Hansen Sensei compared with manually performed ablation is similar when low power settings at the posterior wall are used.

6. Ultrasound

The flexibility and ease of use of ultrasound has made it the imaging modality of choice in many intraoperative surgery rooms and laboratories worldwide. In this section we discuss specific applications of the common ultrasound instrumentation used in the electrophysiology laboratory.

6.1 CARTOSound

An extension to the CARTO mapping technology enabling ultrasound integration was created recently and termed, CARTOSound (*Biosense Webster Inc., Diamond Bar, California, USA*). It creates a three-dimensional image of a specific heart chamber undergoing cardiac ablation by utilizing an intracardiac ultrasound catheter. A first study (Schwartzman, & Zhong, 2010) evaluated the use of CARTOSound for left atrial navigation during atrial fibrillation ablation. The authors first integrated the images obtained from CARTOSound into a preoperative CT (Figure 13) and then assessed the accuracy of the CARTOSound volume representation of the left atrium from each of four different ultrasound positions (RA, left atrium, coronary sinus, and esophagus). It turns out that the most accurate representation of the chamber was obtained with the ultrasound catheter placed in the left atrium. Hence, at first sight, the CARTOSound chamber representation was found to be as accurate as the CT image (LaPage & Saul, 2011).

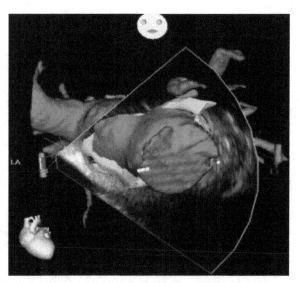

Fig. 13. The CARTOSound mapping technology that fused ultrasound images into the reconstructed volume. Image taken from Knecht et al., 2008. (doi: 10.1093/europace/eun227)

6.2 TEE imaging

Recently, real-time 3D transoesophageal echocardiography (TEE) has become available for clinical practice, offering clear and detailed rendering of the cardiac anatomy. The 3D TEE probe (*Matrix 3DTEE, Philips, Inc., Andover, MA*) allows for both 2D and 3D real-time imaging of both the left atrium and pulmonary veins. 3D TEE also provides excellent visualisation of the interatrial septum (Chierda et al., 2008a). A small study implied that 3D TEE guidance might provide safer trans-septal puncture in patients with unusual anatomy (Chierda et al., 2008b), as it offers the benefit of recognising some shapes of the atrial septum that are not well characterised by conventional two dimensional TEE. Despite these promising features, post-acquisition image processing is necessary and time-consuming. Moreover, general anaesthesia along with endotracheal intubation would be mandatory (Casella et al., 2010).

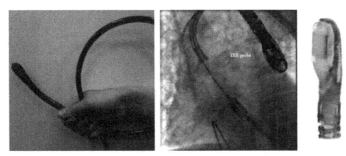

Fig. 14. The TEE probe and its tip sensor used to image left atrium or pulmonary veins during ablation procedures. Also shown is the TEE probe visible in X-ray. Image taken from King et al., 2010.

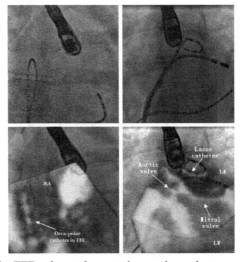

Fig. 15. (*First column*) the TEE volume shows a deca-polar catheter positioned in right atrium and dots highlight the position of the deca-polar catheter in the background of the X-ray image. (*Second column*), a lasso catheter was inserted into the left atrium with TEE volumes registered to X-ray images. Image taken from King et al., 2010.

6.3 ICE imaging

The first catheter-based 2D echocardiography systems were developed in the late 20th century for intracoronary imaging. They had high frequencies (20–40 MHz) and limited depth of penetration, making them suitable only for intravascular applications (Robinson & Hutchinson, 2010). Over the years, there has been a significant improvement in the technology with the advent of low frequency (12.5 - 9 MHz) and more recently the phased array (5.5 - 10 MHz) transducers which have been miniaturized and mounted on the catheters capable of percutaneous insertion (Pandian et al, 1990; Packer et al. 2002). Phased array ICE imaging uses a 64-element transducer on the distal end of an 8-10 French catheter. These catheters are capable of M-mode, pulsed, continuous wave and color Doppler (Daoud, 2005; Ren et al., 2002; Verma et al., 2002; Ferguson et al., 2009; Kabra & Singh, 2010.) During intervention, once transseptal access is achieved, ICE facilitates visualization of the left atrial and pulmonary venous anatomy. It also helps to assess the electrode-tissue contact. The images of ICE can be integrated with the electroanatomic mapping systems (CARTOSound) to generate the geometry of left atrium. A recent study demonstrated the feasibility of catheter ablation of atrial fibrillation without fluoroscopy using intracardiac echocardiography and electroanatomic mapping (Ferguson, 2009). Advances in intracardiac echocardiography include creation of accurate, real time three-dimensional ultrasound geometries that may obviate the need for pre-procedure CT/MRI imaging for catheter ablation of atrial fibrillation (Okumura, 2008). Other advantages over CT and MRI include ICE offering the advantage of showing the real-time detailed anatomy of the cardiac chambers that can be updated multiple times during the procedure. Furthermore, creating a 3D reconstruction without entering the LA may reduce procedural time, enhance the safety of catheter ablation procedures and eliminate geometrical distortion resulting from distension of the tissue. However, this technology bears an important financial burden because of the employment of expensive non-reusable ICE catheters (Casella et al., 2010).

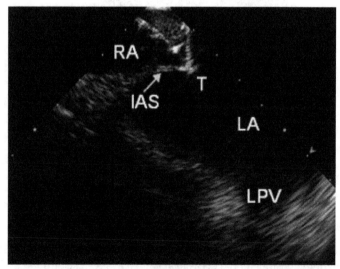

Fig. 16. ICE image showing left and right atriums, interatrial septum, needle tenting and left pulmonary veins. Image taken from Robinson & Hutchinson, 2010.

7. Conclusion

In summary, this chapter presented the latest findings involving several electroanatomical mapping systems that are available to assist electrophysiologists in treating arrhythmias. Techniques are still evolving to address the challenge of a catheter-based cure. The chapter indicates that the registration of MRI/CT images to the existing fluoroscopy image or 3D anatomical map can facilitate navigation of the ablation catheter. In addition, robotic catheter navigation is now available as well. Each method, whether it is the conventional fluoroscopic treatment or the more sophisticated remote navigation systems has its own merits and weaknesses. While all these systems provide a wealth of data and reduce fluoroscopy times slightly, they cannot replace careful interpretation of data and strict adherence to electrophysiologic principles. Although these benefits are achieved at a greater cost, there may be long-term benefits to the community and catheter laboratory staff.

8. Acknowledgment

Dr. Pascal Fallavollita would like to acknowledge the support of the Chair for Computer Aided Medical Procedures & Augmented Reality, Technische Universität München.

9. References

Azizian, M. & Patel, R. (2011). Intraoperative 3D stereo visualization for image-guided cardiac ablation.*SPIE Medical Imaging: Visualization, Image-Guided Procedures, and Modeling*, Vol. 7964, pp. 79640F

Bhakta, D. & Miller, JM. (2008). Principles of Electroanatomic Mapping. *Indian Pacing and Electrophysiology Journal*, (ISSN 0972-6292), Vol.8, Issue 1, pp. 32-50

Casella, M.; Perna, F.; Dello Russo, A.; Pelargonio, G.; Bartoletti, S.; Ricco, A.; Sanna, T.; Pieroni, M.; Forleo, G.; Pappalardo, A.; Di Biase, L.; Natale, L.; Bellocci, F; Zecchi, P.; Natale, A. & Tondo, C. (2009). Right ventricular substrate mapping using the Ensite NavX system: accuracy of high-density voltage map obtained by automatic point acquisition during geometry reconstruction. *Heart Rhythm*, Vol.6, pp. 1598-1605

Casella, M.; Perna, F.; Dello Russo, A.; Moltrasio, M.; Fassini, G.; Riva,S.; Zucchetti, M.; Majocchi,B.; Tundo,F.; Colombo, C.; De Juliis, P.; Giraldi, F.; Carbucicchio, C.; Fiorentini C. & Tondo, C. (2010). Atrial Fibrillation Ablation – New Approaches, New Technologies. *European Cardiology*, Vol.6, Issue 3, pp. 71–6

Chierchia, G.B.; Capulzini, L.; de Asmundis, C.; Sarkozy, A.; Roos, M.; Paparella, G.; Boussy, T.; Van Camp, G.; Kerkhove D. & Brugada, P. (2008a) First experience with real-time three-dimensional transoesophageal echocardiography-guided transseptal in patients undergoing atrial fibrillation ablation. *Europace*, Vol. 10, pp. 1325–8

Chierchia, G.B.; Van Camp, G., Sarkozy, A.; de Asmundis, C. & Brugada, P. (2008b). Double transseptal puncture guided by real-time three-dimensional transoesophageal echocardiography during atrial fibrillation ablation. *Europace*, Vol. 10, pp. 705–6

Chong, D.; Ching, C.K.; Liew, R.; Galalardin; Khin, M.W. & Teo, W.S. (2011a). Outflow tract ventricular tachycardia ablation with a magnetic-guided catheter is effective, safe and reduces radiation exposure. *Europace*, Vol.13, suppl 1, pp. i47-i82, poster 008

Chong, D.; Tan, B.Y.; Liew, R.; Ching, C.K. & Teo, W.S. (2011b). Ablation of incessant ventricular tachycardia using a remote magnetic-guided catheter: a tertiary centre case series. *Europace*, Vol.13, suppl 1, pp. i47-i82, poster 009

Daoud E.G. (2005). Transseptal catheterization. *Heart Rhythm*, Vol.2, pp. 212-214

D'Silva, A. & Wright, M. (2011). Advances in Imaging for Atrial Fibrillation Ablation. *Radiology Research and Practice*. Vol. 2011, Article ID 714864, 10 pages, doi:10.1155/2011/714864

Eitel, C.; Hindricks, G.; Dagres, N.; Sommer, P. & Piorkowski, C. (2010). EnSite Velocity cardiac mapping system: a new platform for 3D mapping of cardiac arrhythmias. *Expert Rev Med Devices*, Vol.7, pp.185–188

Ferguson, J.D.; Helms, A.; Mangrum, J.M.; Mahapatra, S.; Mason, P.; Bilchick, K.; McDaniel, G.; Wiggins, D. & DiMarco, J.P. (2009). Catheter ablation of atrial fibrillation without fluoroscopy using intracardiac echocardiography and electroanatomic mapping. *Circ Arrhythm Electrophysiol*, Vol. 2, pp. 611-619

Kabra, R. & Singh, J. (2010). Recent Trends in Imaging for Atrial Fibrillation Ablation. *Indian Pacing and Electrophysiology Journal*, Vol. 10, Issue5, pp. 215-227, 2010

King, A.P.; Rhode, K.S.; Ma, Y.; Yao, C.; Jansen, C.; Razavi, R. & Penney, G. (2010). Registering preprocedure volumetric images with intraprocedure 3-D ultrasound using an ultrasound imaging model. *IEEE Transactions on Medical Imaging, Vol. 29*, pp. 924 – 937

Knecht, S.; Nault, I.; Wright, M.; Matsuo, S.; Lellouche, N.; Somasundaram, P.E.; O'Neill, M.D.; Lim, K.T.; Sacher, F.; Deplagne, A.; Bordachar, P.; Mélèze, H.; Clémenty, J.; Haissaguerre, M.; & Jais, P. (2008). Imaging in catheter ablation for atrial fibrillation: enhancing the clinician's view. *Europace*, Vol.10, pp. iii2–iii7

Knecht, S.; Wright, M.; Akrivakis, S.; Nault, I.; Matsuo, S.; Chaudhry, GM.; Haffajee, C.; Sacher, F.; Lellouche, N.; Miyazaki, S.; Forclaz, A.; Jadidi, AS.; Hocini, M.; Ritter, P.; Clementy, J.; Haïssaguerre, M.; Orlov, M. & Jaïs, P. (2010). Prospective randomized comparison between the conventional electroanatomical system and three-dimensional rotational angiography during catheter ablation for atrial fibrillation. *Heart Rhythm*, Vol.7, Issue 4, pp. 459-65

Kwong, W.; Neilson, AL.; Hamilton, RM.; Chiu, CC.; Stephenson, EA.: Gross, GJ.; Soucie, L. & Kirsh, JA. (2011). NavX mapping reduces ablation fluoroscopy times in paediatric catheter ablation. *Europace*, Vol.13, suppl 1, pp. i47-i82, poster 001.

LaPage, MJ. & Saul, JP. (2011).Update on rhythm mapping and catheter navigation. *Current Opinion in Cardiology*, Vol.26, pp.79–85

Liu, XQ.; Zhou, X.; Yang,G.; Zhong, GZ.; Shi, L.; Tian, Y.; Li, YB.; Wang, Au. & Yang XC. (2011). Radiofrequency catheter ablation for atrioventricular nodal re-entrant tachycardia without fluoroscopic guidance. *Europace*, Vol. 13, suppl 1, pp. i47-i82, poster 013

Okumura, Y.; Henz, B.D.; Johnson, S.B.; Bunch, T.J.; O'Brien, C.J.; Hodge, D.O.; Altman, A.; Govari, A. & Packer, D.L. (2008). Three-dimensional ultrasound for image-guided mapping and intervention: Methods, Quantitative validation, and clinical feasibility of a novel multimodality image mapping system. *Circ Arrhythm Electrophysiol*, Vol. 1, pp. 110-119

Packer, D.L.; Stevens, C.L.; Curley, M.G.; Bruce, C.J.; Miller, F.A.; Khandheria, B.K.; Oh, J.K.; Sinak, L.J. & Seward, J.B. (2002). Intracardiac phased-array imaging: methods and initial clinical experience with high resolution, under blood visualization-initial experience with intracardiac phased-array ultrasound. *J Am Coll Cardiol*. Vol.39, pp. 509-516

Pandian, N.G.; Kreis, A.; Weintraub, A.; Motarjeme, A.; Desnoyers, M.; Isner, J.M.; Konstam, M.; Salem, D.N. & Millen, V. (1990). Real-time intravascular ultrasound imaging in humans. *Am J Cardiol*. Vol. 65, pp. 1392-1396

Rajnish, J. (2009). Radiofrequency ablation for cardiac tachyarrhythmias: principles and utility of 3D mapping systems. *Current Science*, Vol.97, No.3, (August 2009), pp. 416-424

Ren, J.F.; Marchlinski, F.E.; Callans, D.J.; Zado, E.S. (2002). Intracardiac Doppler echocardiographic quantification of pulmonary vein flow velocity: an effective technique for monitoring pulmonary vein ostia narrowing during focal atrial fibrillation ablation. *J Cardiovasc Electrophysiol*, Vol.13, pp. 1076–1081

Rossillo, A.; Indiani, S.; Bonso, A.; Themistoclakis, S.; Corrado, A. & Raviele, A. (2009). Novel ICE-guided registration strategy for integration of electroanatomical mapping with three-dimensional CT/MR images to guide catheter ablation of atrial fibrillation. *J Cardiovasc Electrophysiol*, Vol 20,pp. 374–378

Schmitt, C.; Zrenner, B.; Schneider, M.; Karch, M.; Ndrepepa, G.; Deisenhofer, I.; Weyerbrock, S.; Schreieck, J. & Schömig, A. (1999). Clinical Experience with a Novel Multielectrode Basket Catheter in Right Atrial Tachycardias. *Circulation*. Vol. 99, pp. 2414-2422

Schmidt, S.; Tilz, R.R.; Neven, K.; Chun, J.K.R.; Fuernkranz, A. & Ouyang, F. (2009). Remote robotic navigation and electroanatomical mapping for ablation of atrial fibrillation: considerations for navigation and impact on procedural outcome. *Circ Arrhythmia Electrophysiol*, Vol. 2, pp. 120–128

Schneider, H.E.; Kriebel, T.; Jung, K.; Gravenhorst, V.D. & Paul, T. (2010) Catheter ablation of idiopathic left and right ventricular tachycardias in the pediatric population using noncontact mapping. *Heart Rhythm*, Vol. 7, pp.731–739.

Schwartzman, D. & Zhong, H. (2010). On the use of CartoSound for left atrial navigation. *J Cardiovasc Electrophysiol*; Vol. 21, pp. 656–664

Thornton, A.S.; Rivero-Ayerza, M. & Jordaens, L. (2008) Ablation of a focal left atrial tachycardia via a retrograde approach using remote magnetic navigation. *Europace*, Vol. 10, Issue 6, pp. 687-689

Thornton, A.S.; De Castro, C.A.; van Deel, E.; van Beusekom, H.M. & Jordaens, L.(2010). An in vivo comparison of radiofrequency cardiac lesions formed by standard and magnetically steered 4mm tip catheters. *Neth Heart J,Vol*. 18, pp. 66–71

Verma, A.; Marrouche, N.F.; Natale, A. (2002). Pulmonary vein antrum isolation: intracardiac echocardiography-guided technique. *J Cardiovasc Electrophysiol*, Vol. 15, pp. 1335–1340

Wielandts, JY.; De Buck, S.; Ector, J.; LaGerche, A.; Willems,R.; Bosmans, H. & Heidbuchel, H. (2010). Three-dimensional cardiac rotational angiography: effective radiation dose and imagequality implications. *Europace, Vol*.12, pp.194–201

Wu, J.; Pflaumer, A.; Deisenhofer, I.; Hoppmann, P.; Hess, J. & Hessling, G. (2010) Mapping
    of atrial tachycardia by remote magnetic navigation in postoperative patients with
    congenital heart disease. *J Cardiovasc Electrophysiol*, Vol. 21, pp. 751–759

Xu, D.; Yang, B.; Shan, Q.; Zou, J.; Chen, M.; Chen, C.; Hou, X.; Zhang, F.; Li, W.Q.; Cao, K.
    & Tse, H.F. (2009). Initial clinical experience of remote magnetic navigation system
    for catheter mapping and ablation of supraventricular tachycardias. *J Interv Card
    Electrophysiol*, Vol.25, pp. 171–174

Zvereva, V.; Rillig, A.; Meyerfeldt, U. & Jung, W. (2011). Incidence of oesophageal lesions
    using either a remote robotic navigation system or a manual approach for *Europace*,
    Vol.13, suppl 1, pp. i47-i82, poster 009

8

Electromagnetic Mapping During Complex RF Ablations

Shimon Rosenheck, Jeffrey Banker, Alexey Weiss and Zehava Sharon
Hadassah Hebrew University Medical Center, Jerusalem,
Israel

1. Introduction

Electromagnetic mapping has made possible the routine approach to complex arrhythmia mapping. Originally, it was developed to facilitate accessory pathway location, but it only complicated solitary pathway ablation. Especially, with the introduction of atrial fibrillation ablation, the electromagnetic mapping has become an irreplaceable component of this procedure. Latter, this 3-dimentional mapping method facilitated ventricular foci ablation in patients with ventricular tachycardia. During the last decade, the application of this mapping method is continuously extended and applied to a large number of complex arrhythmia cases. The electromagnetic mapping is based on minimal magnetic field generation around the tip of the catheter and several antennas, located in a special hardware, called location pad, detect this field. In the near future the location pad will be replaced by an intracardiac detection system. As multiple antennas record the signal, the location pad precisely localizes the catheter tip. By apposition of a location on the endocardial surface and the catheter tip, a virtual map of the cardiac chamber is obtained. Multiple points are represented in space and finally, a continuous wall is completed. Moreover, the catheter records the electrical activity in its vicinity, and the electrical flow can be superimposed on the location in the space. A color-coding localizes the starting point of the arrhythmia and the current flow from it.

As of today, an advanced generation is used and data from other imaging systems are merged with the electromagnetic picture. First, magnetic resonance data was merged with the electroanatomic mapping, but today cardiac computed tomography and echo picture might also be merged. Using these merged pictures the anatomical presentation more accurately represents the anatomical structure.

2. A brief history of catheter ablation

The first type of energy used for catheter ablation to cure cardiac arrhythmias was the direct current (DC) shock delivered through the catheter tip in apposition to the desired site of ablation. By ablating the AV junction in supraventricular tachycardia, a reasonable rate control was achieved (Scheinman MM et al, 1982). The ablation of well-defined positioned accessory pathways could also be achieved by DC ablation (Morady F & Scheinman MM, 1984). The DC shock can be adjusted by delivering different amplitude of shocks, but as soon as it was delivered there was no more way to titrate or cancel it. To achieve a titratable energy, a different source is needed and the radiofrequency energy has fulfilled this condition. At the end of 1980's the radiofrequency energy has been introduced into the clinical electrophysiology. With the advent of specific pathways ablation, the clinical electrophysiology has become a continuously extending brunch of the cardiology. The radiofrequency energy in opposite to the direct current shock, can be titrated, limited, suddenly discontinued and reapplied. For this reason, the RF energy is easily applied in clinical practice. The first accessory pathways ablations and AV Nodal pathways ablations were performed during the late 1980's and published for the first time in 1991 (Jackman WM et al, 1991: Calkins H et al, 1991). Since than, a vast amount of literature was published on this subject and almost all type of arrhythmia has become feasible for ablation. In Table 2.1 a list of ablatable arrhythmic substrates is presented.

Arrhythmia Type	Fist performed	Publication
WPW	1989	Jackman WM et al 1991; Clakins H at al, 1991
ANRT	1989	Lee MA at al, 1991
A Flutter	1992	Feld GK et al, 1992; Cosio FG et al, 1993
A Tachycardia	1992	Kall JG& Wilber DJ, 1992; Walsh EP et al, 1992
VT idiopathic	1991-1992	Kuck KH et al, 1991; Klein LS et al, 1992
VT in Heart Disease	1992	Morady F et al, 1993
A Fibrillation	1996	Haissaguerre M et al, 1998
VF idiopathic	2001	Takatsuki S et al, 2001, Haissaguerre M et al, 2002

Abbreviations: WPW-Wolf Parkinson White Syndrome; AVNRT- AV Nodal Reentrant Tachycardia; A Flutter-Atrial Flutter; A Tachycardia-Atrial Tachycardia; VT-Ventricular Tachycardia; A Fibrillation-Atrial fibrillation; VF- Ventricular Fibrillation

Table 2.1. The table summarizes the types of arrhythmia treated with catheter ablation.

In accessory pathway ablation, the presumed location is meticulously mapped with a special developed steerable tip catheter. The pathways are located on the mitral or tricuspid rings, or in the septum separating the left and right heart. When the recoding from this site is satisfactory, RF energy is delivered for certain duration. If the accessory pathway conducts electricity in both directions, or at least, in the antegrade direction (from the atrium to the ventricle), the resting ECG shows a typical preexcitation pattern. Short PR interval and a widening of the QRS characterize this preexcitation. A typical delta wave is preceding the QRS and its direction depends on the location of the pathway. Wolf, Parkinson and White described this type of ECG in 1930 and if it is associated with palpitation is called Wolff-Parkinson-White syndrome (Wolff L et al, 1930). During the RF energy delivery the preexcitation disappears and the ECG becomes normal. After the ablation, during temporary blockage of the AV node with intravenous adenosine injection, AB block is achieved, demonstrating the remaining conduction only through the AV junction.

However, in 50% of the patients the resting ECG is normal, but still the patient can develop supraventricular tachycardia. In this case, the accessory pathway conducts the electricity only in the retrograde direction (from the ventricle to the atrium) and is called concealed Wolff-Parkinson-White syndrome. The mapping is completed either during tachycardia or ventricular pacing. RF energy application eliminates the retrograde conduction without affecting the resting ECG.

Patients with dual AV Nodal conduction may develop supraventricular tachycardia based on reentry circuit in the AV Node. One of the pathways has slow conduction of the electricity and the other has fast conduction. If the refractoriness of these pathways and the conduction times are appropriate, the electric impulse may be conducted in a circuit constituted by this two pathways and the clinical expression will be supraventricular tachycardia with short VA time. A premature beat during unidirectional block in one of the pathways initiates the tachycardia. Different duration of refractoriness of these pathways creates the unidirectional block. Blocking one of these pathways will prevent induction of the tachycardia. RF ablation is based on the same principle: selective elimination of the conduction on one of these pathways. In the late 1980's the fast pathway was ablated (Lee MA et al, 1991). These fast pathways are located in the anterior site of the AV node very near to the proximal His Bundle. Although the success rate was very high, special attention was needed to avoid complete AV Block. After a year, the slow pathway ablation was described (Jackman WM et al, 1992). The slow pathway is located in the posterior AV nodal area, relatively far from the His Bundle. The ablation of these slow pathways is safer and today is routinely performed in most of the electrophysiology laboratories. After the ablation, the AV refractoriness prolongs and the AH interval (atrial-His conduction time) remains short immediately before the blocking.

The third classical ablation is that of typical atrial flutter (Feld GK et al, 1992, Cosio FG et al, 1993). In typical atrial flutter, a single electrical wavefront circulates in the perimeter of the right atrium. The area between the lower pole of the tricuspid valve and the inferior vena cava is called isthmus. A multipolar catheter on the lateral wall of the right atrium demonstrates the counter-clockwise or clockwise rotation during the flutter. Complete blocking of the isthmus, terminates the flutter. After the successful ablation, pacing at the coronary sinus osteum demonstrates the block, by conduction to the lateral wall only from above the tricuspid annulus.

In atrial tachycardia, idiopathic or peri-scar, and idiopathic ventricular tachycardia from right outflow tract or the basal left ventricle (fascicular), the atrial or the ventricular foci are ablated. The first three ablations, the accessory pathway (WPW) ablation, the selective or non selective AV Nodal pathways ablation and typical atrial flutter ablation are the classical ablations, which rarely if at all need other mapping methods, like the three-dimensional mapping methods. The atrial and ventricular tachycardia foci ablation is feasible in the majority of cases with "simple" electrophysiology mapping, like early activity, bracketing, entrainment, pace mapping, multi-pole catheter mapping, etc. However, occasionally, this mapping is not sufficient and three-dimensional mapping is needed (Marchlinski FE et al, 1998; Leonelli FM et al, 2001; Peichl P et al, 2003; Dong J et al, 2005). As we can notice, in the classical ablations, both the diagnostic test and the ablation procedure are focused on electrophysiology parameters. In atrial and ventricular tachycardia, although there are well defined electrophysiology maneuvers as previously mentioned, the more exact location of the focus and the demonstration of the ablation results demands the advanced electroanatomic mapping.

3. The development of the electroanatomic mapping and the electroanatomic mapping guided ablation

In the early 1990's, Ben Haim and his colleagues developed a new method of three-dimensional mapping of a tubular or spherical organ. First it was presented in the NASPE meeting in 1996 (Smeets J et al, 1996; Ben-Haim SA et al, 1996a; Hayam G et al, 1996; Gepstein L et al, 1996), than published as a new method evaluated in animal model and human subjects (Ben-Haim SA et al, 1996b; Gepstein L et al, 1997, Shpun S et al, 1997; Gepstein L et al, 1998). In this method, the locator pads, located beneath the operating table, generate a week magnetic field. The magnetic field strength is between 5×10^{-6} and 5×10^{-5} tesla. A miniature sensor embedded in the body of the distal catheter collects these magnetic fields. As the fields vectors have different directions, computer integration of the data resolves the location and orientation of the sensor in space. During the same time, the distal electrodes, located on the catheter tip, record the electrical activity behind it. By collecting multiple points, the heart chamber anatomy and the local electrical impulse in amplitude and timing are superimposed. With higher number of points added, higher precision is achieved. The resolution of the sensor location in space is < 1 mm. Finally, the electrical field propagation is presented on the virtual reconstruction of the heart chamber anatomy. If the amplitude is expressed, scar anatomy is obtained based on very low electrical activity on the scar. Moreover, a transitional region with increasing amplitude will interpose between the scar and normal tissue. In this type of mapping, invagination of conducting tissue in the scar, gaps and marginal zones may present the substrate of arrhythmias. Early in the development of the electroanatomic mapping, the scar mapping contributed to the understanding of the arrhythmia substrate and made possible non-specific scar ablation (Stevenson WG et al, 1998a; Stevenson WG et al, 1998b; Marchlinski FE et al, 2000; Sra J et al, 2001). However, the main development of the electroanatomic mapping happened with the use in atrial fibrillation ablation. After discovery of the triggers in the pulmonary veins, focal ablation was suggested, but the application of this ablation is limited and associated with an increased incidence of complication (Haissaguerre M et al, 1998). The use of electro-anatomic guided ablation offered ablation lines in the antrum of the veins and in this way the ablation is far from the vein itself and also significant debalking is added (Pappone C et al, 1999; Pappone C et al, 2000; Oral H et al, 2003). The ablation was extended to persistent atrial fibrillation and even to long-standing persistent cases (Nademanee K et al, 2004; Oral H et al, 2006; Takahashi Y et al, 2007). This addition contributed to development of this mapping. Additional mapping methods were developed and promoted in parallel with the original electromagnetic mapping, the CARTO mapping. Finally, the list of ablatable substrates has continuously increased and today includes beside atrial fibrillation and ventricular tachycardia in patients with or without structural heart disease, also atrial tachycardia, recurrent and refractory atrial flutter, idiopathic ventricular fibrillation (Knecht S et al, 2009) and more recently, the substrate of Brugada syndrome (Nademanee K et al, 2011). The following sections will describe in details the use of the mapping in each of these indications.

4. Right atrial tachycardia

The mechanism of right atrial tachycardia may be an autonomic focus or reentry around a physical obstacle, most commonly an iatrogenic scar or a post-infectious scar.

4.1 Right atrial tachycardia-reentrant type

For mapping the scar, bipolar voltage mapping is needed. Figure 4.1 shows two views obtained during atrial tachycardia ablation in a 32 year old man, who had a remote atrial septal closure surgery. During the surgery the lateral wall in the right atrium was opened and the septal defect was closed. On a recent echo, no interatrial shunt could be seen demonstrating lack of atrial septal defect and late success of the surgery. However the patient developed incessant and persistent atrial tachycardia. During the electrophysiology study, the right atrium was mapped using bipolar voltage mapping. This technique allows determination of the scar, as on the scar the electrical activity is practically non-existent. We defined everything bellow 0.04V as scar and assigned with red color. The normal tissue is defined everything above 0.47V and assigned with purple. The tissue in between them is the transition zone. As evident from the picture, the two red areas were connected with a continuous ablation line obtained with a point-by-point ablation.

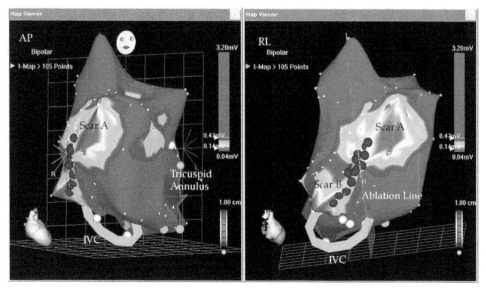

Fig. 4.1. The picture shows the voltage mapping of the right atrium with two scars on the lateral wall, a large (Scar A) and a small one (Scar B). The small one (Scar B) is connected to the Inferior Vena Cava. A small strip on normal myocardium separates the scars and this strip was transected with the ablation line. Annotations: AP- antero-posterior (the left picture); RL- Right lateral (the right picture). For further explanation see the text.

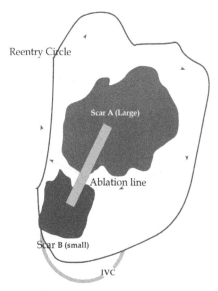

Fig. 4.2. Schematic presentation of picture 4.1; the picture shows the two scars, a large and a small one. The IVC ring limits the small one. To interrupt to reentry circle the ablation line connects the two scars.

During two-year follow-up the patients is free of any arrhythmia. This case demonstrates the of electro-anatomic mapping used for scar dependent atrial tachycardia ablation.

4.2 Right atrial tachycardia-automatic focus type

The next case will exemplify the ablation of automatic paroxysmal atrial tachycardia. The patient is a 17-year-old male patient with a history of palpitation and documented supraventricular tachycardia. Electrophysiology study demonstrated supraventricular tachycardia with long VA time and the ventricular rate was dictated by the atrial rate. Occasionally 2:1 AV conduction and even Wenkebach conduction was documented. The final diagnosis was right atrial tachycardia originating in the inferior third of the crista terminalis. Ablation was focused on the earliest atrial activity using a duodecapolar catheter. The tachycardia terminated during the RF application and has become noninducible. However, after 2 weeks the patient again experienced palpitation and again a similar arrhythmia was documented. The patient was referred for a second ablation this time CARTO guided. The tachycardia was again easily induced with atrial overdrive pacing, but not with atrial premature beats. Figure 4.3 shows the CARTO mapping.

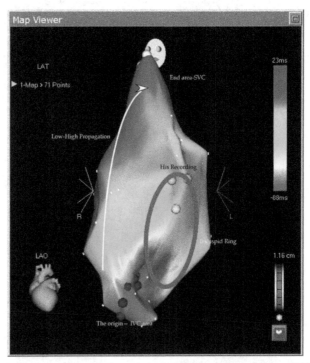

Fig. 4.3. Right Atria Tachycardia with the origin at the Inferior Vena Cava (IVC) area and the activation terminating at the Superior Vena Cava (SVC) area. This is a propagation map and the colors define the timing at each area. The red is the earliest time (-88 msec) and the purple the latest time (+23 msec) compared to the reference catheter. The white line with the arrow shows the activation direction. The red points in the origin area show the Radiofrequency application sites, which terminated the tachycardia rendering it non-inducible.

In this case, voltage mapping cannot be used as no scar could be mapped and the patient had no any previous cardiac procedure except the ablation procedure. For this reason, a propagation mapping was used. During this mapping the virtual reconstruction of the right atrium is completed parallel with accurate timing detection by comparing the activation time with the timing on a reference catheter, in this case in the coronary sinus osteum. The timing of the points located with the mapping catheter is compared with the reference catheter and is assigned with red color if it is early and purple if it is late. In between are the other colors like yellow, green and blue. Finally, a cine presentation shows the flow of the electrical activity, starting at the red point and terminating at the blue points. The red points are the area focused for ablation. As evident in Figure 4.3, the origin is well determined and ablation at this point again terminated the tachycardia leaving it noninducible. During the follow-up the patient is asymptomatic, practicing non-professional sportive activity.

These two cases exemplify not only two types of right atrial tachycardia, but also two methods of mapping. If a scar is to be mapped, the amplitude of the electrical activity will discriminate it from the normal tissue with clear demarcation. The reentry can be completed around a scar and by connecting the scar to a non-conducting tissue will prevent the reentry. This map is called, voltage-map, or scar mapping. In contrary, if the tachycardia is generated by an automatic focus, the earliest activation will reveal the origin of the tachycardia and the ablation may be focused to it. This is achieved by determining the timing at each point and the map is called, flow-map.

These two cases are presenting the classical types of atrial tachycardias. However, occasionally the diagnosis is not so simple and the first impression may be misleading. The electro anatomic mapping may elucidate the diagnosis and make possible the correct ablation. In the next subsection such a complex case is presented.

4.3 Atrial flutter or not flutter that is the question

A 28-year-old man presented with an ECG showing typical atrial flutter and was referred to radiofrequency ablation. He was in sinus rhythm when admitted for the ablation and the inferior isthmus (between the tricuspid ring and the inferior vena cava) was ablated using a 10 mm tip ablation catheter, a duodeca mapping catheter on the lateral wall and a quadripolar pacing-mapping catheter in the proximal coronary sinus. The ablation was performed during coronary sinus pacing and the original collision on the lateral wall was abolished demonstrating the block bellow the valve. Pacing from the coronary sinus and from above the inferior vena cava approved the block in the isthmus. Although the bidirectional block was persistent the patient had additional episode of "typical atrial flutter". In a second electrophysiology study the block in the isthmus was persistent and the patient had still inducible arrhythmia (Figures 4.4 and 4.5). Although the diagnosis of atrial flutter was attempting the duodeca catheter recording showed a big delay in the isthmus area during the tachycardia. This is not acceptable in typical atrial flutter or at least during an isthmus dependent flutter. Figure 4.5 shows details of the duodeca catheter recording during the atrial tachycardia-the last 10 tracings on Figure 4.4. The earliest point on the lateral wall is on pole D5-6. Pole D1-2 records from the median site of the isthmus block and pole D3-4 from the lateral site. The double arrow shows the big delay demonstrating the isthmus block during the tachycardia and non-isthmus dependent tachycardia. For this reason, CARTO mapping was initiated.

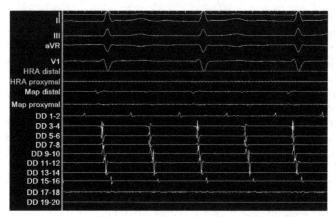

Fig. 4.4. The tracing shows a regular tachycardia, recorded at 100 mm/sec. The first 5 tracing are surface electrograms L_1, L_2, L_3, AVR and V_1. The next two belong to the right atrial tracing as reference for the CARTO mapping (not recording temporarily), than the mapping catheter and finally 10 tracings from the duodeca catheter deployed on the right lateral wall of the right atrium. The tracing on the duodeca catheter reveals unidirectional conduction suggesting atrial flutter. However, the tracing at DD1-2 is extremely delayed. As DD1-2 is medial to the isthmus block line and DD3-4 lateral, this delay demonstrates isthmus block during the tachycardia (See also Fig 4.5)

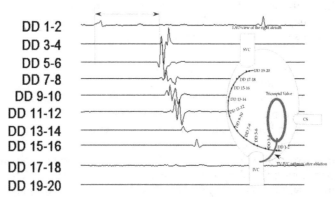

Fig. 4.5. The figure shows the tracing on the duodeca catheter at 200 ms/min recording speed. The cartoon inserted on the tracing shows the right atrium, IVC, SVC and CS. The isthmus block line is also depicted. The position of 10 bipolar poles is also shown. DD 1-2 is medial to the block line and all the other 9 poles are lateral to the line. On the tracing, a long delay is between DD 1-2 and 3-4 demonstrating the persistence of the block during the tachycardia, which is not compatible with typical atrial flutter.

A CARTO mapping demonstrated tachycardia originating from the lateral border of the block line in the isthmus (Figure 4.6) and was abolished by focal ablation using the area determined by the flow-map (Figure 4.7 and 4.8). The surface ECG was misleading and the real arrhythmia was atrial tachycardia and not atrial flutter! The electro-anatomic mapping made possible the correct diagnosis and finally the appropriate treatment.

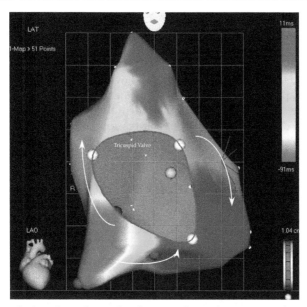

Fig. 4.6. Flow map during the tachycardia showing the early activation lateral to the isthmus line (purple color). The white arrows depict the current flow, simulating the flutter activation pattern except in the area between the origin (red color) and isthmus line (purple color) where a slow conduction in the opposite direction is clearly revealed. The isthmus is invaded from both sites.

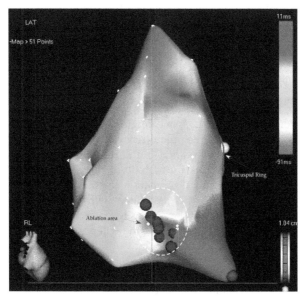

Fig. 4.7. The flow map from right lateral view is superimposed with the ablation mark signs. During the applications in this area the tachycardia terminated as shown in Figure 4.8.

This is an illustration of the importance of electro-anatomic mapping in this case as the surface ECG suggested typical atrial flutter and apparent recurrence after successful ablation of the cavo-tricuspid isthmus. At the first glance, the recording suggests atrial flutter, but there is a sudden delay between DD 3-4 and DD 1-2. This is possible only if the isthmus block is persistent and the catheter is laid over the block line with the tip over the line and the rest of poles before the block line. If the tachycardia can continue despite the block in the isthmus, it cannot be isthmus-dependent flutter. The electro-anatomic mapping revealed the correct diagnosis and made possible the appropriate ablation.

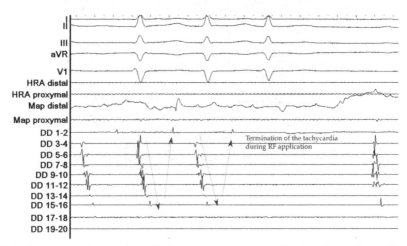

Fig. 4.8. In this tracing during the radiofrequency energy application, the tachycardia terminates and at the right side of the tracing the first sinus beat is seen. Of note, the tachycardia termination is sudden and not caused by ectopic activity, but only by the ablation. During the termination the last recording is from DD 1-2, demonstrating that the origin was between DD 3-4 and 5-6 and the last activation is on DD 1-2 (See Figure 4.6).

5. Left atrial tachycardia

Left atrial tachycardia may be of the same origin like the right atrial tachycardia. The automatic form mostly originates in the pulmonary veins, but the reentry forms originate in the atrial tissue like the reentry tachycardia in the right atrium. The most common form today is related to catheter ablation of atrial fibrillation, which will be discussed and presented within a next section on atrial fibrillation ablation. A rare form is the para-septal atrial tachycardia, which interestingly is associated with patent foramen ovale. For this reason, to map and ablate it, the septum is easily passed and the left atrium is easily mapped. The next presentation will exemplify it and will present the use of electro-anatomic mapping to determine the earliest activation point.

A 48 year old woman was referred because a persistent form of atrial tachycardia. First right atrium was mapped and the earliest activation was on the septal area. The activation time was at about zero time when compared to the reference catheter located in the coronary sinus osteum. By mapping the septum at the fosa ovalis, the catheter passed to the left atrium without need for standard septal puncture. The left atrium was mapped. A fast map was obtained, than the activation was superimposed on it. An early activation was mapped on the anterior wall, immediately above the mitral ring (Figure 5.1). At this point the ablation terminated the incessant atrial tachycardia.

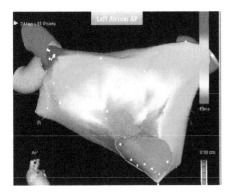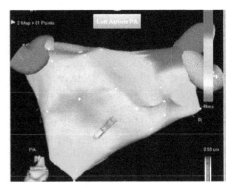

Fig. 5.1. The picture shows the left atrial flow map during incessant tachycardia. The activation time in the anterior wall and above the mitral ring was -43 msec (red color). On the posterior wall the activation times were all longer than 0 msec (compared to the reference catheter at the coronary sinus osteum. The area above the right pulmonary vein is as late as 53 msec after the activation on the reference catheter (purple color).

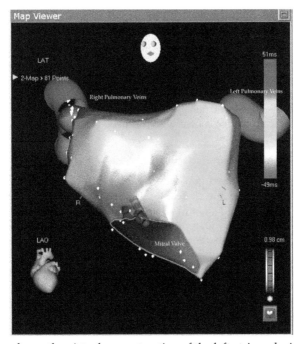

Fig. 5.2. The figure shows the virtual reconstruction of the left atrium during the tachycardia with the earliest point in red color. The catheter tip is pointing to that area. The ablation sites are shown. The tachycardia terminated with these ablation points.

As of today, the published information on electro-anatomic mapping during atrial tachycardia ablation is scars and limited. However, the clinical application is well known and rich and the accumulated and published knowledge is worth to mention. Atrial tachycardia is encounter in both pediatric and adult patients. We have information on the use of electro-magnetic mapping in both groups. In right atrial tachycardia, the use of this mapping adds a significant degree of accuracy and, just like in our patient described in subsection 4.3, rarely the electro-magnetic mapping adds to the correct diagnosis. In patients with incessant focal tachycardia, the electrophysiological maneuvers may be enough but in patients with scar related tachycardia, this mapping has irreplaceable value. In incessant focal tachycardia, the earliest activation in the Crista Terminalis area or along the tricuspid ring will reveal the origin and radiofrequency energy application will terminate it and total cure is achieved. However, if the tachycardia persists or reoccurs, 3D mapping is justified (Subsection 4.2). As previously mentioned, the activation map helps to localize the origin of the tachycardia. In scar related reentrant tachycardia, the scar is delineated and a narrow isthmus in between them is ablated (Subsection 4.1). Voltage mapping delineates the scar, and amplitude lower than 0.14 mV suggests scar.

The published studies involved a limited number of patients, 7 to 120. Focal tachycardias in the right atrium are ablatable with success rate >90% (Kottkamp H et al, 1997; Marchlinski F et al, 1998; Iwai S et al, 2002). The same success rate may be achieved in macroreentrant atrial tachycardia related to post-surgical scar (Iwai S et al, 2002). In the left atrium, focal tachycardias were localized to mitral annulus, roof, posterior wall, appendage and septum (Dong J et al, 2005). Left septal atrial tachycardia is rare and the electroanatomic mapping facilitates its ablation (Marrouche NF et al, 2002). Atrial tachycardia originating in the mitral annulus is also rare and the electro-anatomic mapping also facilitates its ablation (Kistler PM et al, 2003). Our patient presented in section 5 had also tachycardia originating from the mitral annulus (Figures 5.1 and 5.2). In pediatric patients, the acute success is significantly higher with the electro-anatomic mapping compared to standard electrophysiological mapping and the recurrence rate was lower (Cummings RM, 2008).

In all these conditions, the electroanatomic mapping for ablation of all types of atrial tachycardia in the clinical practice is firmly established.

6. Atrial fibrillation ablation

Atrial fibrillation is the most common arrhythmia an presents a great challenge for any cardiologist and even more for the clinical electrophysiologist. This arrhythmia has a very erratic response to antiarrhythmic treatment and for this reasons a non-medical treatment is demanded. Device therapy did not prove to be an effective alternative to the mediocre medical treatment. For this reason, the ablative opinion is an attractive alternative.

Haissaguerre and his colleagues, by investigating the mode of initiation of paroxysmal atrial fibrillation, discovered that the trigger for this type of arrhythmia originates, in the majority of the cases, in the pulmonary veins (Haissaguerre M et al, 1998). Focal ablation of these foci, as a logical next step, turned to be complicated with damage to the vein, narrowing with significant and symptomatic increase in the pulmonary pressure. The electrical connection between the pulmonary vein and left atrium is through distinct pathways (Ehrlich JR et al, J Physiol 2003). Electrical disconnection of these veins avoided this damage and offered the same result. However, the recurrence and occasional pulmonary stenosis were still encountered. In 1999, Pappone and his colleagues suggested a different approach to disconnect electrically the pulmonary veins (Pappone C et al, 1999; Pappone C et al, 2000; Pappone et al, 2004). This method is based on electroanatomic mapping. The left atrium is approached by passing the inter atrial septum using the Brockenbrough method and the left atrial mapping is completed by virtual reconstruction of the atrial walls and tagging the veins and the mitral annulus. The ablation includes circles around the pulmonary veins and lines connecting the mitral annulus with the ablation line around the left lower pulmonary vein and lines connecting the left and right ablation rings around the veins. In patients with paroxysmal atrial fibrillation, this type of ablation was superior to the pulmonary vein disconnection, with higher success rate and lower recurrence rate after one year (Oral H et al, 2003). Moreover, in patients with persistent atrial fibrillation, circumferential pulmonary vein ablation was superior to amiodarone treatment in preventing recurrence of the fibrillation (Oral H et al, 2006; Pappone C et al, 2006). Multiple escalated methods exemplify the problematicity of the ablation in patients with long persistent atrial fibrillation (Oral H et al, 2006; Takahashi Y et al, 2007; Satomi K et al, 2008). However, consensus was achieved on the necessity of catheter ablation of atrial fibrillation (Calkins H at al, 2007).

Following we will present several patients with atrial fibrillation and electro-anatomic guided ablation.

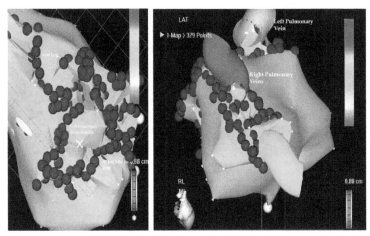

Fig. 6.1. The picture shows the ablation lines around the common left entrance and the two right veins. The lines are continuous.

SB 74 year old woman with a long history of paroxysmal atrial fibrillation on multiple antiarrhythmic medication including beat blockers, calcium channel blockers, Propafenon, Flecainide, Amiodarone all turned to be ineffective. The etiology of the atrial fibrillation was hypertension treated with multiple drugs. Finally she was referred to catheter ablation of atrial fibrillation. In the mean time the fibrillation converted to persistent. An ECHO showed normal systolic left ventricular function with decreased diastolic function, enlarged left ventricle with minimal mitral regurgitation. Patten Foramen Ovale with small left to right shunt was demonstrated. During the ablation, the septum was easily passed and the left atrium was reconstructed using anatomical map as she was in atrial fibrillation. The veins were tagged and the mitral annulus was reconstructed. The veins were circumvented with ablation points and the roofline and mitral isthmus lines were completed. When the radiofrequency was delivered in the junction between the roofline and right superior pulmonary vein the patient converted to sinus rhythm after 2 months of atrial fibrillation. Figure 6.1 shows the ring around the left veins and the right veins; Figure 6.2 shows the posterior view of the left atrium after the ablation. The mapping and ablation were done with CARTO EXP 7. She was in sinus rhythm 5 years after the ablation and during her last follow-up 3 years ago.

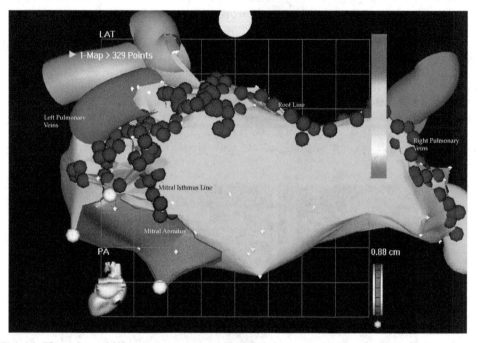

Fig. 6.2. The enlarged left atrium in a posterior view shows the rings around the pulmonary veins, the roofline and the mitral isthmus line. At least two lines connect the peri venous ring to the mitral annulus. There are 3 large left veins with a common entrance to the left atrium. The mapping is an anatomical map different from the mappings in atrial tachycardia ablation (Sections 4 and 5).

MD is 81-year-old man with persistent atrial fibrillation failing multiple medical treatments. He had long history of supraventricular tachycardia and had a successful slow pathway ablation 8 years ago. Two years ago presented with symptomatic atrial fibrillation. Medical treatment with beta-blockers, Propafenon, Flecainide were not effective and Amiodarone was discontinued because hyperthyroidism. As medical treatment had to discontinued because lack of efficacy or side effects he was referred to catheter ablation. At the admission he was in persistent atrial fibrillation for 3 months and without antiarrhythmic treatment. The transseptal catheterization was performed safely under intra cardiac echo guidance. After the ablation he converted to sinus bradycardia. Figure 6.3 shows the ablations lines in the left atrium and presents new modes of mapping (fast map).

SS is a 68-year-old man with long history of atrial flutter and fibrillation and hypertension. In 2002 he had a successful atrial flutter ablation. In 2004 he had catheter ablation of atrial fibrillation using the point-by-point method. Until recently he was in stable sinus rhythm when 3 months ago presented in the follow-up clinic with atrial fibrillation. Anticoagulation was started and referred for a second ablation. In the new mapping there was no electrical activity in the veins, on the posterior wall, but at several points around the veins was a low amplitude regular activity and all this places were ablated again. In the next figures the two mappings will be compared in the same patients emphasizing the advance in the mapping methods. The patient has common entrance of both left and right pulmonary veins. The intracardiac echo used during the second ablation in 2011 approved this anatomical variance.

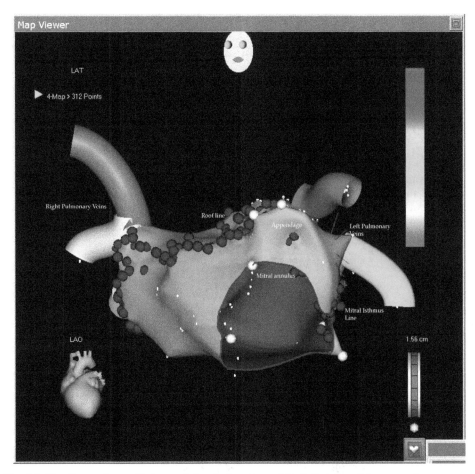

Fig. 6.3. The figure shows 20 degree left anterior view of the left atrium. The appendage covers the ablation ring around the left veins. The atrium is minimally enlarged. There is a common right entrance and two separate left veins. This map was performed using the fast map mode, a new future of the electro-anatomic mapping. The atrial anatomy much more resembles the other imaging models. The lines are continuous and the veins are completely isolated with no residual electrical activity in the veins or posterior wall. The mode is new and for this reason the follow up after the ablation is only 3 months, however the patient is in sinus rhythm.

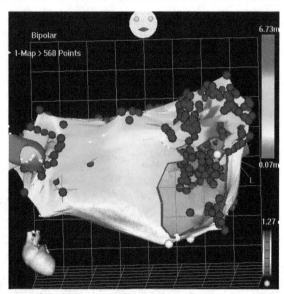

Fig. 6.4. The figure shows the anterior view of the left atrium recorded in 2004 using the point-by point method. The patient was in sinus rhythm during the procedure. A large number of ablation sites are seen through the mitral valve from inside the atrium. The left atrium is not enlarged. The left ablation lines are heavy and the right ablation lines are discrete. The roofline is slightly posterior an not present in this picture.

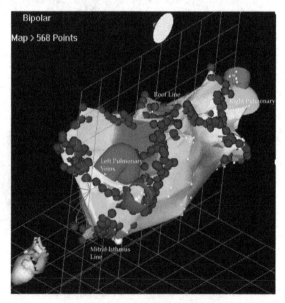

Fig. 6.5. This is a posterior view recorded during the first ablation procedure. The ablation lines are clearly seen and are heavy in the left side and discrete in the right side. The voltage amplitude in the posterior wall is low (red color).

The next figure (6.5) shows the ablation lines in the posterior view and also the roofline not seen in Figure 6.4. Following the ablation the atrial fibrillation was not inducible. The areas around the veins were quiescent from any electrical activity. As the patient had a previous cavo-tricuspid isthmus line ablation, atrial flutter could also not be induced. As mentioned above, after 7 years the patient developed again atrial fibrillation, this time persistent and not paroxysmal. The following pictures will exemplify the second ablation procedure, with a more advanced electro-anatomic mapping system (Figures 6.6 and 6.7).

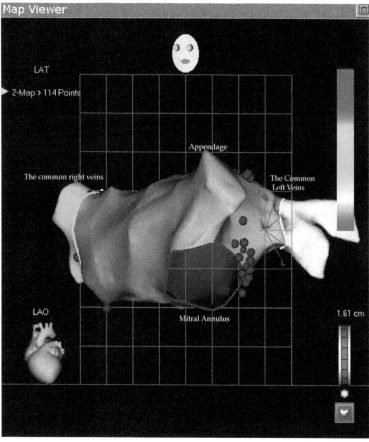

Fig. 6.6. The picture shows the left atrium using the fast map technique. This is the same left atrium like in Figures 6.4 and 6.5, just obtained 7 years latter and using more advanced method of mapping. The veins with common entrance are in colors, left with yellow and right with green. The mitral isthmus was reinforced with several ablation points and the left upper vein is also reinforced at the junction with the roofline were low amplitude relatively slow and regular activity was recorded. The ablation canceled this activity and the entire vein was free of any electrical activity. The next figure will show the areas with residual activity on the right side.

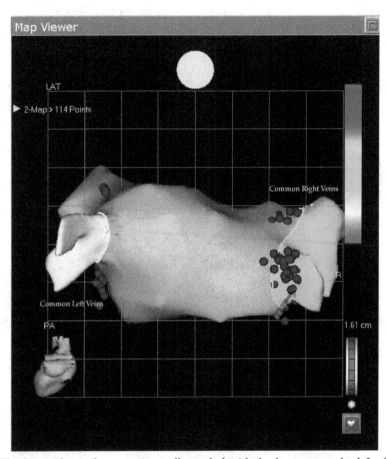

Fig. 6.7. The figure shows the posterior wall recoded with the fast map method. In the lower-posterior border of the right vein and on the junction point with the roofline additional application eliminated the activity and left the entire vein free of any electrical activity. The right vein different from the left, had multiple brunches and with common entrance into the left atrium. The anatomy was approved with the intra-cardiac echo recorded simultaneously with CARTO mapping. The posterior wall also free of electrical activity like in box-ablation (lines anterior to the veins completed with roofline and another line in the low atrium on the posterior wall).

7. Ventricular tachycardia ablation

A vast amount of information was accumulated during the last decades of the 20th Century supporting the superiority of implantable defibrillators (ICD) over any medical treatment in saving patients with high risk for sudden cardiac death (Ezekowitz JA et al, 2003). However, the defibrillator cannot guaranty the quality of life especially in patients with frequent ICD therapy. Moreover, patients may develop clusters of ventricular fibrillation, called VT storm. Some studies even suggest that repeated shock is associated with increased death rate

(Exner DV et al, 2001; Poole JE et al, 2008; Daubert JP et al, 2008; van Rees JB et al, 2011). It is still not clarified if the presence of high number of VT or the shocks signals the imminent death. When both the ICD and adjuvant antiarrhythmic treatment (mainly Sotalol or Amiodarone) cannot prevent frequent recurrence of VT, the only option is the ablation (Sra J et al, 2001). The next step in the strategy is ablation before the storm or frequent recurrence of VT (Reddy V et al, 2007; Stevenson WG et al, 2008; Tung R et al, 2010; Kuck KH et al, 2010; Natale A et al, 2010). The main problem is that patients with structural heart disease have multiple VT foci, large scars with many possible reentry circles. For this reason, focal ablation may be only a temporary step. Occasionally, these patients with reduced left ventricular function may not tolerate hemodynamically the VT and focal ablation may not be feasible. To resolve this problem, scar ablation was suggested (Marchlinski FE et al, 2000; Sra J et al, 2001). The following 4 patients will exemplify these methods in different types of structural heart disease.

AA is a 60-year-old patient with coronary artery disease, large anterior myocardial infarction in the recent past, and ventricular tachycardia. A cardioverter-defibrillator was implanted. As the tachycardia reoccurred, amiodarone treatment was added. Amiodarone did not control the tachycardia and the symptomatic cardioverter-defibrillator therapy and the patient was frequently re-hospitalized.

For this reason, the patient was brought to the electrophysiology laboratory in purpose to study the ventricular tachycardia and to attempt an ablation procedure. The tachycardia was easily and reproducible induced with two premature beats. Although the tachycardia, on chronic amiodarone treatment, was relatively slow, the patient did not tolerate it hemodynamically. Propagation mapping was not applicable and the only option remained the scar/voltage mapping. Interestingly, the mapping revealed two scars, a large one and a small one with a small and narrow strip of myocardium between them. The small scar extended until the mitral annulus and no continuous myocardium surrounded it. The only reentry circuit for the slow tachycardia could be the large scar and by blocking the narrow myocardial strip between the scars necessarily will interfere with the current wave passage around the large scar, too.

The flowing pictures exemplify the scars and the ablation (Figures 7.1, 7.2 and 7.3)

The tachycardia has become not inducible after the ablation and during the 1 year follow-up since the ablation the patient was free of ICD therapies. As we can see, in this case a clear delineation of the reentry circle was revealed by the scar mapping without an intend to map the activation. Scar mapping is the option when the patient cannot tolerate the tachycardia (Marchlinski FE et al, 2000; Sra J et al, 2001). A narrow conduction tissue in the scar serves the tachycardia (Figure 7.2 and 7.3). The strategy is to block this tissue, however it is important to connect the scar to a non-conducting structure like valve annulus, otherwise the ablation will only increase the reentry circle and may render the tachycardia more incessant. In our patient the smaller scar was already connected to the mitral annulus (Figure 7.3) leaving the only possible reentry circle around the large scar and the target of the ablation the narrow myocardial strip in between them. This patient presents an ideal ablatable reentry circle. Eliminating the conduction only on a single possible pathway eliminates also the VT substrates and the patient continues to be without ICD therapy for one year. Identification of the channel was crucial in this procedure and is discussed in recent published literature (Arenal A et al, 2004; Hsia HH et al al, 2006).

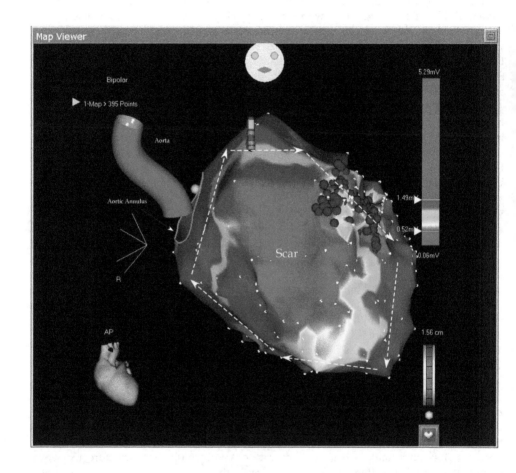

Fig. 7.1. The picture shows the antero-posterior projection of the enlarged left ventricle with a large scar on almost all the anterior wall. Any voltage bellow 0.5 mV (red color) was considered scar and any voltage above 1.5 mV were considered normal myocardium (purple color). In between them three transitional tissues are collared in yellow, green and blue. No tissue penetrated the scar and no central pathways could be mapped. The arrows show the large reentry cycle around the scar. Normal myocardium is around the scar and constitutes the reentry circle. The ablation points (red dots) block the isthmus between two scars (see Figure 6.2)

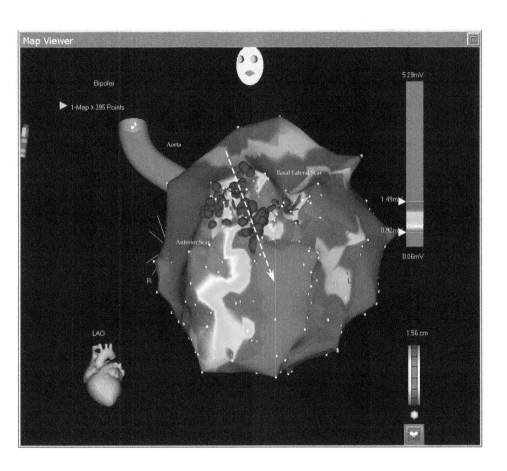

Fig. 7.2. The picture shows the antero-lateral projection of the left ventricle. In this voltage mapping two scars are evident: the large anterior scar and a smaller basal lateral scar. The scars delineate in between them a slowly conducting myocardial tissue called isthmus (arrow). The isthmus is blocked by the ablation points. As we will see in the next picture, the basal scar is extending until the mitral annulus the reason why the reentry could not be closed around it.

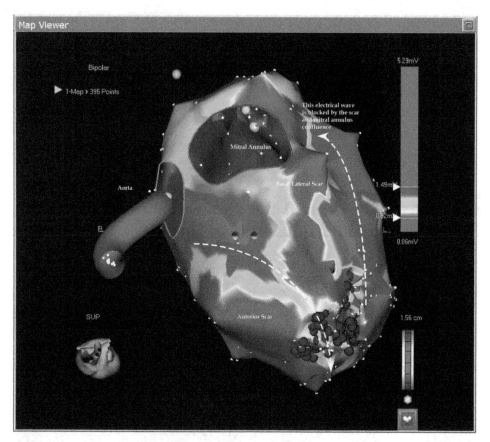

Fig. 7.3. This picture shows the superior projection of the left ventricle with the aortic and mitral annuli. The basal lateral scar is confluent with the mitral ring and this confluence prevents closure of the reentry around this lateral scar leaving only the anterior scar open to permit the reentry. The ablation blocked the isthmus leaving the tachycardia non inducible.

Scar ablation is an accepted approach to ablate ventricular tachycardia. Electromagnetic mapping is indispensable in delineating the scar and magnetic resonance imaging (MRI), three-dimensional computer topographies (CT) and positron emission topographies combined with CT (PET/CT) pictures may enhance it and makes possible evaluation of the exact trans-mural dispersion (Codreanu A et al, 2008; Dickfeld T et al, 2008, Tian J et al. 2010).

The second patient is AG; 61-year-old man with dilated cardiomyopathy, sustained ventricular tachycardia and was referred for CRTD (cardiac resynchronization therapy-defibrillator) implantation. Interestingly, during the implantation, at the left lead pacing threshold measurement, the patient developed ventricular tachycardia. This suggested a tachycardia focus near the pacing area in the left basal posterior-lateral wall.

After the implantation he developed frequent episodes of VT not suppressed by adjuvant medical treatment with amiodarone and mexiletine (Figure 7.4). For this reason he was taken to the electrophysiology laboratory and the left ventricle was mapped during ventricular tachycardia (Figure 7.5 and 7.6). Only a partial mapping was needed (overall 27 points) and the tachycardia origin was located on the basal posterior wall (Figure 7.6), just like suggested by the induction during the implantation. After 4 radiofrequency application on this site the tachycardia terminated and has become non inducible. Of note, the ECG (Figure 7.4 and 7.5) suggested the basal posterior location of the origin and the QRS during the tachycardia had RBBB (Right Bundle Brunch Block), inferior and rightward axis (Figure 7.4 and 7.5).

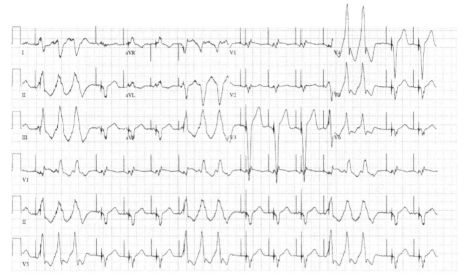

Fig. 7.4. The clinical VT in non-sustained form, but with the same morphology of RBBB, inferior and rightward axis

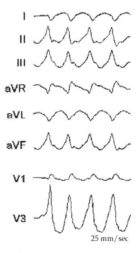

25 mm/sec

Fig. 7.5. The figure shows the ECG of the VT during the ablation. This VT had RBBB configuration and inferior and rightward axis. This configuration is suggesting a left ventricular VT with the origin in the basal area.

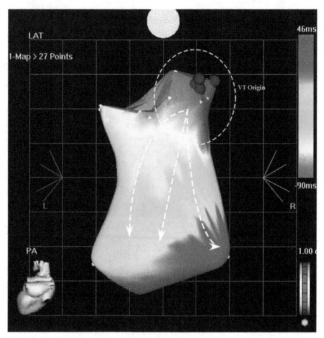

Fig. 7.6. The picture shows the potero-anterior projection of a part of the left ventricle during the VT. The earliest points are located on the basal posterior wall (red area) and the VT is propagated to the apical are as shown by the arrows (blue area). Ablation in this area terminated the VT and rendered it non-inducible.

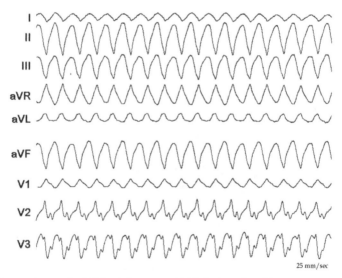

Fig. 7.7. The figure shows the ECG of the second VT during the ablation two weeks after the first one. The QRS has an RBBB configuration and superior axis. When compared with the

first VT (Figure 7.5), the rightward axis is less expressed (L1 compared in the two ECGs, and AVL in the first ECG is negative and in the second is positive). There are also differences in the chest leads available (V3 is strongly positive in the first VT and clearly negative in the second VT). The rates of the VTs are similar.

Although the ablation was successful as exemplified by the previous pictures, the patient presented after two weeks with a second VT (Figure 7.7). He was taken again to the electrophysiology laboratory and the VT was mapped, again with CARTO (Figure 7.8). This time the VT had an RBBB configuration and superior axis! (Figure 7.7)

It was evident that the two VTs are not coming from the same area and again a limited map was completed (to avoid hemodynamic compromise during prolonged mapping). As Figure 7.8 exemplifies, the second VT originated from the apical septum. This are was ablated (Figure 7.9) and interestingly, after the ablation at the earliest point the tachycardia terminated, but was reinduced. This time the second ablation site at this procedure was more inferior, but after termination of the VT by the ablation, it has become noninducible.

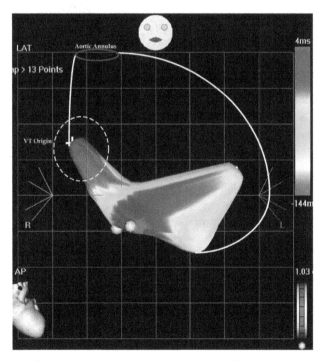

Fig. 7.8. The picture shows an antero-posterior projection of the left ventricular flow map during VT at the second ablation procedure. The left ventricular perimeter is shown with the white lines, including the aortic annulus. The earliest points are originating on the septal area and propagate in the anterior and posterior wall. There is collision on the inferior wall (pink color) and is tagged. The earliest points are -144 msec before the reference catheter in the right ventricle and the collision is 4 msec after the reference catheter.

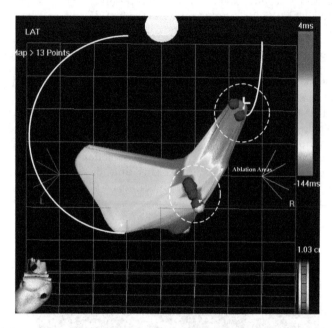

Fig. 7.9. The picture shows the flow map of the left ventricle in postero-anterior projection. Two areas had to be ablated to terminate the VT, first the higher area and earliest one was ablated than the second more inferior are which has become early (not shown) and finally terminated the VT and left it non-inducible.

At the end of the second ablation procedure a very fast VT (200 msec cycle length) was induced requiring DC shock termination (through the implanted ICD which was immediately activated). Two years after the second ablation the patient was free of any ICD therapy. Only rare non-sustained VT was stored by the ICD. In this patient we made several clinical decisions and observations during and around the ablation procedures:

1. The left ventricle mapping was not completed, was quickly achieved and culminated with ablation
2. Propagation mapping was done as this patient has dilated cardiomyopathy and no discrete scar can be mapped
3. Although the ICD was deactivated during the procedure to prevent early termination of the VT during the mapping, it was immediately activated with the induction of the rapid VT (200 msec cycle length- ventricular flutter)
4. The rapid VT-ventricular flutter was not clinical as was not recorded by the ICD during the long follow-up.
5. The proarrhythmic effect of biventricular pacing, well known from the current literature (Nayak HM et al, 2008; Gasparini M et al, 2008, Nordbeck P et al, 2010)

CH was a 59-year-old patient with a large anterior wall myocardial infarction, ventricular tachycardia and implantable defibrillator.

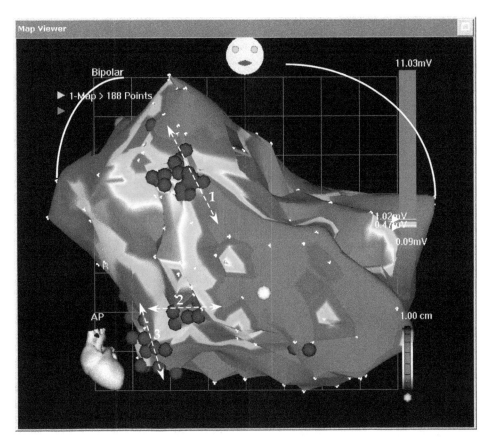

Fig. 7.10. The picture shows the extremely enlarged left ventricle, scar mapping and multiple isthmuses ablation (3 shown on this antero-posterior projection). All the procedure was completed during sinus rhythm, without ventricular pacing. The defibrillator was deactivated during the procedure.

The defibrillator was upgraded to CRTD. Two years after the upgrading, he presented with "VT storm" (more than 150 episodes of VT, majority treated with overdrive pacing and two of them with ICD shock). As medical treatment was not effective and the tachycardia has become resistant to overdrive pacing (including pacing from the RV lead, LV lead and biventricular), he was taken to the electrophysiology laboratory for catheter ablation. It was understood that no mapping during the VT can be completed because the hemodynamic imbalance. Scar mapping was attempted. The left ventricle was extremely enlarged and no catheter was available to complete to basal area mapping. After the ablation the VT frequency was significantly reduced, but not completely abolished and the patient had ventricular assist device implantation, but not survived until appropriate donor heart was available for him.

BN is a 75 year-old-man with a history of a large anterior infarction at the end of 1980's. He was treated with intravenous Streptokinase and despite apparent reperfusion the laboratory tests suggested a large infarction. In the early 1990's he developed aborted sudden cardiac death and a defibrillator was implanted. Occasionally, he had successfully treated episodes of ventricular tachycardia and was resolved with adjuvant amiodarone treatment. In 2008 the defibrillator was upgraded to cardiac resynchronization therapy-defibrillator (CRT-D). Recently he was admitted with incessant tachycardia with a rate between 135-140 beats per minute with relative hemodynamic stability. No medical treatment could suppress the tachycardia, including amiodarone reloading, additional mexiletine, beta-blockers and carvedilol. A coronary angiogram revealed no new coronary lesions and no target for revascularization. As the tachycardia was still incessant, the patient was taken to the electrophysiology laboratory for an ablation attempt. The left ventricle was approached through the aortic valve and the left ventricle was mapped using the fast map technique. The patient was all this time in his slow ventricular tachycardia. As evident in Figure 7.11, the left ventricle is enlarged with a large apical aneurysm and a large scar on the antero-lateral wall. The origin of the tachycardia was in the apical area at the border of the large scar (Figure 7.11). Ablation in this site terminated the tachycardia and was returned to the Cardiology Ward in sinus rhythm.

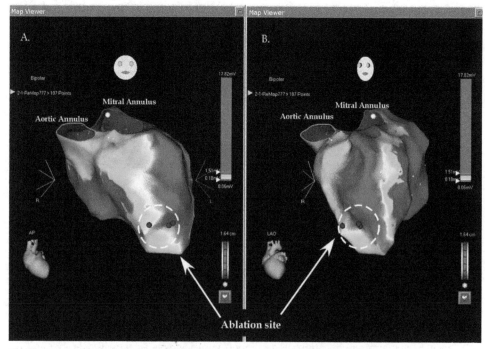

Fig. 7.11. The picture shows the voltage mapping of the left ventricle in two projections: A. antero-posterior; B. left anterior oblique; the ventricle is enlarged with a large apical aneurysm and a large antero-lateral scar. The ablation site is shown in both projections and the ablation was completed during incessant ventricular tachycardia (135 BPM) and propagation mapping. With the two lateral applications the tachycardia terminated spontaneously.

Although the tachycardia was not anymore incessant, the patient still had episodes of tachycardia at a faster rate (150-160 beats per minute). As this tachycardia was not tolerated, he was returned to the electrophysiology laboratory for a "scar ablation". This time the tachycardia was not induced and the mapping was completed in sinus rhythm (paced rhythm). Using slightly different definitions (scar in the first mapping was defined as <0.18 mV and during the second mapping as <0.54 mV), a large golf of myocardial tissue was revealed in the anterior basal area (Figure 7.12). This area was isolated from the surrounding normal tissue and the ablation area was continued until the mitral annulus to avoid any possible large reentry around the whole scar. Although the endocardial surface was completely blocked, the tachycardia was still inducible with impression of multiple breakthrough points suggesting epicardial origin. However, no real mapping could be completed because the hemodynamic instability during the VT. For this reason, he was scheduled for an epicardial ablation. During the epicardial mapping the origin of the VT was on the apical area and wide area ablation terminated the tachycardia. This epicardial site was almost the same with the successful site during the first mapping. During 3 months follow up the defibrillator recorded and stored only 4 episodes of VT successfully treated with overdrive pacing and not recalled by the patient. He continued the combination of amiodarone and carvedilol treatment. This patient also exemplifies the presence of multiple VT foci in a patient with ischemic cardiomyopathy and a large post myocardial infarction scar.

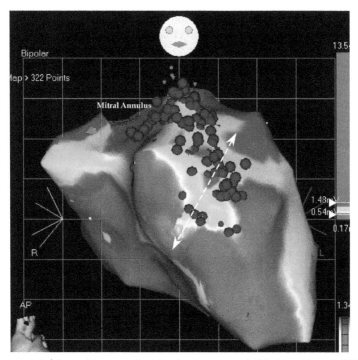

Fig. 7.12. The picture shows the mapping during the second ablation attempt. This is an antero-posterior projection of the left ventricular voltage mapping. The normal tissue was defined as >1.5 mV (like in Figure 6.11), but the scar was defined as <0.5 mV. A large invagination of myocardium into the basal scar was revealed and ablated (see text).

In this patient, with poor left ventricular function and resynchronization therapy, a combined endocardial focal ablation, scar ablation and finally epicardial ablation completed the procedure and achieved an acceptable clinical outcome. The electro-anatomic mapping exemplifies the complexity of the ablation in this patient, and it was possible only using this advanced mapping.

Four patients were presented, each one with a different condition and different mapping. The first patient had a well-defined scar with a clear narrow strip of myocardium dividing it into a large scar and a smaller basal scar limited by the mitral annulus. The second patient has dilated cardiomyopathy without discrete scar and two different foci ablated in two consecutive procedures. The third patient had an extreme ischemic cardiomyopathy, with uncontrollable ventricular tachycardia storm and labile hemodynamic condition. Only scar ablation was possible, because the extremely dilated left ventricle. The fours patient had an enlarged left ventricle, with a large apical aneurysm. The same patient has endocardial focal ablation, scar ablation and finally epicardial ablation.

8. Theoretical aspects

As mentioned in the introduction, first DC shock ablations than RF ablation of solitary pathways in the AV Node or outside it is practiced in clinical electrophysiology. However, DC was used for the first AV Nodal ablation, well-defined origin of WPW and ventricular tachycardia foci. Radiofrequency replaced the DC shock. During 2-3 years first the AV Nodal and AV pathways were ablated. Subsequently, idiopathic VT foci and atrial flutter and focal tachycardia were ablated. In the early 1990's, ventricular tachycardia in structural heart disease, atrial fibrillation and idiopathic ventricular fibrillation were not considered candidates for ablation. Electro-anatomic mapping open the possibility to ablate this complex arrhythmia foci. (Exception was atrial fibrillation where first focal ablation than point ablation guided by special catheters- lasso- preceded the electro-anatomic mapping).

8.1 Atrial tachycardia ablation

In large branching scar, the ablation requires electroanatomic mapping. Patients after corrective surgery of congenital heart disease may develop large scars in the atrium and frequently develop incisional reentry tachycardia. As early as in 2001, several institutions reported small groups or case reports describing the use of electroanatomic mapping (Leonelli FM et al, 2001; Peichl P et al, 2003). Before the use of this mapping, electrophysiological definition of the slow isthmus, called central pathway, was needed. This was a long procedure with limited success. The electro-anatomic mapping delineates the scar, and delineates the isthmus in between scars or in the scar itself. Blocking these pathways, or as occasional called, channels, will prevent induction or spontaneous recurrence of the tachycardia. Interestingly, the number of publication describing the use of electroanatomic mapping for ablation of focal tachycardia ablation is much larger (Kottkamp H et al, 1997; Marchlinski FE et al, 1998; Cummings RM et al, 2008). There is also ample of information on the use of this mapping in the ablation of different left atrial tachycardias (Iwai S et al, 2002; Marrouche NF et al, 2002; Kistler PM et al, 2003; Dong J et al, 2005). Left atrial tachycardias may originate on the septum, along the mitral annulus and from the pulmonary veins. Correct mapping may localize the origin and ensure successful ablation.

Two arrhythmias were extensively discussed in the literature: atrial fibrillation ablation and ablation of ventricular tachycardia in patients with structural heart disease.

8.2 Atrial fibrillation ablation

After the description of the pulmonary vein as trigger in atrial fibrillation, ablation was attempted, first focal, than pulmonary vein isolation (Haissaguerre M et al, 1998). A special catheter was developed- the lasso catheter- to permit mapping of the pulmonary vein osteum and to localize the pathway connecting electrically the vein with the left atrium. This site was ablated and pacing from the coronary sinus could prove the electrical disconnection of the veins (Takahashi Y et al, 2007). This treatment was indicated for patients with paroxysmal atrial fibrillation and not for the other forms of chronic atrial fibrillation, like persistent and permanent. Atrial fibrillation ablation based on electro-anatomic mapping has become an accepted alternative to the pulmonary vein disconnection (Pappone C et al 1999; Pappone C et al, 2000; Pappone C et al 2004; Oral H et al 2006, pappone et al, 2006). Developed at the beginning of this century, this approach offered already at the beginning of its implementation, a possible ablation also for persistent atrial fibrillation and even for long standing persistent type (more then 1 year). The pulmonary vein isolation is achieved by circle ablation in the antrum of the veins. Line ablations in the roof and in the mitral isthmus (between the mitral annulus and the left lower pulmonary vein) completes the procedure and are necessary to avoid left atrial flutter/tachycardia around the ablation rings in the pulmonary vein antrum. One first advantage of the left atrial ablation is the sparing of the vein and by this to reduce to minimum the possible damage to the vessel. This damage may result in pulmonary vein stenosis/occlusion, pulmonary hypertension and symptomatic shortness of breath. The correct and exact reconstruction of the left atrium and its appendages is a prerequisite not only for successful isolation of the pulmonary veins, but also for preventing the above-mentioned damage. Following the original introduction of the electro-anatomic approach to atrial fibrillation ablation, this method was compared with the original pulmonary vein disconnection and both the acute success and the recurrence rate after 1 year was in advantage of the left atrial ablation (Oral H et al, 2003). Moreover, the method was evaluated in patients with long-persistent atrial fibrillation and a significantly higher number of patient in the ablation group was in sinus rhythm after 1 year-77% versus 53% (Oral H et al, 2006a). A large percent of the control group moved to the ablation group and the symptomatic improvement was significantly higher in the ablation group. An additional approach to atrial fibrillation ablation was targeted to complex atrial electrograms. This method is accepted as adjuvant to the left atrial ablation. Finally, even if the first method is use to disconnect the pulmonary veins, the procedure is escalated and elements of the second and third procedure are added (Oral H et al, 2006b; Takahashi Y et al, 2007). Although, we are still not at the end of the way in the development of atrial fibrillation ablation methods, the place of the electroanatomic mapping is well established. The most complex ablation is probably that of ventricular tachycardia in patients with structural heart disease.

8.3 Ventricular tachycardia ablation

Ventricular tachycardia ablation is going back to 1983 when DC shock was delivered to the ablation site (Hartzler GO, 1983). Soon after the presentation of ablation using radiofrequency energy, it was applied to patients with idiopathic ventricular tachycardia (Kuck KH et al, 1991; Klein LS et al, 1992) and subsequently to ventricular tachycardia in structural heart disease (Morady F et al, 1993). Different methods of pacing helped to localize a critical area in the tachycardia circle or focus pending on the type of heart disease. Although this method was successful, the procedure was prolonged, required a long time to be in ventricular tachycardia and the recurrence rate or new tachycardias generation were high. It has become accepted as an adjuvant to other treatments and focused to the tachycardia causing repeated defibrillator therapy, ventricular tachycardia storm or intolerable shock therapy. The electroanatomic mapping opened to possibility to delineate the scar and reveal any narrow strips of myocardium bridging through the scar. These strips are targeted in the ablation and they are necessary parts of the tachycardia circle. In patients with tolerated tachycardia, the propagation map points to the tachycardia origin. This origin may be the exit point of the reentry circle or the other non-reentry focus (like in patients with dilated or hypertrophic cardiomyopathy). The ablation may be targeted to this early point. There is no need to hold the patient in prolonged tachycardia and no need for the pacing techniques. Moreover, in patients with non-tolerated tachycardia the scar is mapped and is isolated and connected to the valve annulus. Ablation, before defibrillation implantation, may reduce significantly the defibrillator therapy, when compared to non-ablation control group. This approach was called SMASH-VT (Reddy V et al, 2007, Kuck KH et al, 2010). Finally, endocardial ablation may be completed with epicardial ablation (Tedrow U & Stevenson WG, 2009; Sacher F et al, 2010). In patients with post myocardial infarction scars, most of the tachycardia reentry circle is endocardial, but in patients with dilated cardiomyopathy it may be epicardial (Nakahara S et al, 2010).

8.4 Future ablations

There are several other ablation targets recently added to the electrophysiology treatment armamentarium. The first arrhythmia is the idiopathic ventricular fibrillation. Patient with idiopathic ventricular fibrillation may need daily shock therapies and no medical treatment can suppress it. For these patients ablation of the initiating beats origin may reduce the number of treatments needed. These sites are characterized by high density of Purkinje fibers. Clinically, fascicular spikes may be recorded at the successful site in the ventricle (Knecht S et al, 2009; Natale A et al, 2010). If this approach will be applicable in patients with aborted sudden cardiac death and structural heart disease is still on evaluation. The second group with possible future application of electro-anatomic mapping is in patients with Brugada Syndrome. Epicardial fractionated electrograms in the RV outflow may be targeted and after the ablation, the ECG normalizes (Nademanee K et al, 2011). Occasionally, the site may be approached from the endocardium. Of note, the ventricular wall in the RV outflow is relatively thin.

If these two ablations will be implemented in routine practice, the future years will let us know.

9. Conclusions

Complex ablation has become routine in the clinical electrophysiology. Although these arrhythmias originally were approached with classical electrophysiology methods, the electroanatomic mapping simplified them and opened these ablations before rapidly increasing number of electrophysiology centers.

10. References

Arenal A, del Castillo S, Gonzalez-Torrecilla E, Atienza F, Ortiz M, Jimenez J, Puchol A, Garrcia J 7 Almedral J. (2004). Tachycardia-related channel in the scar tissue in patients wuth sustained monomorphic ventricular tachycardia: Influence of the voltage scar definition. *Circulation* Vol. 110:2568-2574

Ben Haim SA, Gepstein L, Hayam G, Ben David J & Josephson MM. (1996a). A new nonfluoroscopic Electroanatomic mapping system. Pacing Clin Electroanatomic mapping system. *Pacing Clin Electrophysiol* Vol. 19:709

Ben-Haim SA, Osadchy D, Schuster I, Gepstein L, Hayam G & Josephson MM. (1996b). Nonfluoropscopic, in vivo navigation and mapping technology. *Nature Med* Vol. 2:1393-1395

Codreanu A, Odille F, Aliot E, Marie PY, Angnin-Poull I, Andonache M, Mandry D, Djaballah W, Regent D, Felblinger J & de Chillou C. (2008). Electroanatomic characterization of post-infarction scars. Comparison with 3-dimensional myocardial scar reconstruction based on magnetic resonance imaging. *J Am Coll Cardiol* Vol. 52:839-42

Cosio FG, Lopez-Gil M, Goicolea A, Arribas F & Barroso JL. (1993). Radiofrequency ablation of the inferior vena cava-tricuspid valve isthmus in common atrial flutter. *Am J Cardiol* Vol. 71:705-709

Cummings RM, Mahle WT, Stieper MJ, Cambell RM, Costelo L, Balfour V, Burchfeld A, Frias PA. (2008). Outcome following electroanatomic mapping and ablation for the treatment of ectopic tachycardia in the pediatric population. *Pediatr Cardiol* Vol. 29:393-397

Daubert JP, Zareba W, Cannom DS, McNit S, Rosero SZ, Wang P, Schuger C, Steinberg JS, Higgins SL Wilber DJ, Klein H, Andrews ML, Hall J, Moss AJ & the MADIT II investigators. (2008). Inappropriate implantable cardioverter defibrillator shock in MADIT II. Frequency, mechanism, predictors, and survival impact. *J Am Coll Cardiol* Vol. 51:1357-1365

Dickfeld T, Lei P, Dilsizian V, Jeudy J, Dong J, Voudouris A, Peters R, Saba M, Shekhar R & Shorofsky S. (2008). Integration of three-dimensional scar maps for ventricular tachycardia ablation with positron emission tomography-computer tomography. *JACC: Cardiovascular Imaging* Vol. 1:73-82

Dong J, Zrenner B, Schreieck J, Deisenhofer I, Karch M, Schneider M, Von Bary C, Weyerbrock S, Yin Y & Schmitt C. (2005). Catheter ablation of left focal atrial tachycardia guided by electroanatomic mapping and new insights into interatrial electrical conduction. *Heart Rhythm* Vol. 2:578-591

Ehrlich JR, Cha TJ, Zhang L, Chartier D, Melnyk P, Hohnloser S & Nattel S. (2003). Cellular electrophysiology of canine pulmonary vein cardiomyocytes: action potential and ionic current properties. *J Physiol* Vol. 551:801-813

ExnerDV, Pinski SI, Wyse G, Renftoe EG, Follman D, Gold M, Beckman KJ, Coromilas J, Lancester S, Hallstrom AP & the AVID investigators. (2001). Electrical storm presages nonsudden death: The Antiarrhythmic Versus Implantable Defibrillators (AVID) Trial. *Circulation* Vol. 103:2066-2071

Ezekowitz JA, Amstrong PW & McAlister FA. (2003). Implantable cardioverter defobrillators in primary and secondary prevention: a systematic review of randomized trials. *Ann Intern Med* Vol. 138:445-452

Feld GK, Fleck P, Chen PS, Boyce K, Bahnson TD, Stein JB, Calisi CM & Ibarra M. (1992) Radiofrequency catheter ablation for the treatment of human type 1 atrial flutter. *Circulation* Vol. 86:1233-1240

Gasparini M, Lunati M, Landolina M, Santini M, Padaletti L, Perego G, Vincenti A, Curnis A, Carboni A, Denaro A, Spotti A, Grammatico A, Regoli F, Boriani G & on behalph of the InSync ICD Italian Registry Investigators. (2008). Electrical storm in patients with biventricular implantable cardioverter defibrillator: incidence, predictors, and prognostic implications. *Am Heart J* Vol. 156:847-854

Gepstein L, Hayam G, Josephson ME & Ben-Haim SA. (1996). A new method for cardiovolumetric measurement based on nonfluoroscopic electrophysiological electroanatomic. *Pacing Clin Electrophysiol* Vol. 19:724

Gepstein L, Hayam G & Ben Haim SA. (1997). A novel model for nonfluoroscopic catheter-based electroanatomic mapping of the heart: in vitro and in vivo accuracy results. *Circulation* Vol. 95:1611-1622

Gepstein L, Goldin A, Lessick J, Hayam G, Shpun S, Schwartz Y, Hakim G, Shofty Turgeman A. Kirshenbaum D & Ben Haim SA. (1998). Electromechanical characterization of chronic myocardial infarction in the canine coronary occlusion model. *Circulation* Vol. 98:2055-2064

Hassaguerre M, Shoda M, Jais P, Nogami A, Shah DC, Kautzner J, Arentz TKalushe D, Lamaison D, Griffith M, Cruz F, de Paola A, Gaita F, Hicini M, Garrigue S, Macle L, Weerasooriya R & Clementi J. (2002). Mapping and ablation of idiopathic ventricular fibrillation. *Circulation* Vol. 106:962-967

Haissaguerre M, Jais P, Shah DC, Takahashi A, Hocini M, Quinou G, Garrigue S, Le Mouroux A, Le Metayer P & Clementy J. (1998). Spontaneous initiation of atrial fibrillation by ectopic beats originating in the pulmonary veins. *N Engl J Med* Vol. 339:659-666

Hartzler GO. (1983). Electrode catheter ablation of refractory focal ventricular tachycardia. *J Am Coll Cardiol* Vol. 2:1107-1113

Hayam G, Gepstein L & Ben-Haym. SA. (1996). Accuracy of the In Vivo Determination of location using non fluoroscopic electroanatoamical mapping system. *Pacing Clin Electrophysiol* Vol. 19:712

Hsia HH, Lin D, Sayer WH, Callans DJ & Marchlinski FE. (2006). Anatomic characteristics of endocardial substrate for hemodynamic stable reentrant ventricular tachycardia: identification of endocardial conducting channels. *Heart Rhythm* Vol. 3:503-512

Iwai S, Markowitz SM, Stein KM, Mittal S, Slotwiner DJ, Das MK, Cohen JD, Hao SC & Lerman BB. (2002). Response to adenosine differentiates focal from macroreentrant atrial tachycardia. Validation using three-dimensional electroanatomic mapping. *Circulation* Vol. 106:2793-2799

Jackman WM, Beckman KJ, NcClelland JH, Wang X, Friday KJ, Roman CA, Moulton KP, Twidale N, Hazlitt HA, Prior MI, Oren J, Overholt ED, Lazzara R. (1992). Treatment of supraventricular tachycardia due to atrioventricular nodal reentry, by radiofrequency catheter ablation of slow-pathway conduction. N Engl J Med Vol. 327:313-318

Kistler PM, Saders PB, Hussin A, Morton JB, Vohra JK, Sparks PB & Kalman JM. (2003). Focal atrial tachycardia arising from the mitral annulus. Eelctrocardiographic and electrophysiologic characterization. *J Am Coll Cardiol* Vol. 41:2212-2219

Klein LS, Shih HT, Hackett K, Zipes DP & Miles WM. (1992). Radiofrequency catheter ablation of ventricular tachycardia in patients without structural heart disease. *Circulation* Vol. 85:1666-1674

Knecht S, Sacher F, Wright M, Hocini M, Nogami A, Arentz T, Petit B, Frank R, De Chillou C, Lamison D, Farre J, Lavergne L, Weerasooriya R, Cauchemez B, Lellouche N, Derval N, Narayan SM, Jais P & Clementy J, Haissaguerre M. (2009). Long-term follow-up of idiopathic ventricular fibrillation ablation: a multicenter study. *J Am Coll Cardiol* Vol. 54:522-528

Kottkamp H, Hindricks G, Breithardt G & Borggrefe M. (1997). Three-dimentional electromagnetic catheter technology: Elecroanatomical mapping of the right atrium and ablation of ectopic tachycardia. *Pacing Clin Electrophysiol* Vol. 8:1332-1337

Kuck KH, Schluter M, Geiger M & Siebels J. (1991). Successful catheter ablation of human ventricular tachycardia with radiofrequency current guided by an endocardial map of the area of slow conduction. *Pacing Clin Electrophysiol* Vol. 14:1060-1071

Kuck KH, Schamann A, Eckhardt L, Willems S, Ventura R, Delacretaz E, Pitcschner HF, Kautzner J, Schumacher B, Hansen PS & for the VTACH study group. (2010). Catheter ablation of stable ventricular tachycardia before defibrillator implantation in patients with coronary artery disease (VTACH): a multicenter randomized controlled trial. *Lancet* Vol. 375:31-40

Kumagai K, Muraoka S, Mitsutake C, Takashima H & Nakashima H. (2007). A new approach for complete isolation of the posterior left atrium including pulmonary veins for atrial fibrillation. *J Cardiovasc Electrophysiol* Vol. 18:1047-1052

Lee MA, Morady F, Kadish A, Schamp DJ, Chin MC, Scheinman MM, Griffin JC, Pederson D, Goldberger J, Calkins H, deBuitleir M, Kou WH, Rosenheck S, Sousa J & Langberg J. (1991). Catheter modification of the atrioventricular junction with radiofrequency energy for control of atrioventricular nodal reentry tachycardia. *Circulation* Vol. 83:827-835

Leonelli FM, Tomassoni G, Richey M & Natale A. (2001). Ablation of incisional atrial tachycardias using three-dimensional nonfluoroscopic mapping system. *Pacing Clin Electrophysiol* Vol. 24:1653-1659

Marchlinski F, Callans D, Gottlieb C, Rodriguez E, Coyne R & Kleinman D. (1998). Magnetic electroanatomic mapping for ablation of focal atrial tachycardias. *Pacing Clin Electrophysiol* Vol. 21:1621-1635

Marchlinski FE, Callans DJ, Gottlieb CD & Zado E. (2000). Linear ablation lesions of unmappable ventricular tachycardia in patients with ischemic and nonischemic cardiomyopathy. *Circulation* Vol. 101:1288-1296

Marrouche NF, Groenewegen AS, Yang Y, Dibs S & Scheinman MM. (2002). Clinical and electrophysiologic characteristics of left septal atrial tachycardia. *J Am Coll Cardiol* Vol. 40:1133-1139

Morady F & Scheinman MM. (1984). Transvenous catheter ablation of posteroseptal accessory pathway in patients with Wolff-Parkinson-White syndrome. *N Engl J Med* Vol. 310:705-707

Morady F, Harvey M, Kalbfleisch SJ, El-Atassi R, Calkins H & Langberg JJ. (1993) Radiofrequency catheter ablation of ventricular tachycardia in patients with coronary artery disease. *Circulation* Vol. 87:363-372

Nademanee K, McKenzie J, Kosar E, Schwab M, Sunsaneewitayakul B, Vasavakul T, Khunnawat C & Ngarmukos T. (2004). A new approach for catheter ablation of atrial fibrillation: mapping of the electrophysiologic substrate. *J Am Coll Cardiol* Vol. 43:2044 –2053

Nademanee K, Veerakul G, Chandanamattha P, Chaothawee L, Ariyachaipanich A, Jirasirirojanakorn K, Likittanasombat K, Bhuripanyo K & Ngarmukos T. (2011). Prevention of ventricular fibrillation episodes in Brugada Syndrome by catheter ablation over the anterior right ventricular outflow epicardium. *Circulation* Vol. 123:1270-1279

Nakahara S, Tung R, Ramirez RJ, Michowitz Y, Vasedhi M, Buch E, Gima J, Wiener I, Mahajan A, Boyle NG & Shivkumar K. (2010). Characterization of the arrhythmogenic substrate in ischemic and nonischemic cardiomyopathy. Implications for catheter ablation of hemodynamically unstable ventricular tachycardia. *J Am Coll Cardiol* Vol. 55:2355-2365

Natale A, Raviele A, Al-Ahmad A et al. (2010). Venice Chart international consensus document on ventricular tachycardia/fibrillation ablation. *J Cardiovasc Electrophysiol* Vol. 21:339-379

Nayak HM, Verdino RJ, Russo AM, Gerstenfeld EP, Hsia HH, Lin D, Dixit S, Cooper JM, Callans D & Marchlinski FE. (2008). Ventricular tachycardia storm after initiation of biventricular pacing: incidence, clinical characteristics, management, and outcome. *J Cardiovasc Electrophysiol* Vol. 19:708-715

Nordbeck P, Seidl B, Fey B, Bauer WR & Titter O. (2010). Effect of cardiac resynchronization therapy on the incidence of electrical storm. *Int J Cardiol* Vol. 143:330-336

Oral H, Scharf C, Chugh A, Hall B, Cheung P, Good E, Veerareddy S, Pelosi F & Morady F. (2003). Catheter ablation for paroxysmal atrial fibrillation. Segmental pulmonary vein ostial ablation versus left atrial ablation. *Circulation* Vol. 108:2355-2360

Oral H, Pappone, Chugh A, Good E, Bogun F, Pelosi F, Bates ER, Lehmann MH, Vicedomini G, Augello G, Agricola E, Sala S, Santinelli V & Morady F. (2006a). Circumferential pulmonary-vein ablation for chronic atrial fibrillation. *N Engl J Med* Vol. 354:934-941

Oral H, Chugh A, Good E, Sankaran S, Reich SS, Igic P, Elmouchi D, Tschopp D, Crawford T, Dey S, Wimmer A, Lemola K, Jongnarangsin K, Bogun F, Pelosi F & Morady F. (2006b). A tailored approach to catheter ablation of paroxysmal atrial fibrillation. *Circulation* Vol. 113:1824-1831

Pappone C, Oreto G, Lamberti F, Vicedomini G, Loricchio ML, Shpun S, Rillo M, Calabro MP, Conversano A, Ben-Haim SA, Cappato R & Chierchia S. (1999). Catheter ablation of paroxysmal atrial fibrillation using a 3D mapping system. *Circulation* Vol. 100:1203-1208

Pappone C, Rosanio S, Oreto G, Tocchi M, Gugliotta F, Vicedomini G, Sakvati A, Dicandia C, Mazzone P, Santinelli V, Gulletta S & Chiechia S. (2000). Circumferentia radiofrequency ablation of PV ostia. *Circulation* Vol. 102:2619 –28

Pappone C, Manguso F, Vicedomini G, Gugliotta F, Santinelli O, Ferro A, Gulletta S, Sala S, Sora N, Paglino G, Augello G, Agricola E, Zngrillo A, Alfieri O & Santinelli V. (2004). Prevention of iatrogenic atrial tachycardia after ablation of atrial fibrillation: a prospective randomized study comparing circumferential pulmonary vein ablation with a modified approach. *Circulation* Vol. 110:3036-3042

Pappone C, Augello G Sala S, Gugliotta F, Vicedomini G, Gulletta S, Paglino G, Mazzone P, Sora N, Greiss I, Santagostino A, LiVolsi L, Pappone N, Radinovic A, Manguso F & Santinelli V. (2006). A randomized trial of circumferential pulmonary vein ablation versus antiarrhythmic drug therapy in paroxysmal atrial fibrillation. The APAF Study. *J Am Coll Cardiol* Vol. 48:2340-2347

Peichl P, Kautzner J, Cihak R, Vancura V & Bytesnik J. (2003). Clinical application of electroanatomic mapping of "incisional" atrial tachycardia. *Pacing Clin Electrophysiol* Vol. 26:420-425

Poole JE, Johnson GW, Hellkamp AS, Anderson J, Callans DJ, Raitt MH, Reddy RK, Marchlinski FE, Yee R, Guarnieri T, Talajic M, Wilber DJ, Fishbein DP, Oacker DL, Matk DB, Lee KL & Bardy GH. (2008). Prognostic importance of defibrillation shocks in patients with heart failure. *N Engl J Med* Vol. 259:1009-1017

Reddy V, Reynolds MR, Neuzil P, Richardson AW, Taborsky M, Jongnarangsin K, Kralovec S, Sediva L, Ruskin JN & Josephson ME. (2007). Prophylactic catheter ablation for the prevention of defibrillator therapy. *N Engl J Med* Vol. 357:2657-2665

van Rees JB, Borleff JW, de Bie MK, Stijnen T, van Erven L, Bax JJ & Schlij MJ. (2011). Inappropriate Implantable cardioverter-defibrllator shocks. Incidence, predictors, and impact on mortality. *J Am Coll Cardiol* Vol. 57:556-562

Sacher F, Roberts-Thomson K, Maury P, Tedrow U, Nault I, Steven D, Hocini M, Koplan B, Leroux L, Derval N, Seiler J, Wright MJ, Epstein L & Haisaaguerre M. (2010). Epicardial ventricular tachycardia ablation. A multicenter safety study. *J Am Coll Cardiol* Vol. 55:2366-2376

Scheinman MM, Morady F, Hess DS & Gonzalez R. (1982). Catheter-induced ablation of the atrioventricular junction to control refractory supraventricular arrhythmias. *JAMA* Vol. 248:851-855

Shpun S, Gepstein L, Hayam G & Ben Haim SA. (1997). Guidance of radiofrequency endocardial ablation with real-time three-dimentional magnetic navigation system. *Circulation* Vol. 96:2016-2021

Smeets J, Ben Haim S, Ben David J, Gepstein L & Josephson MM. (1996). Non-fluoroscopic endocardial mapping: first experience in patients. *Pacing Clin Electrophysiol* Vol. 9:627

Sra J, Bhatia A, Dhala A, Blanck Z, Deshpande S, Cooley R & Akhtar M. (2001). Electroanatomically guided catheter ablation of ventricular tachycardia causing multiple defibrillation shocks. *Pacing Clin Electrophysiol* Vol. 24:1645-1652

Stevenson WG, Delacretaz E, Friedman PL & Ellison KE. (1998). Identification and ablation of macroreentrant ventricular tachycardia with CARTO electroanatomic mapping system. *Pacing Clin Electrophysiol* Vol. 21:1448-1456

Stevenson WG, Friedman PL, Kocovic D, Sager PT, Saxon LA & Pavri B. (1998). Radiofrequency catheter ablation of ventricular tachycardia after myocardial infarction. *Circulation* Vol. 98:308-314

Stevenson WG, Wilber DJ, Natale A, Jackman WM, Marchlinski FE, Talber T, GonzalesMD, Worley SJ, Daoud EG, Hwang C, Schuger C, Bump TE, Jazayeri M, Tomassoni GF, Koplelman HA, Soejima K, Nakagawa H & for the Multicenter Thermocool VT Ablation Trial Investigators. (2008). Irrigated radiofrequency catheter ablation guided by electroanatomic mapping for recurrent ventricular tachycardia after myocardial infarction. The Multicenter Thermocool Ventricular Tachycardia Ablation Trial. *Circulation* Vol. 118:2773-2782

Takatsuki S, Mitamura H & Ogawa S. (2001). Catheter ablation of monfocal premature ventricular complex trigerring idiopathic ventricular fibrillation. *Heart* Vol. 86:E3

Takahashi Y, O'Neill MD, Hocini M, Reant P, Jonsson A, Jaïs P, Sanders P, Rostock T, Rotter M, Sacher F, Laffite S, Roudaut R, Clémenty J, MD & Haïssaguerre M. (2007). Effect of stepwise ablation of chronic atrial fibrillation on atrial electrical and mechanical properties. *J Am Coll Cardiol* Vol. 49:1306-1314

Tedrow U & Stevenson WG. (2009). Strategies for epicardial mapping and ablation of ventricular tachycardia. *J Cardiovasc Electrophysiol* Vol. 20:710-713

Tian J, Jeudy J, Smith MF, Jimenez A, Yin X, Bruce PA, Lei P, Turgeman A, Abbo A, Shenkhar R, Saba M, Shorofsky S & Dickfeld T. (2001). Tree-dimensional contrast-enhanced CT for anatomic, dynamic, and perfusion characterization of abnormal myocardium to guide ventricular tachycardia ablation. *Circ Arrhythm Electrophysiol* Vol. 3:496-504

Tung R, Josephson ME, Reddy V, Reynolds MR & on behalf of the SMASH-VT investigators. (2010). Influence of clinical and procedural predictors on ventricular tachycardia ablation outcomes: An analysis from the substrate mapping and ablation in sinus rhythm to halt tachycardia trial (SMASH-VT). *J Cardiovasc Electrophysiol* Vol. 21:799-803

Wolff L, Parkinson J & White PD. (1930) Bundle-brunch block with short P-R interval in healthy young people prone to paroxysmal tachycardia. *Am Heart J* Vol. 5:685-704

Part 3

Miscellaneous

9

Arrhythmias in Pregnancy

Marius Craina[1], Gheorghe Furău[2], Răzvan Nițu[1], Lavinia Stelea[1],
Dan Ancușa[1], Corina Șerban[1], Rodica Mihăescu[1] and Ioana Mozoș[1]
[1]*"Victor Babeș" University of Medicine and Pharmacy, Timișoara,*
[2]*"Vasile Goldiș" Western University of Arad,*
Romania

1. Introduction

Pregnancies, as well as the post-partum period, are characterized by important metabolic changes. A lot of physiological changes affect the circulating blood volume, peripheral vascular compliance and resistance, myocardial function, heart rate and the neuro-hormonal system. These changes are well known in normal pregnancies, due to thorough examination and intense study; however there are still some questions related to the differences between women with and without structural diseases. Tocolitic medication used in pregnancy can cause cardiac complications in a healthy woman.

The presence of cardiovascular diseases in pregnancy must not be ignored because:

- Cardiovascular diseases are top causes of non-obstetrical maternal death (Sullivan, 1990).
- The modern possibilities of investigation improved diagnosis of cardiac diseases.
- The modern therapy can help women with cardiovascular diseases to have a good pregnancy outcome. Until recently, pregnancy was forbidden in those women.
- Women with repaired congenital heart defects. These women will have an increased risk of arrhythmias during pregnancy (Tateno, 2003). These types of patients usually have fragile hemodynamics and need additional therapy in most of the cases.

2. Physiological changes during pregnancy

The antepartum period is characterized by three main changes: an increased blood volume and heart rate and a reduction in the systemic vascular resistance. The increased blood volume can be estimated by examining ventricular diastolic volume and pressure. The increase starts gradually in the 6th week of gestation and by the end of the pregnancy it will reach 50% more than in the pre-pregnant state (Lind, 1985). However, this value is not constant. Studies have shown that there are increases from 20% to 100% above pre-pregnant blood volume (Pirani, 1973). It has been demonstrated that the blood volume increases at least until mid-pregnancy. The period, when the blood pressure plateaus, is arguable: some studies consider that it plateaus in the third trimester (Rovinsky, 1965), others have found a continuous increase until term (Lund, 1967). Blood volume increases considerably in a twin pregnancy (Thomsen, 1994). The increase in the end-diastolic volume can be noticed after 10 weeks of gestation and it will peak during the third trimester (Campos O, 1996). Pregnancy is associated with "physiological anemia", as a consequence of hemodilution (there is a proportional greater increase in the plasma volume than in the red blood cell mass, the latter being around 40% above pre-pregnancy levels) (Pirani 1973). Hypervolemia is caused by hormonal factors like: prolactin, placental lactogen, growth hormone, and estrogen or peptides like the prostaglandins. Considering women without heart disease, the cardiac filling pressures are not higher in women at term compared to women 11-13 weeks' postpartum (Clark, 1989). The vascular resistance differs from one pregnancy state to another. A fall in systemic vascular resistance has been described in the 5th week of gestation; a nadir between the 20th and 32nd week was followed by a slowly increase. The overall fall in the systemic vascular resistance occurs because of the changes in the resistance and flow in multiple vascular beds, such as the uteroplacental, renal, muscular, cutaneous and mammary bed. There are no changes in the hepatic or the cerebral blood flow. Variations in the renal and unteroplacental blood flow are primarily caused by positional changes (Jurkovic, 1991). For example, in the supine position in case of a pregnant woman, there is a compression of the inferior vena cava. An obstruction of the abdominal aorta and iliac arteries may also occur because of the uterus (Bieniarz, 1969). The resistance of these vascular beds is decreased due to the great amount of secreted vasodilators for example prostacyclin.

The systemic arterial pressure has a similar behavior: it decreases in the first semester and reaches its nadir at mid-pregnancy. Thereafter it increases and, in some cases, its level is higher than the pre-pregnancy level. The cardiac output is the most common measure of cardiac performance. Cardiac output, which is dependent on the heart rate and stroke volume, is gradually increasing by about 30-50% (Clark, 1989; and Rubler S, 1977) in the 5th week of gestation, reaching its peak at approximately the end of the second trimester (Robson, 1989) or in the third trimester (Bader, 1955). Afterwards, it is either constant until term or it decreases slightly near term. Although the amount of the oxygen in the blood is proportional with the cardiac output; there is no relation between the cardiac output and oxygen consumption, the last, increasing progressively by 20-30% at term (Elkus, 1992). Studies show different results when the ejection fraction is debated: some indicate that there are no alterations in the left ventricular ejection fraction (Katz, 1978 and Geva T, 1997), meanwhile other demonstrate increases in ejection fraction (Robson, 1989). This may be a result of the different loading conditions. The ratio of early to late diastolic flow velocity has been shown to be lower during the third semester compared with postpartum (Sadaniantz, 1992).

There is a wide individual variation of heart rate; however it usually increases by 10-20 beats; peaking in the late second trimester or early third trimester. Most pregnant women remain in sinus rhythm; but premature atrial and ventricular complexes may frequently occur.

Hemodynamic changes are also a cause of neurohormonal responses. The most important are the vasodilators: nitric oxide and prostaglandins, which cause, on one hand decreases in the peripheral resistance and, on the other hand, changes in the uterine and renal blood flow. Decreased cerebral blood flow activates the sympathetic nervous system. Conversely, plasma volume expansion suppresses catecholamine levels.

Neurohormones also activate the renin-angiotensin-aldosterone system that is responsible for the regulation of the salt and water homeostasis in the body (August, 1990). Pregnancy is characterized by increased levels of renin and angiotensin. The increased level of renin is not dependent on the extracellular volume.

Natriuretic peptides (also activated by neurohormones) are associated with cardiovascular and renal functions. The level of the two main natriuretic peptides (the atrial natriuretic-ANP and the brain natriuretic-BNP) is increased during pregnancy (Yoshimura, 1994). Their release is caused by atrial and ventricular distension.

During the peripartum period the hemodynamics will radically change, due to pain, anxiety and uterine contractions. For example, uterine contractions will increase the blood volume up to 500 mL (Ueland, 1969). The blood loss will be associated to the type of delivery. If in vaginal delivery there is a 10% blood loss; in caesarian delivery there may be a loss of up to 29% of the total blood volume (Ueland, 1976). Research has demonstrated that the circulation is not influenced by the placental separation. With every contraction the cardiac output increases up to 7-15%, consequently increasing the basal blood pressure. Early after delivery, cardiac output may continue to increase to as much as 80% above pre-labour values. Cardiac output will return to pre-labour levels about 1 hour post-partum. In labour the amount of the catecholamine increase. As a result, the heart rate will have high values. These values are not constant, and depend on many factors such as: position or anesthesia. Hemodynamic parameters need around 6 months to return to their normal values. Immediately after delivery, the cardiac output increases by as much as 80%, followed by a decrease in 24 weeks. Within the first 3 days after delivery the blood volume will decrease by 20%, however the hematocrit needs 2 weeks to be stabilized. Also, within 2 weeks after delivery the systemic vascular resistance increases by 30 % (Robson, 1987), and the heart rate will return to baseline levels. Stroke volume decreases for the first 24 weeks after delivery. Systolic and diastolic blood pressures remain unaltered from late pregnancy until 12 weeks post-partum (Campos, 1996).

2.1 Prevalence of arrhythmias in pregnancy

The elevated levels of estrogen and b-choral gonadotropine appear, from experimental models, to affect the expression of cardiac ion channels. By functioning in a proarrhythmic way, pregnancy gives rise to significant problems concerning the diagnosis and treatment of certain arrhythmias, especially when drugs and/or non pharmaceutical therapeutic methods are required (Mark, 2002).

Palpitations, fatigue and syncope are common in pregnancy. The sinus rate increases by about 10 beats/minute during pregnancy, and sinus tachycardia greater than 100 beats/min is common (Conti, 2005). Extrasystoles, intermittent sinus tachycardia and non-sustained arrhythmia are encountered in more than 50% of pregnant women are investigated for symptoms of arrhythmia (Gowda, 2003). Some arrhythmias occuring during pregnancy represent a recurrence of a pre-existing problem, but a substantial number of cases appear for the first time in pregnancy. Bradyarrhythmias presenting during pregnancy are rare with a prevalence of about 1–20 000, and are usually caused by sinoatrial disease or congenital complete heart block (Lee, 1995). Atrial fibrillation and flutter are rarely encountered during pregnancy unless organic heart disease or endocrine disorders are present. Episodes of such arrhythmias appearing for the first time during pregnancy require further evaluation for possible congenital heart disease, rheumatic valvular disease or hyperthyroidism (Leung, 1998).

3. Mechanisms of arrhythmia in pregnancy

The management of the arrhythmia is not different in pregnant women. However, hemodynamic conditions should be considered.

The cardiovascular system undergoes significant changes in adaptation to pregnancy, including an increased heart rate and cardiac output, reduced systemic resistance, increased plasma catecholamine concentrations and adrenergic receptor sensitivity, atrial stretch and increased end-diastolic volumes due to intravascular volume expansion, as well as hormonal and emotional changes (Adamson, 2007). Pregnancies with abnormal uterine perfusion and subsequent pathological outcomes are paralleled by changes in ventricular repolarization, that precede clinical symptoms (Baumert, 2010). Repolarization of the ventricular myocardium might be affected in pregnancy due to changes in circulating hormones, electrolyte imbalances and increased sympathetic tone.

It is important to determine if the arrhythmia has clinical conequences such as deterioration of the underlying cardiac condition. Arrhythmogenic effects are linked to the type of arrhythmia. There is a high risk of maternal and fetal morbidity in women with repaired CHD (chronic heart diseases). Studies have demonstrated that simple tachyarrhythmia does not lead to death. However, death may occur if this type of arrhythmia is associated with structural diseases. New research suggests that women with cyanosis and CHD may experience still birth or miscarriage. In this situation, the best case scenario is a low birth weight infant.

4. Signs, investigations and diagnosis

4.1 Symptoms
Palpitations, the most common presenting symptom, are usually intermittent and only rarely indicate a serious problem. Patients with arrhythmia may also present with fatigue, breathlessness, peripheral edema and chest discomfort resulting from cardiac failure. Symptoms of thromboembolism may be the presenting feature of atrial fibrillation or atrial flutter. Patients complaining of palpitations, but without documented arrhythmia, have a low likelihood for having a life-threatening arrhythmia, and no further evaluation is warranted (Andreson, 1997). A history of previous heart disease increases the likelihood of life threatening arrythmias. Inquiry should be made about the family history, particularly with reference to cases of premature sudden death.

The severity of the symptoms allows the physician to judge whether the risks of therapy outweigh the benefits. The only difference in pregnancy is that the physician must consider the risk/benefit ratio for both the mother and the fetus. An arrhythmia that is hemodynamically compromising to the mother constitutes a major concern because of inadequate maternal, as well as placental, blood flow (Anderson, 1997).

4.2 Examination
The pulse may be abnormal during symptoms; the clinician should focus on looking for signs of heart disease that may be associated with arrhythmia, including scars from previous surgery, murmurs of structural heart disease and signs of cardiac failure. It is also important to look for systemic problems such as thyrotoxicosis that may cause arrhythmia. The diagnosis of heart disease in pregnancy is often difficult due to the anatomical and physiological changes in the cardiovascular system. Many symptoms and signs of normal pregnancy can mimic heart disease. Dyspnea is especially common, with 75% of women complaining of breathlessness by 31 weeks (Elkos, 1992). Orthopnea may also occur in the advanced stages of pregnancy and is due to pressure exerted on the diaphragm by the gravid uterus. Light-headedness and syncope can result from venocaval compression by the enlarged uterus causing supine hypotensive syndrome. Palpitations are common and are related to the increased heart rate and to women being more aware of their heart beat.

Abnormal findings which may warrant further evaluation include the following: (1) a laterally displaced apex beat (more than 2 cm beyond the mid-clavicular line) and (2) non-physiological murmurs such as diastolic murmurs, pan-systolic murmurs, late systolic murmurs, ejection systolic murmurs with intensities of grade 3 or more or those associated with ejection clicks. The radiation dose associated with a chest X-ray is very small (<0.005 rads) and the risk to the fetus is minimal with proper shielding. There should be no hesitancy in performing a chest X-ray when it is clinically indicated.

4.3 ECG

Several electrocardiographic changes have been described in pregnant patients (Gowda, 2003). Caution should be exercised when interpreting the electrocardiographic abnormalities in pregnant women, and must account for the normal physiological changes occuring in pregnancy. This may results in decreased PR, QRS, and QT intervals, but usually there is no change in the amplitude of the P wave, QRS complex, and T wave. There is an increase of the heart rate (about 10 beats/minute). The electrical axis shift can occur, more commonly leftward, due to rotation of the heart secondary to the enlargement of the gravid uterus. Premature atrial and ventricular contractions are common during pregnancy (Stein, 1999). Supraventricular tachycardia may occur as new onset paroxysmal supraventricular tachycardia or exacerbation during pregnancy, cause probably by the hyperdynamic state (Gowda, 2003). Wolf-Parkinson White (WPW) syndrome may first occur during pregnancy or the frequency of episodes may increase in women with previously diagnosed WPW syndrome. Atrial fibrillation and flutter are rare in pregnant patients and are secondary to congenital or valvular heart disease, electrolyte imbalances or metabolic disorders. Ventricular tachycardia raises usually the suspicion of underlying cardiovascular disease, but physical or physiological stresses may precipitate ventricular arrhythmias in pregnant women without structural heart disease. Bradyarrhythmias are uncommon in pregnancy.

A patient without previous heart disease will usually have a normal ECG between episodes of arrhythmia. Infrequently, a patient may have 12-lead ECG abnormalities indicative of primary 'electrical' disease, such as frequent ectopic beats or Wolff–Parkinson–White syndrome. A patient with previous heart disease may have an abnormal resting ECG, reflecting their condition and any surgical intervention they may have received in the past.

Arrhythmia symptoms are typically intermittent and a 12-lead ECG recording during symptoms may not be available. Prolonged ECG monitoring with either inpatient bedside monitoring or a portable Holter monitor may pick up an episode in a patient with frequent symptoms. Where symptoms are less frequent, it is appropriate for the patient to wear a cardiac rhythm event monitor for 7 days or longer, with a patient-activation function for use during episodes of symptoms. It is helpful for the patient to keep a diary of symptoms, which can then be related to the recorded rhythm. Most types of devices will also record asymptomatic episodes when the heart rate falls outside certain preprogrammed limits. The patient should be encouraged to pursue all her normal activities during the recording, in particular those activities that previously triggered her symptoms.

4.4 Echocardiography and Doppler

Echocardiography is of undisputed value in the diagnosis and follow-up of structural and functional heart disease, and should be considered an integral part of the investigation of any pregnant patient with arrhythmia. It is noninvasive and poses no risk to the fetus. It is the best way to exclude puerperal cardiomyopathy. Changes include slight increases in systolic and diastolic left ventricular dimensions, moderate increases in the size of the right atrium, right ventricle and left atrium, progressive dilatation of the pulmonary, tricuspid and mitral valve annuli with functional regurgitation (Campos, 2009).

4.5 Genetic testing
Several cardiac conditions increase the vulnerability to arrhythmias and have a defined genetic basis. Although routine genetic testing for these conditions is not currently available for the evaluation of arrhythmia risk in pregnancy, a detailed family history should always be taken, and include specific questioning about premature sudden death. Counseling about the risk of transmission of these conditions to offspring is essential, and it is likely that there will be an increasing role for pre-implantation diagnosis of these conditions in affected families (Ueda, 2004).

4.6 Laboratory tests
Laboratory tests are not effective in diagnosis of syncope, but it can reveal some of its causes. Blood tests like complete blood count, electrolyte panel, and chemistry panel can lead to causes of arrhythmia. The blood test count is used to detect anemia or acute blood loss. Electrolyte panel may reveal the level of hydration. As far as the chemistry panel is concerned, thyroid stimulating hormone and serum drug levels should be assessed. Studies have shown that routine blood tests are not always necessary or fruitful (Olshansky, 2008). Besides blood tests, there are more precise diagnostic tests, like HUTT used by clinicians to assess patients who present syncope (Bendit et al. 1996). Used first by the NASA, HUTT emerged in cardiology in 1980 (NASA 1999, Baron-Esquivas et al 2003). The design of the HUTT was based on the following physiological mechanism: due to gravity, in a up-ward position, the blood will be displaced downwards. Consequently, the venous system will expand. The sympathetic system will increase the PVR and the skeletal muscle tone, the latter being an important component in maintaining the upright posture and also helping the venous blood to return to the heart and brain (Brignole, 2005). The role of the HUTT is to inhibit the skeletal muscle pump in the extremities that are responsible for the upright posture or orthostatic stress. In normal conditions; skeletal muscles contraction does not occur when venous pooling starts. However, individuals presenting excessive venous pooling, difficulty with PVR or sensitivity to diminish venous return, may experience difficulty in maintaining the upright posture on HUTT. The number of HUTT protocols varies, but the main idea is to induce venous pooling either through passive upright position or using vasodilators (protenerol, nitroglycerin, and adenosine) which inhibit the innate skeletal muscle pump. Guidelines (American College of Cardiology 1996) state that HUTT is efficient in cases such as: recurrent syncope or single episode in a high-risk patient; no evidence of the structural heart disease; structural heart diseases, as long as other causes have been excluded by the diagnostic testing. There are also conditions in which HUTT has proved to be inefficient. The most common are syncope episodes without injury and not in high risk setting and syncope with identified cause and identification of NCS would not alter therapy. There are some cases in which the use of HUTT is forbidden (syncope with ventricular outflow obstruction, critical mitral stenosis, and critical cerebral vascular stenosis).

5. Treatment

Due to the fact that physiological changes of pregnancy affect drug absorption as well as the metabolism in several ways, it may be difficult to obtain adequate therapeutic drug levels and to avoid toxicity. This may explain why some women experience recurrence of symptoms of arrhythmia during pregnancy despite continuing therapy that had previously been effective (Tan, 2001).

Arrhythmias in pregnancy are treated conservatively. After determining the type of arrhythmia, the physician will evaluate for underlying causes. If symptoms are minimal, rest and vagal maneuvers may be used to help slow the heart rate. Vagal maneuvers include carotid massage, applying ice to the face, and the Valvsalva maneuver, which is the most successful in stopping tachycardias (Zu-Chi, 1998). When the arrhythmia causes symptoms or a drop in blood pressure, antiarrhythmic medications may be used. No anti-arrhythmic medication is completely safe during pregnancy; therefore medications are avoided during the first trimester, if possible, to limit risk to the fetus. Drugs with the longest safety record should be tried first. Propranolol, metoprolol, digoxin, and adenosine have been tested and shown to be well tolerated and safe during the second and third trimester (Ferrero, 2004).

When a cardiac disease is identified in a pregnant woman, we must keep in mind the following (ACOG, 1992):

- The blood volume and the cardiac output increase with approximately 50% at the beginning of the first trimester of pregnancy.
- There are big changes of the circulated volume and of the cardiac output during the birth and in the period after.
- The peripheral vascular resistance decreases in pregnancy and returns to minimum in the second trimester. After that it increases, up to 20% referred to normal, during late pregnancy.
- Hypercoagulability is present in pregnancy. This is very important, particularly in patients requiring anticoagulant therapy outside the pregnancy.

Pregnancies with any cardiac problem must be managed by a complex team, consisting of an obstetrician, a cardiologist and, if necessarily, an intensive therapy specialist and/or a fetal medicine specialist. The aforementioned are compulsory in order to obtain an excellent outcome both for mother and for the child.

5.1 Arrhythmia prevention

In pregnancy, risk of cardiac disease or arrhythmias should be eliminated by:

- *Making healthy lifestyle choices*

Living a "heart healthy" life is the best way to decrease the chances of developing heart disorders. Exercising regularly (brisk walking, running, bicycling, swimming) and eating healthy are the most important. According to the American Heart Association, a heart-healthy diet includes high amounts of fruits and vegetables (at least five servings a day) and of whole grain foods. It includes lean protein sources like fish, beans, and low-fat dairy products, derives most of its fat from unsaturated fats like olive oil, and avoids saturated fats, trans-fats, and cholesterol.

- *Maintaining a healthy weight*

It's important to balance the eaten calories with burned calories through daily activity and exercise. Obesity is linked to heart disease.

- *Smoking cessation and limiting the intake of caffeine or alcohol*

Tobacco contributes to as much as one-third of all cardiovascular disease. It is necessary to avoid or limit the intake of caffeine, alcohol, and other substances that may contribute to arrhythmias or heart disease. The American Heart Association recommends restriction of the use of alcohol to one drink a day for women and two a day for men (a drink equals 12 ounces of beer, 4 ounces of wine or 1 ounce of 100-proof spirits). A single episode of heavy consumption can trigger arrhythmias like atrial fibrillation. Stimulants, both legal and illegal, can contribute to the development of heart arrhythmias. Caffeine and nicotine may, in some cases, cause premature ventricular contractions, which, over time, may develop into more serious arrhythmias. Cocaine and amphetamines also accelerate the heart rate, in some cases leading to ventricular fibrillation and sudden death. Supplements or some herbal remedies may increase the risk of arrhythmias. For instance, Ephedra, the herbal supplement once promoted as a diet aid and energy booster, increases the risk of arrhythmia. In 2004 the FDA pulled it from the shelves for that very reason.

-   *Avoiding unnecessary stress*, such as anger, anxiety or fear, and finding ways to manage or control stressful situations that cannot be avoided.
-   *Avoiding stimulant medications*

Many drugs may cause arrhythmias. Over-the-counter cough and cold medicines may speed up the heart. And approximately 50 FDA-approved medications have the potential to prolong the QT interval—the measure of time it takes for the electrical system in the ventricles to recharge after each heartbeat—and thus cause the acquired form of long QT syndrome (LQTS), in which the heart's mechanical or pumping function is normal but its recharging system is slow or ineffective. Those medications include certain antibiotics, antidepressants, antifungal, antihistamines, psychotropic medications, oral hypoglycemic (medications for diabetes), anesthetic agents, and even drugs used to treat heart disease like lipid-lowing drugs and diuretics. Patients with inherited LQTS should always ask physicians and pharmacists if a prescribed drug has the potential to aggravate the condition. Women have a longer QT interval on the electrocardiogram compared to men, despite higher heart rates.

Tocolitics may induce arrhythmias. Corrected QT and Tpeak-Tend intervals were unchanged from pre-operative values after induction of spinal anaesthesia in women undergoing caesarian section, but increased significantly after oxytocin injection. The risk-benefit balance of oxytocin bolus during caesarean delivery should be discussed with women with a history of long QT syndrome. (Guillon, 2010). Women with a long QT syndrome are more susceptible to ventricular arrythmias during pregnancy, labour, delivery and postpartum (Drake, 2007; Seth, 2007).

-   *Having regular physical exams* and promptly reporting any unusual symptoms to a physician. The Centers for Disease Control and Prevention suggests that families with a history of arrhythmias or sudden cardiac arrest consider screening younger family members.
-   *Seeking treatment for underlying health problems* that may contribute to arrhythmias and heart disease.

Any of the following conditions can increase the likelihood of developing arrhythmias: coronary artery disease, congenital heart disease, heart failure, stroke, atherosclerosis, heart valve damage, high blood pressure, high cholesterol, diabetes, obesity, thyroid disease, advancing age

5.2 Monitoring and treating existing heart disorders

Effectively treating any existing heart disorder is the best way to prevent it from becoming more severe. This can be done by:

-   Having regular check ups
-   Understanding how various conditions increase the risk of arrhythmias.

- Learning about heart disorders, tests, and treatment options, and discussing them with caregivers.
- Finding out if the heart's electrical system and its ability to pump blood efficiently have been affected by heart muscle damage from a heart attack or another cause.
- Learning the importance of an ejection fraction (EF). EF is a measure of the proportion, or fraction, of blood the heart pumps out with each beat. An abnormally low EF is the single most important factor in predicting the risk of Sudden Cardiac Arrest (SCA).
- Following treatment plans.
- Reporting any new symptoms or changes in existing symptoms to physicians as soon as possible.

5.3 Treatment
When the treatment plan is conceived, the physician has to consider factors like: the severity of the arrhythmia, the severity of patient's symptoms, if the patient has other health problems/medications that the patient takes, patient's age, overall health, and personal and family medical history of the patient.
Arrhythmia treatments may include one or more of the following:
1. Medicine to prevent and control arrhythmias and to treat related conditions such as high blood pressure, coronary artery disease and heart failure
2. Anticoagulant medication to reduce the risk of blood clots and stroke
3. A pacemaker that uses batteries to help the heart to beat more regularly
4. Cardiac defibrillation and implanted cardioverter defibrillators (ICDs)
5. Cardiac ablation; cryoablation (the defective cells are detected with the help of computerized mapping techniques and destroyed with a cold probe).
6. Surgery
7. Cardioversion
8. Other therapies.
In association with the effect on the human body, heart medication is categorized into two groups: "rate control" medicines, are used to slow the heart rate to less than 100 beats per minute or "rhythm control" medications (antiarrhythmic/cardioversion drugs) used in order to restore your heart's normal sinus rhythm. The aforementioned drugs are being used less, with more care and often in conjunction with implantable cardioverter defibrillators (ICDs) or cardiac ablation.
Many of the prescription medications reviewed here are also used to treat other kinds of heart-related conditions, including heart failure, high blood pressure, and angina (chest pain).

5.3.1 Rate control heart medication
Rate control heart medicine may include beta or calcium channel blockers. The first group of medication reduces the heart rate and cardiac output by lowering the blood pressure by blocking adrenalin. The most used beta blockers are: Acebutolol, Atenolol, Betaxolol, Bisoprolol/hydrochlorothiazide, Carteolol, Esmolol, Metoprolol, Nadolol, Penbutolol, Pindolol, Propranolol and Timolol. Calcium channel blockers, also called "calcium antagonists", work by interrupting the movement of calcium into heart and blood vessel tissue, slowing the heart rate. They are used in other disorders like: angina and arrhythmias. Examples of calcium channel blockers: Amlodipine, Diltiazem, Felodipine, Isradipine, Nicardipine, Nifedipine, Nimodipine, Nisoldipine and Verapamil.

5.3.2 Rhythm control heart medications

Rhythm control medication includes sodium channel blockers, beta blockers, class III antiarrhythmics that slow the electrical conductivity of the heart to improve rhythm problems. This type of medication can be administrated intravenously in emergency situations and orally in long term situations: Amiodarone, Bepridil Hydrochloride, Disopyramide, Dofetilide, Flecainide, Ibutilide, Lidocaine, Procainamide, Propafenone, Propranolol, Quinidine, Sotalol and Tocainide.

5.3.3 Drug administration

All medications have potential side effects and risks. Antiarrhythmic drugs must be taken daily and indefinitely. There are also side effects that are hard to manage. These side effects may include proarrhythmia, which means drug-related arrhythmia. When medication proves unsuccessful, the American College of Cardiology and the American Heart Association suggest catheter (cardiac) ablation or surgical ablation as a safe and effective treatment option.

The greatest risk is however drug-induced congenital malformation, that is most prone to occur during fetal organogenesis, a process which is completed by the end of the first trimester. Thereafter, the risk is mainly of impaired growth and functional development, or direct toxicity to fetal tissues. Drugs given shortly before term or during labour may have adverse effects on labour or the neonate after delivery. Most antiarrhythmic drugs are categorized by the US Food and Drug Administration (FDA) as category C during pregnancy which signifies that: risk (to the fetus) cannot be ruled out. Adequate well-controlled human studies are lacking, and animal studies have shown a risk to the fetus or are lacking as well. There is a chance of fetal harm if the drug is administered during pregnancy; but the potential benefits may outweigh the risks (Blomstrom-Lundqvist, 2003).

Drug treatment is not required for a benign tachycardia that is well tolerated. A low dose should be used initially with titration according to response, and this must be accompanied by regular monitoring. The selection of an appropriate drug depends on knowledge of the arrhythmia mechanisms, and only drugs with a safe track record in pregnancy should be used. The most common drugs are: Adenosine, Digoxine, and Beta Blockers.

Research showed that Adenosine is useful for the emergency management of SVT and broad QRS complex tachycardias, and has been used safely in pregnant women (Blomstrom-Lundqvist, 2003). It is administered as a bolus dose and it has a very short duration of action of no more than 5–10 s. The role of this medication is to depress sinus and AV nodal function causing transient bradycardia and AV block in the mother, but it has no detectable effect on the fetal cardiac rhythm. Adenosine is contraindicated in patients with brittle asthma, in whom it may cause bronchospasm, and in those taking dipyridamole because of the risk of prolonged asystole.

There is a long history of digoxin use during pregnancy and it is considered to be safe (Blomstrom-Lundqvist, 2003). It crosses the placenta, but is not teratogenic. It is cleared by the kidney, although renal excretion is inhibited by concomitant use of amiodarone. It is mainly used for the control of ventricular rate in patients with persistent atrial fibrillation, but may also be effective in some cases of focal atrial tachycardia.

Propranolol is the beta blocker with the longest track record and is considered safe in pregnancy (Blomstrom-Lundqvist, 2003). Beta blockers are not teratogenic, but beta1-selective blockers, such as atenolol or metoprolol, may be preferred because they may interfere less with beta2-receptor-mediated uterine relaxation. However, beta1-selective agents achieve less complete cardiac beta blockade because there are functional beta2-

receptors on cardiac myocytes, and these may, therefore, be less effective anti-arrhythmic agents. There have been reports linking beta blockers to fetal bradycardia, hypotonia, hypoglycemia and intrauterine growth retardation.

Sotalol is a combined beta blocker and class III anti-arrhythmic drug. It does cross the placenta and is excreted renally. It has achieved class B classification with the FDA and its use in pregnant patients has been reported with no adverse outcome (Blomstrom-Lundqvist, 2003).

Flecainide has been used frequently during pregnancy and is a reasonable choice for patients with a structurally normal heart (Blomstrom-Lundqvist, 2003). It should probably be avoided in those with myocardial disease, and in particular patients with ventricular tachycardia or vulnerability to myocardial ischemia.

The conflict between the interests of the mother and the well-being of the fetus is thrown into sharp relief with Amiodarone. Amiodarone is a very effective anti-arrhythmic drug to treat and prevent life-threatening ventricular arrhythmias in patients with ventricular disease. Amiodarone crosses the placenta and achieves fetal concentrations of around 10% of maternal serum values (Ovadia, 1994). Maternal amiodarone use may cause a goiter, which in turn compromises the upper airway in the neonate. Amiodarone is prone to cause, neonatal hypothyroidism, and fetal growth retardation. For these reasons, amiodarone should be used only when the mother's life is significantly threatened and no other agent will do (Chow, 1998).

There are no reports of teratogenicity, but verapamil does cross the placenta and may have fetal cardiovascular effects (Klein, 1984). Intravenous verapamil is a useful alternative to adenosine for emergency termination of SVT, and oral verapamil may be used in patients to prevent SVT recurrence when beta blockers are contraindicated or not tolerated (Klein, 1984).

Anticoagulant medications help to prevent new clots appearance in the blood or existing clots from getting larger. They are often prescribed for patients with atrial fibrillation to help reduce stroke risk. Aspirin also is often recommended for these patients in addition to or instead of prescription anticoagulants.

The pacemaker is a small device that's surgically placed under the skin at the collarbone; wires lead from it to the atrium and ventricle(s). The pacemaker sends small electric signals through the wires to control the speed of the heartbeat. Most pacemakers contain a sensor that activates the device only when the heartbeat is abnormal.

An ICD (Implantable Cardioverter Defibrillator) provides automatic electrical therapy on a chronic basis for patients suffering from recurrent tachycardias. (When an episode of fast, irregular heartbeat begins, the device delivers a shock to end the tachycardia, preventing the heart from going into ventricular fibrillation, which is frequently fatal). The device is connected to leads positioned inside or on the surface of the heart. These leads sense cardiac rhythm, provide necessary electrical shocks when necessary, and at times - pace the heart as needed. Various leads are connected to a pulse generator implanted in a pouch beneath the skin of the chest or abdomen. Newer devices are smaller, with simpler lead systems and can be installed through blood vessels.

Women with an implanted cardioverter defibrillator (ICD) may undergo pregnancy successfully with a good reported outcome. Potentially threatening arrhythmias are promptly detected and automatically terminated by an ICD by, either a series of rapid pacing impulses delivered via an endocardial right ventricular pacing lead, or delivery of a synchronized shock between a coil electrode in the right ventricular cavity and a second electrode formed by the ICD box, which is located in the pre-pectoral position on the left. Prompt detection and termination of an arrhythmia by an ICD minimize the hemodynamic disturbance and thereby limit the risk of harm to the fetus. ICDs are configured to concentrate the maximal electrical field strength to the mother's ventricular myocardium, and the electrical energy to which the fetus is exposed is minimal. Delivered energies (2–40 J) are about a tenth of those used for external DC cardioversion. Research found Cardioversion safe for the entire pregnancy state therefore, it can be used, if necessary (Blomstrom, 2003). Also, there is not additional risk (excepting patients with underlying heart condition) to develop ICD complications, during pregnancy (Natale, 1997).

Ablation is a nonsurgical technique that neutralizes parts of the abnormal electrical pathway (tissue) that is causing the arrhythmia. The technique utilizes a variety of imaging and monitoring systems that navigate flexible wires (catheters) to the heart through an artery or vein, locate the abnormal electrical activity (where ablation is needed), and evaluate their progress.

Once in the heart, one or more catheters are used to pinpoint the source of the abnormal electrical signals. When the source of the arrhythmia is located, the catheter delivers bursts of high-energy waves that eliminate the abnormal areas.

There are two techniques of ablation: radiofrequency ablation and transcatheter technique. In this first technique, a catheter with an electrode at its tip is guided to the damaged portion of heart muscle and mild, painless radiofrequency energy is transmitted to the site of the pathway, killing a few cells (about 1/5 of an inch). Consequently, these cells stop conducting the extra impulses that caused the rapid heartbeats. This non-surgical procedure is used to treat patients suffering from atrial fibrillation, atrial flutter, atrial tachycardia and supraventricular tachycardia. The second technique, however, electrocauterization is performed at a targeted spot in the heart. This technique is generally used to treat supraventricular tachycardia.

Most patients who receive this treatment experience a long-term reduction in the number of episodes of arrhythmia and the severity of symptoms, or a permanent return to normal heart rhythm.

Sometimes, surgery is used to treat arrhythmia. Often this is done when surgery is already being performed for another reason, such as repair of a heart valve. One type of surgery for atrial fibrillation is called "maze" surgery. In this operation, the surgeon makes small cuts or burns in the atria, which prevent the spread of disorganized electrical signals. Ventricular resection implies the removal of a part of the heart's muscle, where the arrhythmia originates.

Coronary artery bypass surgery may be needed for arrhythmias caused by coronary artery disease. The operation improves blood supply to the heart muscle.

Cardioversion treatment can be chemical (implemented through fast-acting drugs) or electric (implemented through a direct current using paddles over the chest) and is used to restore the heart's normal rhythm. DC cardioversion may be used to terminate sustained tachycardias. It should be carried out with general anesthesia, or deep sedation with midazolam or diazepam. Traditionally, the cardioversion electrodes are placed at the right sternal edge and cardiac apex, but for atrial fibrillation, it may be more effective to use an anterior–posterior configuration. Firm downward pressure on the sternal paddle reduces the electrode separation and increases the intensity of the electrical field, thus maximizing the chance of success. A waveform that reverses polarity during delivery (biphasic waveform) achieves cardioversion at energy thresholds that are half those required when a monophasic waveform is used. For all tachyarrhythmias, except ventricular fibrillation, the shock should be synchronized to the R wave, to minimize the risk of inducing ventricular fibrillation. Patients with atrial flutter or fibrillation are particularly vulnerable to systemic thromboembolism after restoration of sinus rhythm. DC cardioversion should not be carried out on patients who have been in atrial fibrillation for longer than 24 hours unless the arrhythmia results in serious cardiovascular compromise, or the patient has been fully anticoagulated since the onset of arrhythmia, or the absence of thrombus in the left atrium has been verified by transesophageal echocardiography. Anticoagulation should be continued for a minimum of 4 weeks after DC cardioversion. DC cardioversion seems to be quite safe in all stages of pregnancy because the intensity of the electrical field to which the fetus is exposed is low. Nevertheless, the fetus should be carefully monitored throughout the procedure. In the later stages of pregnancy, full general anesthesia and intubation are used, considering the increased risk of gastric aspiration.

Vagal maneuvers are another arrhythmia treatment. These are simple exercises that sometimes can stop or slow down certain types of supraventricular arrhythmias. They stop the arrhythmia by affecting the vagus nerve, which controls the heart rate. Some vagal maneuvers include:

- Gagging
- Holding breath and bearing down (Valsalva maneuver)
- Immersing the face in ice-cold water
- Coughing
- Putting the fingers on the own eyelids and pressing down gently.

6. Management of specific arrhythmias during pregnancy, labour and delivery

Dynamic changes in maternal physiology, as well as concern for the fetal well-being, are factors that complicate the treatment of arrhythmia. Premature atrial and ventricular contractions associated with a structurally normal heart are considered to be benign. However, in order to prevent them, exacerbating factors (dehydration, caffeine, sleep deprivation) should be avoided. Also, nonpharmacologic vagal maneuvers are recommended in atrial tachycardias. In the aforementioned case, drug therapy is indicated as long as the patient present refractory symptoms. In order to prevent recurrence, digoxin and beta-blockers are recommended. If the patient does not respond to these, flecainide and propafenone should be taken into consideration. Cardioversion or intravenous adenosine is indicated in acute management. Arrhythmias in association with the Wolf-Parkinson-White syndrome should be treated with Prosainamide, during pregnancy.

Records demonstrating the safety usage of digoxin and beta-blockers have determined the specialists to use these drugs in diseases like atrial flutter and fibrillation. In these cases, there are some who appeal to a rate or rhythm control strategy, similar to the nonpregnant state.

The management of ventricular arrhythmias is closely associated to the underlying heart condition; for instance patients suffering from idiopathic ventricular tachycardia (VT), but whith a structurally normal heart will receive, as first line therapy, beta-blockers, with IC agents or sotalol as second-line agents.

In pregnancy, congenital heart diseases have a complex prognosis. In most cases, long QT or hypertrophic cardiomyopathy are associated with ventricular arrhythmias. Sustained VT can develop into peripartum cardiomyopathy or vasospastic coronary artery disease. In each case daily evaluation is compulsory. If VT is unstable hemodynamically, emergent cardioversion is recommended. Well tolerated VT is treated with lidocaine, however if VT is sustained or recurrent, procainamide, flacainide, propafenone, sotalol or amiodarone are required.

Conservatory management is the best option for asymptomatic bradycardia. In pregnancy, pacemakers' insertions are tolerated.

During labour as well as delivery, hemodynamic changes occur, due to pain, anxiety. These hemodynamic changes increase the risk of arrhythmia.

Holter monitorization of the pregnancies with arrhythmias showed a high incidence of ventricular and/or atrial extrasystoles, with no consequences on the future mother or on the child. They will gradually disappear in post-partum.

7. Conclusion

Pregnancy increases cardiac output, heart rate and prevalence of dysrrhythmias in normal healthy women. The factors that can promote arrhythmias during pregnancy are: the direct electrophysiological effects of the hormones, the increased sympathetic tone and sensitivity, hemodynamic changes, electrolyte imbalances, atrial stretch, increased end-diastolic volumes and underlying heart diseases.

The most important problem in patients diagnosed with cardiac arrhythmia in pregnancy is the early detection, a multidisciplinary monitorization and an adequate therapy. The purpose is to decrease the cardiovascular complications in pregnancy and to have a good pregnancy outcome.

8. References

Abbott, G.W.; Federico, S.; Splawski, S.I.; Marianne E Buck, Michael H Lehmann, et. al. MiRP1 forms I_{Kr} potassium channels with HERG and is associated with cardiac arrhythmia, *Cell*, Vol.97, No.2, (Aprilie, 1999), pp.175-187.

Anderson, M.H. Heart disease in pregnancy. (1997). In: Oakley C, ed. Heart disease in pregnancy. London: BMJ Publishing Group, pp. 248-81.

Adamson, D.L.; Nelson-Piercy, C. (2007). Managing palpitations and arrhythmias during pregnancy. *Heart*, Vol. 93, No.12, (December, 2007), pp. 1630-1636.

August, P.; Lenz, T.; Ales, K.L, et al. (1990). Longitudinal study of the renin–angiotensin-aldosterone system in hypertensive pregnant women: deviations related to the development of superimposed preeclampsia. *American Journal of Obstetrics and Gynecology*, vol. 163, (November, 1990), pp. 1612–1621.

Bader, R.A.; Bader, M.E.; Rose DF, Braunwald E. (1955). Hemodynamics at rest and during exercise in normal pregnancy as studies by cardiac catheterization. *Journal of Clinic Investigation*, Vol. 34, (October, 1955), pp. 1524–1536.

Baumert, M.; Seeck, A.; Faber, R., et al. (2010). Longitudinal changes in QT interval variability and rate adaptation in pregnancies with normal and abnormal uterine perfusion, *Hypertension Research*, Vol. 33, No. 6, (June, 2010), pp.555-560.

Bieniarz, J.; Yoshida, T.; Romero-Salinas, G.; Curuchet, E.; Caldeyro-Barcia, R.; Crottogini, J.J. (1969). Aortocaval compression by the uterus in late human pregnancy. IV.

Circulatory homeostasis by preferential perfusion of the placenta. *American Journal of Obstetrics and Gynecology*, Vol. 103, (January, 1969), pp. 19–31.

Blomstrom-Lundqvist, C.; Scheinman, M.M.; Aliot, E.M. et al. (2003) ACC/AHA/ESC guidelines for the management of patients with supraventricular arrhythmias. *Circulation*, Vol. 108, (October, 2003), pp. 1871–909.

Brodsky, M.; Doria, R.; Allen, B.; Sato, D.; Thomas, G.; Sada, M. (1992). Newonset ventricular tachycardia during pregnancy. *American Heart Journal*, Vol. 123, No.4, (April, 1992), pp. 933–941.

Campos, O. (1996). Doppler echocardiography during pregnancy: physiological and abnormal findings. *Echocardiography*, Vol. 13, (Mars, 1996), pp. 135–146.

Chow, T.; Galvin, J.; McGovern, B. (1998). Antiarrhythmic drug therapy in pregnancy and lactation. *American Journal of Cardiology*, Vol. 82, (August, 1998), pp. 58I–62I.

Clark, S.L.; Cotton, D.B.; Lee, W. et al. (1989). Central hemodynamic assessment of normal term pregnancy. *American Journal of Obstetrics and Gynecology*, Vol. 161, (December, 1989), pp.1439–1442.

Conti, J.B.; Curtis, A.B. (2005). Arrhythmias during pregnancy. In: Saksena S, Camm AJ (eds), Electrophysiological Disorders of the Heart. Philadelphia: Elsevier, pp. 517–532.

Drake, E.; Preston, R.; Douglas, J. (2007). Brief review: Anesthetic implications of long QT syndrome in pregnancy. *Canadian Journal of Anesthesia*, Vol. 54, No.7, (July, 2007), pp. 561-72.

Eliahou, H.E.; Silverberg, D.S.; Reisin, E.; Romem, I.; Mashiach, S.; Serr, D.M. (1978). Propranolol for the treatment of hypertension in pregnancy. *British Journal of Obstetrics and Gynaecology*, Vol. 85, No.6, (June, 1978), pp. 431–436.

Elkus, R.; Popovich, J. (1992). Jr. Respiratory physiology in pregnancy. *Clinics in Chest Medicine*, Vol. 13, No.4. (December, 1992), pp. 555–565.

Ferrero, S.; Colombo, B.M.; Ragni, N. (2004). Maternal arrhythmias during pregnancy. *Archives of Gynecology and Obstetrics, Vol.* 269, No. 4 (May, 2004), pp. 244-253.

Geva, T.; Mauer, M.B.; Striker, L.; Kirshon, B.; Pivarnik, J.M. (1997). Effects of physiologic load of pregnancy on left ventricular contractility and remodeling. *American Heart Journal*, Vol. 133, (January, 1997), pp. 53–59.

Gowda, R.M.; Khan IA, Mehta NJ, Vasavada BC, Sacchi TJ. (2003). Cardiac arrhythmias in pregnancy: clinical and therapeutic considerations. *International Journal of Cardiology*, Vol. 88, (April, 2003), pp.129-133.

Guillon, A.; Leyre, S.; Remerand, F.; et al. (2010). Modification of Tp-e and QTc intervals during caesarean section under spinal anaesthesia. *Anaesthesia*, Vol. 65, no. 4, (February, 2010), pp. 337-342.

Jurkovic, D.; Jauniaux, E.; Kurjak, A.; Hustin, J.; Campbell, S.; Nicolaides, K.H. (1991). Transvaginal color Doppler assessment of the uteroplacental circulation in early pregnancy. *Obstetrics and Gynecology*, Vol. 77, No.3. (March, 1977), pp. 365–369.

Katz, R.; Karliner, J.S.; Resnik, R. (1978). Effects of a natural volume overload state (pregnancy) on left ventricular performance in normal human subjects. *Circulation*, Vol. 58, (September, 1978), pp. 434–441.

Ueda, K.; Nakamura, K.; Hayashi, T. et al. (2004). Functional characterization of a trafficking- defective HCN4 mutation, D553N, associated with cardiac arrhythmia. *Journal of Biological Chemistry*, Vol. 279, No.26, (April, 2004), pp. 27194-27198.

Klein, V.; Repke, J.T. (1984). Supraventricular tachycardia in pregnancy: cardioversion with verapamil. *Obstetrics and Gynecology*, Vol. 63, Suppl. 3, (March, 1984), pp. 16S-18S.

Lee, S.H.; Chen, S.A.; Wu, T.J. et al. (1995). Effects of pregnancy on first onset and symptoms of paroxysmal supraventricular tachycardia. *American Journal of Cardiology*, Vol. 76, No.10, (October, 1995), pp.675–678.

Leung, C.; Brodsky, M. (1998). Cardiac arrhythmias and pregnancy, in Elkayam U (ed.): Cardiac Problems in Pregancy. Wiley-Liss, New York 1998; pp. 155-174.

Lind, T. (1985). Hematologic system. Maternal physiology. *Washington: CREOG*, Vol. 25, pp. 7–40.

Lydakis, C.; Lip, G.Y.; Beevers, M.; Beevers, D.G. (1999). Atenolol and fetal growth in pregnancies complicated by hypertension. *American Journal of Hypertension*, Vol.12, No.6. (June, 1999), pp. 541–547.

Mark, S.; Harris, L. (2002). Arrhythmias in pregnancy, in Wilansky S (ed.): Heart Disease in Women. Churchill Livingstone, Philadelphia, 2002; pp. 497-514.

Mashini, I.S.; Albazzaz, S.J.; Fadel, H.E. et al. (1987). Serial noninvasive evaluation of cardiovascular hemodynamics during pregnancy. *American Journal of Obstetrics and Gynecology*, Vol. 156, (May, 1987), pp. 1208–1213.

Natale, A.; Davidson, T.; Geiger, M.J.; Newby, K. (1997). Implantable cardioverter-defibrillators and pregnancy: a safe combination? *Circulation*, Vol. 96, No.9, (November, 1997), pp.2808-2012.

Onuigbo, M.; Alikhan, M. (1998). Over-the-counter sympathomimetics: a risk factor for cardiac arrhythmias in pregnancy. *South Medical Journal*, Vol.91, (December, 1998), pp.1153–1155.

Campos, O. (1996). Doppler echocardiography during pregnancy: physiological and abnormal findings. *Echocardiography*, Vol. 13, (March, 1996), pp. 135–146.

Ovadia, M.; Brito, M.; Hoyer, G.L.; Marcus, F.I. (1994). Human experience with amiodarone in the embryonic period. *American Journal of Cardiology*, Vol. 73, No.4, (February, 1994), pp. 316–317.

Pirani, B.B.; Campbell, D.M.; MacGillivray, I. (1973) Plasma volume in normal first pregnancy. *The Journal of obstetrics and gynaecology of the British Commonwealth*, Vol. 80, No.10, pp. 884-7.

Pritchard, J.A.; Rowland, R.C. (1964). Blood volume changes in pregnancy and the puerperium. III. Whole body and large vessel hematocrits in pregnant and nonpregnant women. *American Journal of Obstetrics and Gynecology*, Vol. 88, (April, 1964), pp.391–395.

Robson, S.C.; Hunter, S.; Boys, R.J.; Dunlop, W. (1989). Serial study of factors influencing changes in cardiac output during human pregnancy. *American Journal of Physiology*, Vol. 256, (April, 1989), pp. H1060–1065.

Robson, S.C.; Hunter, S.; Moore, M.; Dunlop, W. (1987). Haemodynamic changes during the puerperium: a Doppler and M-mode echocardiographic study. *British Journal of Obstetrics and Gynaecology,* Vol. 94, pp. 1028–1039.

Rovinsky, J.J.; Jaffin, H. Cardiovascular hemodynamics in pregnancy. I. (1965). Blood and plasma volumes in multiple pregnancy. *American Journal of Obstetrics and Gynecology,* Vol. 93, (September, 1965), pp. 1–15.

Rubler, S.; Damani, P.M.; Pinto, E.R. (1977). Cardiac size and performance during pregnancy estimated with echocardiography. *American Journal of Cardiology,* Vol. 40, (October, 1977), pp. 534–540.

Sadaniantz, A.; Kocheril, A.G.; Emaus, S.P.; Garber, C.E.; Parisi, A.F. (1992). Cardiovascular changes in pregnancy evaluated by two-dimensional and Doppler echocardiography. *Journal of the American Society of Echocardiography,* Vol.5, (May-Jun, 1992), pp. 253–258.

Seth, R.; Moss, A.J.; Mc Nitt, S. et al. (2007). Long QT syndrome and pregnancy. *Journal of the American College of Cardiology,* Vol. 49, No. 10, (Mars, 2007), pp. 1092-1098.

Stein, P.K.; Hagley, M.T.; Cole, P.L.; Domitrovich, P.P.; Kleiger, R.E.; Rottman, J.N. (1999). Changes in 24-hour heart rate variability during normal pregnancy. *American Journal of Obstetrics and Gynecology,* Vol. 180, No.4, (April, 1999), pp. 978–985.

Tan, H.L.; Lie, K.I. (2001). Treatment of tachyarrhythmias during pregnancy and lactation. *European Heart Journal,* Vol. 22, No.6, (March, 2001), pp. 458–464.

Tateno, S.; Niwa, K.; Nakazawa, M.; Akagi, T.; Shinohara, T.; Usda, T. (2003). A Study Group for Arrhythmia Late after Surgery for Congenital Heart Disease (ALTAS- CHD). Circulation Journal. Vol. 67, no. 12, (December, 2003), pp. 992-997.

Tawam, M.; Levine. J.; Mendelson. M.; Goldberger, J.; Dyer, A.; Kadish, A. (1993). Effect of pregnancy on paroxysmal supraventricular tachycardia. *American Journal of Cardiology,* Vol. 72, No.11 (October, 1993), pp. 838–840.

Taylor, D.J.; Lind, T. (1979). Red cell mass during and after normal pregnancy. *British Journal of Obstetrics and Gynaecology,* Vol. 86, No.5, (May, 1979), pp. 364–70.

Thomsen, J.K.; Fogh-Andersen, N.; Jaszczak. P. (1994). Atrial natriuretic peptide, blood volume, aldosterone, and sodium excretion during twin pregnancy. *Acta Obstetica et Gynecologica Scandinavica,* Vol. 73, No.1, (January, 1994), pp. 14–20.

Ueland, K.; Hansen, JM. (1969). Maternal cardiovascular dynamics. 3. Labour and delivery under local and caudal analgesia. *American Journal of Obstetrics and Gynecology,* Vol.103, No.1, (January, 1969), pp.8–18.

Ueland, K. (1976). Maternal cardiovascular dynamics. VII. Intrapartum blood volume changes. *American Journal of Obstetrics and Gynecology,* Vol. 126, No.6, (November, 1976), pp. 671–677.

Yoshimura, T.; Yoshimura, M.; Yasue, H. et al. (1994). Plasma concentration of atrial natriuretic peptide and brain natriuretic peptide during normal human pregnancy and the postpartum period. *Journal of Endocrinology,* Vol. 140, No.3. (March, 1994), pp. 393–397.

Wen, Z.C.; Chen, S.A.; Tai, C.T.; Chiang, C.E.; Chiou, C.W.; Chang, M.S. (1998). Electrophysiological mechanisms and determinants of vagal maneuvers for termination of paroxysmal supraventricular tachycardia. *Circulation*, Vol. 98, No.24, (December, 1998), pp. 2716 –2723.

10

Mild Induced Therapeutic Hypothermia for Survivors of Cardiac Arrest

Kevin Baker, John Prior, Karthik Sheka and Raymond A. Smego, Jr.
The Commonwealth Medical College
USA

1. Introduction

Despite advances in emergency response and critical care, good neurologic outcome after cardiac arrest is difficult to achieve, and interventions during the resuscitation phase and treatment within the first hours after the event are crucial. Although recommended by organizations such as the American Heart Association (AHA) and the International Liaison Committee on Resuscitation (ILCOR), implementation of induced mild therapeutic hypothermia for survivors of cardiac arrest in the United States has been slow, at least in part, because of the perception that this therapy is technically difficult, especially at the community level. In this chapter, we review the pathophysiology, cooling techniques, clinical evidence and uses (including costs), and effectiveness of induced mild therapeutic hypothermia in adult patients after cardiopulmonary resuscitation, using any cooling method applied within six hours of arrest. Neurologic outcome, survival and adverse events are the main outcome parameters outlined here. In addition, we also include a discussion of the applicability of mild therapeutic hypthermia for both academic health centers and community hospitals, as well as areas of uncertainty, guidelines, and recommendations.

2. Epidemiology of cardiac arrest

The incidence of out-of-hospital sudden cardiac arrest in industrialized countries is about 62 cases per 100,000 a year making sudden cardiac arrest a major cause of death in the United States amounting to more than 300,000 occurrences of cardiac arrests outside of hospital each year (Adler et al, 2011). Resuscitation is attempted on roughly 100,000 of these arrest patients but results in only 40,000 patients who survive upon arrival to the hospital (Holzer, 2010).

Despite advances in emergency medical services the mortality and morbidity associated with out-of hospital cardiac arrest is high. In 2006, the National Registry of Cardiopulmonary Resuscitation (CPR) published statistics on 19,819 adults and 524 children with return of spontaneous circulation after cardiac arrest. The mortality rates were 67% among adults and 55% among children (Jacobshagen et al, 2010). Currently, less than half of cardiac arrest patients survive to discharge and less than a third of those discharged have a good neurologic outcome as defined by the Cerebral Performance Category (CPS) Scale (Adler et al, 2011). The cost of caring for patients with poor neurologic function within the first six months alone can range anywhere from $10,000 to $300,000, with an increasing morbidity generally associated with increasing cost (Merchant et al, 2009).

3. Pathophysiology of induced mild therapeutic hypothermia

The brain receives approximately 15% of the human resting cardiac output despite comprising 1-2% of our total body weight, illustrating the high metabolic demands associated with the brain. During cardiac arrest the blood supply is interrupted leading to global cerebral ischemia.

Ischemic events are especially detrimental to the brain and are a major cause of morbidity in cardiac arrest survivors. Areas such as the hippocampus, neocortex, cerebellum, corpus striatum, and thalamus are the most vulnerable to global ischemia. Necrosis and apoptosis have both been reported in cardiac arrest victims and it still is unclear the extent to which each of these processes contribute to neuronal cell death. The brain is damaged through an ischemic cascade of events occurring on a time scale of minutes-to-days after cardiac arrest and is summarized below.

A lack of oxygen hinders the neurons ability to produce ATP. Consequently, cells switch to anaerobic metabolism which consumes glucose and produces lactic acid. As glucose concentrations are exhausted, ion transporters using ATP fail to function. Cells become depolarized allowing ions, including calcium, to flow into the cell. Due to the lack of ATPase activities, cells cannot pump calcium out of the intracellular space, and as intracellular calcium levels rise they trigger the release of excitatory neurotransmitters. Glutamate, one of the excitatory neurotransmitters, acts on AMPA and NMDA receptors to allow more calcium into cells and thereby increases the intracellular calcium leading to production of neurotoxic chemicals such as free radicals, reactive oxygen species and calcium-dependent enzyme (Sinclair & Andrews, 2010). This process is referred to as excitotoxicity. Calcium-dependent enzymes such as calpain, endonucleases, and phospholipases break down cells making them more permeable to harmful chemicals and leads to damage of the mitochondrial membrane, ultimately causing release of pro-apoptotic factors that stimulate the caspase cascade and inducing cell suicide. Cells that die due to necrosis cause a release of glutamate and other neurotoxic compounds that act on surrounding cells and perpetuate excitotoxicty.

Hypothermia exerts its effect on the ischemic cascade mentioned above to improve neurologic outcome after cardiac arrest. The following discussion will elaborate on mild therapeutic hypothermia and how it mitigates the pathologic processes involving: 1) blood-brain barrier permeability and edema, 2) inflammation, 3) metabolism, 4) excitotoxicity, 5) intracellular calcium-dependent signaling 6) cerebral vascular effects, and 7) neuronal cell death.

3.1 Blood-brain barrier permeability and edema

The blood-brain barrier displays increased permeability after ischemia and allows the entrance of water, electrolytes, and potentially toxic substances into the brain parenchyma. Hypothermia has been shown to decrease the extravasation of certain protein markers such as horseradish peroxidase from the serum into the brain. Studies have also demonstrated that treatment with hypothermia in focal ischemia results in a decrease in brain water content as measured by MRI, and leads to a reduction in the diffusion of water into the brain and a consequent reduction in vasogenic edema by alleviating blood-brain barrier injury (Sinclair & Andrews, 2010). Vasogenic edema is a result of damage to the blood-brain barrier and the passage of large osmotically-active proteins like albumin into the brain.

The attenuation of matrix metalloproteases is another effect of hypothermia that reduces the permeability of the blood-brain barrier. Matrix metalloproteases are important for the extravasation of several substances into the brain including immunologic and other inflammatory cells. Reducing movement of these cells into the brain decreases deleterious edema associated with inflammatory immune responses to ischemia and neuronal cell injury.

3.2 Inflammation and immune response

Hypothermia mitigates the inflammation response by reducing the leukocyte extravasation as well as the endogenous inflammatory response of the brain to ischemia. Astrocytes and microglia respond to tissue damage in the brain by proliferating and secreting large quantities of pro-inflammatory cytokines such as tumor necrosis factor-α and interleukin-1 which recruit cells of the immune system. Hypothermia reduces the activation of astrocytes and microglia thereby reducing the pro-inflammatory signaling and the ensuing immune response (Sinclair & Andrews, 2010).

The inflammatory response in the brain also results in the release of reactive oxygen species by astrocytes and microglia. Hypothermia, therefore, also reduces the levels of potentially damaging free radicals such as superoxide, nitric oxide, and hydroxyl radicals within the brain by decreasing their secretion from microglia and astrocytes. Hypothermia also increases the levels of superoxide dismutase, the enzyme that clears superoxide from the body, and decreases nitric oxide synthase, the enzyme responsible for production of nitric oxide. This reduction in reactive oxygen species production and increase in reactive oxygen species scavenger enzymes results in decreased neuronal damage.

3.3 Metabolism

Hypothermia has been proven to decrease glucose utilization. Studies implementing 2-deoxyglucose, a glucose analog that can be taken up by glucose transporters but not digested, has shown that hypothermia decreases utilization of glucose when compared to normothermia. Global ischemia affects the brain more than the liver due to the small stores of glycogen found in the brain compared to large stores found in the liver. Therefore, any reduction in glucose utilization will attenuate the damaging effects of poor cerebral perfusion. Hypothermia reduces the metabolic demands of the cell, preserving cellular ATP concentration more effectively when compared to normothermia. Reducing core temperature 1°C decreases metabolic rate by approximately 6%-8% (Adler et al, 2011).

The cell's ability to maintain electrochemical gradients depends heavily upon ATP concentrations. Loss of transmembrane electrochemical gradients directly precedes failure of synaptic transmission and axonal conduction. Hypothermia's ability to reduce metabolic demands, preserve ATP, and potentiate electrochemical gradients translates to better neurologic outcomes after recovery from cardiac arrest.

3.4 Excitotoxicity

The metabolic depletion of ATP associated with ischemia in cardiac arrest results in an inappropriate release of excitatory neurotransmitters such as glutamate. A reduction in the blood flow to the brain allows levels of glutamate to build up in the extracellular space around neurons. This rise in glutamate leads to activation of glutamatergic receptors AMPA (alpha-amino-3-hydroxyl-5-methyl-4-isoxazole-propionate) and NMDA (N-methyl d-aspartate). Glutamate acts through AMPA and NMDA to produce an influx of calcium from the extracellular fluid to the intracellular fluid. This inflow of calcium can injure the cell by initiating several cascades within the cell including, free radical generation, mitochondrial injury, and ultimately apoptosis (Nolan et al, 2008). Hypothermia inhibits the release of glutamine and dopamine while also inducing neurotrophic factors that further reduce glutamine release.

3.5 Intracellular calcium-dependent signaling
Global ischemia leads to an increase in intracellular calcium, thereby affecting normal signaling protein kinases in the cell. Proteins such as calmodulin-dependent kinase II (CaMKII) and protein kinase C (PKC) are rescued by hypothermia (Sinclair & Andrews, 2010). These proteins, as well as other signaling factors, are temperature-sensitive. Controlling signaling factors and proteins such as CaMKII and PKC through hypothermia influences neuronal injury and normal cell signaling.

3.6 Cerebral vascular and cellular effects
Hypothermia affects secretion of vasoactive substances such as endothelin, thromboxane A2, and prostaglandin I2 in the brain. Endothelin and thromboxane A2 have vasoconstrictive effects while prostaglandin I2 is a vasodilator. Thromboxane A2, endothelin, and prostaglandin I2 mediate vascular homeostasis in the brain; during ischemic and traumatic events homeostatic balance is shifted towards vasoconstriction, hypoperfusion, and thrombus formation. Hypothermia has been shown in animal models and small clinical studies to alter the response to injury by attenuating the vasconstrictive response. However, regulation of cerebral perfusion is complex and dependent on several factors including the presence or absence of cerebral autoregulation, ventilator settings, serum blood gas levels, systemic blood pressure, osmotic therapy, etc (Sinclair & Andrews, 2010).

Necrosis and apoptosis are the result of prolonged tissue ischemia and can be influenced by hypothermia. Several gene families associated with apoptosis are temperature-sensitive. Brain cells can sense irreversible injury and begin the process of self-destruction. Hypothermia leads to a delayed response of the cell to injury and this slowed response is mediated by a delay in genetic regulation (Sinclair & Andrews, 2010). Ultimately, hypothermia slows secondary injury and apoptosis through delaying the cells initial reaction to damage. Apoptosis occurs over the time frame of hours-to-days making hypothermia a major factor in mitigating apoptosis during the post-resuscitation phase.

4. Cooling methods

Several different cooling techniques are available for use in therapeutic hypothermia; however, all of the various techniques fall into two general categories: surface cooling and core cooling. Surface cooling can be carried out in two ways; the first utilizes pre-cooled pads while the second makes use of heat-exchanging mattresses or pads. Surface cooling was used in the two hallmark clinical trials carried out in 2003 in Europe and Australia that first demonstrated the beneficial effects of hypothermia on witnessed cardiac arrest survivors (Bernard et al, 2003; Holzer & Sterz, 2003).

Core cooling can be achieved with the use of intravascular cooling catheters filled with cold saline or by intravenous injection of cold fluids. Devices for core cooling and surface cooling have been specifically designed for use in therapeutic hypothermia but the ultimate goal, whether using either surface or core cooling methods, is to rapidly cool the patient and maintain a stable temperature between 32-34°C for at least 24 hours.

Various measurements and devices may be used to monitor relevant core body temperature including esophageal probes, endotracheal tube cuff monitors, and non-invasive continuous cerebral temperature monitoring (Zeiner et al, 2010; Haugk et al, 2010). During the initial phase of head and neck cooling, jugular bulb temperature (Tjb), (which may reflect brain temperature) appears to be lower than esophageal temperature (Wandaller et al, 2009).

4.1 Surface cooling
4.1.1 Ice packs
Ice packs are an inexpensive and easy technique to initiate cooling. However, they can be messy and less effective at cooling and maintaining target temperature. Ice packs can be placed all over the body, but are more effectively placed in anatomic areas that have large heat-exchange capability due to their blood flow. These areas include the head, neck, axillae, and groin. The average temperature drop attained by using ice packs is between 0.03-0.98°C per hour (Adler et al., 2011).

4.1.2 Blankets or surface heat-exchange devices
Conventional surface cooling blankets are not ideal because of poor surface contact with the patient's skin. Generally, water-circulating cooling devices and ice packs used in combination can be effective at rapidly cooling patients. Many clinical studies have used this combination as their cooling technique. The patient is sandwiched between two blankets or cooling devices and ice packs are then applied. Once target temperature is achieved, the ice packs are removed and the blanket or cooling devices are used alone to maintain the target temperature. Newer cooling devices, specific for use in therapeutic hypothermia, use an adhesive gel to facilitate heat exchange that make them more effective at obtaining and maintaining target temperature.

Weihs and coworkers (2011) used adult, human-sized pigs to study the importance of surface area for the cooling efficacy of mild therapeutic hypothermia. Each of five adult, human-sized pigs (88-105 kg) was randomly cooled in three phases with pads that covered different areas of the body surface corresponding to humans (100% or 30% [thorax and abdomen] or 7% [neck]). The cooling pads were effective and safe for rapid induction of mild hypothermia in these porcine simulators. depending on the percentage of body surface area covered. Extrapolating to humans, covering only the neck, chest, and abdomen may achieve satisfactory cooling rates.

Convective-immersion surface cooling using a continuous shower of 2 degrees C water (ThermoSuit System) has also been found to be a rapid, effective method of inducing therapeutic hypothermia (Howes et al, 2010) and demonstrated improvement in survival and neurologic outcome in swine compared to normothermia (Weihls et al, 2008).

4.1.3 Cooling helmet
Helmet cooling devices are also available and have been used in some clinical trials. These helmets contain a solution of glycerol that facilitates heat exchange. Although this method is effective in cooling the brain it is much slower at reducing overall body temperature when compared to other methods.

4.2 Core cooling
4.2.1 Catheter-based technologies
Catheter-based technologies are usually placed in the femoral vein and provide heat exchange between the cooled saline that passes through a large coil in the catheter and the blood. The coiling provides a mechanism to increase surface area, thereby increasing the heat exchange between blood passing over the catheter. Internal cooling and rewarming is much faster and superior to other techniques in tightly regulating target temperature; it is possible to cool patients by 1.46°C - 1.59°C per hour (Jacobshagen et al, 2010). A potential advantage of using catheter-based cooling combined with anxiolytics is that it may avoid the need to use paralytics to decrease the shiver seen in surface cooling techniques.

4.2.2 Cold fluid infusion
Several studies have made use of intravenous cold fluid infusion for the induction of hypothermia. The rates of infusion differ between studies but the overall outcome is rapid cooling of the patient. Cold fluid infusion is a means of inducing hypothermia and cannot be used in the long-term maintenance of hypothermia. Usually, cold fluid infusions are used in conjunction with surface cooling methods to regulate and maintain patient body temperature. Most studies have used either normal saline or lactated Ringer solution as their cooling fluids. Evidence from reports using cold fluid infusion have not been associated with increased venous pressure, left atrial filling pressures, pulmonary pressures, pulmonary edema, cardiac arrhythmia, or other major complications.

Categories of Cooling	Techniques of Cooling	Advantages	Disadvantages
Surface Cooling	Ice packs	Inexpensive can be implemented very quickly.	Slow rate of cooling and provides poor regulation of target temperature.
	Cooling blankets and surface heat-exchange devices	Fair regulation of target temperature once it is obtained.	Slow rate of cooling unless used in conjunction with other techniques.
	Cooling helmet	Fair regulation of target temperature once it is obtained.	Slowest rate of cooling among techniques unless used in conjunction with other cooling methods.
Core Cooling	Catheter-based technologies	Rapid rate of cooling, tight target temperature regulation, minimize shiver and possible avoidance of paralytic usage.	Increased chance of thrombus formation
	Infusion of cold fluids	Rapid rate of cooling	Poor regulation of target temperature

Table 1. Cooling Technique Summary

5. Clinical evidence and uses

5.1 Clinical studies
The abovementioned landmark clinical trials from Europe and Australia, respectively, in 2003 established the benefits of hypothermia and have served as the basis for subsequent therapeutic hypothermia guidelines and clinical trials. Most clinical trials evaluate the

benefits of hypothermia by scoring patients on the CPC Scale, a tool that rates a patient's neurologic status, or by measuring survival rates.

The European trial enrolled 275 patients whose cardiac arrest was caused by ventricular fibrillation or pulseless ventricular tachycardia. Patients were randomly assigned to either hypothermic (n = 137) or normothermic (n = 138) groups. Hypothermic subjects were cooled to between 32-34°C for 24 hours with a cold air mattress. The primary endpoint of this study was to establish a favorable neurologic outcome in patients six months after cardiac arrest. The authors found that 55% of surviving hypothermic patients had a favorable neurologic outcome, as defined by a score of 1 or 2 on the CPC Scale, compared to 39% of surviving normothermic patients. A secondary endpoint was to evaluate complications within the first seven days after cardiac arrest, and mortality rate at six months. The European study demonstrated that neurologic outcome, as well as patient survival at six months (55% vs. 41%), both significantly improved in the hypothermic group as compared to the normothermic group (Holzer, 2002).

In the Australian trial, 77 comatose cardiac arrest survivors with ventricular fibrillation or pulseless ventricular tachycardia as the initial rhythm were similarly assigned to normothermic (n = 34) or hypothermic (n = 43) groups based on randomization. The hypothermic group was cooled to 33°C with ice packs for 12 hours and showed a 49% survival with favorable neurologic outcome (i.e., discharged home or to a rehabilitation facility, with no or moderate disability), while the normothermic group had a 26% survival with favorable neurologic outcome at hospital discharge (Bernard et al, 2002).

In 2009, Arrich and colleagues performed a Cochrane systematic review and meta-analysis to assess the effectiveness of therapeutic hypothermia in patients after cardiac arrest. Neurologic outcome, survival and adverse events were the main outcome parameters. The authors included all randomized controlled trials assessing the effectiveness of the therapeutic hypothermia in patients after cardiac arrest without language restrictions. Studies were restricted to adult populations cooled with any cooling method applied within six hours of cardiac arrest. Four trials and one abstract reporting on 481 patients were included in the systematic review. Quality of the included studies was good in three out of five included studies. For the three comparable studies on conventional cooling methods all authors provided individual patient data. With conventional cooling methods patients in the hypothermia group were more likely to reach a best cerebral performance category score of 1 or 2 (CPC, 5-point scale; 1 -- good cerebral performance, to 5 -- brain death) during hospital stay (individual patient data; RR, 1.55; 95% CI 1.22 to 1.96) and were more likely to survive to hospital discharge (individual patient data; RR, 1.35; 95% CI 1.10 to 1.65) compared to standard post-resuscitation care. Across all studies, there was no significant difference in reported adverse events between hypothermia and control. The authors concluded that conventional cooling methods to induce mild therapeutic hypothermia seem to improve survival and neurologic outcome after cardiac arrest, and their review supports the current best medical practice as recommended by the International Resuscitation Guidelines.

Testori and colleagues (2011) retrospectively studied 347 cardiac arrest survivors aged $\geq$ 18 years suffering a witnessed out-of-hospital cardiac arrest with asystole or pulseless electric activity as the first documented rhythm, for whom hypothermia was induced in 135 patients. They found that subjects who were treated with mild therapeutic hypothermia at a temperature of 32-34°C for 24 hours were more likely to have good neurologic outcomes in comparison to patients who were not treated with hypothermia, with an odds ratio of 1.84 (95% confidence interval: 1.08-3.13). In addition, the rate of mortality was significantly lower in the hypothermia group (odds ratio: 0.56; 95% confidence interval: 0.34-0.93).

While shortening the delay from spontaneous circulation to hypothermic target temperature has been theorized as a way of improving survival and neurologic outcome, randomized controlled trials and clinical registries have not shown evidence of whether the time to target temperature correlates with neurologic outcome. A recent study has reported that in comatose cardiac arrest patients treated with therapeutic hypothermia after return of spontaneous circulation, a faster decline in body temperature to the 34°C target appears to predict an unfavorable neurologic outcome (Haugk, 2011). Among 588 survivors of cardiac arrest managed with therapeutic hypothermia, the median time from restoration of spontaneous circulation to reaching a temperature of less than 34°C was 209 minutes (interquartile range [IQR]: 130-302) in patients with favorable neurologic outcomes compared to 158 minutes (IQR: 101-230) ($p < 0.01$) in patients with unfavorable neurologic outcomes. The adjusted odds ratio for a favorable neurologic outcome with a longer time to target temperature was 1.86 (95% CI 1.03 to 3.38, $p = 0.04$). Whether faster cooling is detrimental or patients with more severe neurologic damage show a faster cooling rate has to be further evaluated.

Animal and human studies have suggested that hypothermia impairs renal function. Zeiner et al (2004) reported that 24 hours of mild therapeutic hypothermia was associated with a delayed improvement in renal function that was not reflected in serum creatinine values, and this transient impaired renal function appeared to be completely reversible within 4 weeks. In trying to determine the relationship between acute kidney injury on survivors of cardiac arrest treated with therapeutic hypothermia we found that the incidence of acute kidney injury in patients with a CPS 1 or 2 score was 13.6% compared to 86.4% in patients with a CPS score > 2 ($p < 0.001$) (J. Prior, personal communication). Stage 3 acute kidney injury correlated with poor neurologic outcome ($p = 0.04$) but there was no correlation between Stages 1 and 2 and neurologic recovery. A longer duration of cardiac arrest was predictive of the subsequent development of acute kidney injury ($p = 0.01$). In summary, the presence of acute kidney injury in survivors of cardiac arrest treated with therapeutic hypothermia appears to be associated with poorer neurologic function determined at the time of hospital discharge. Acute kidney injury in this population may serve as a marker for the severity of anoxic injury incurred during arrest.

5.2 Indications and contraindications
5.2.1 Indications
The AHA has recommended that therapeutic hypothermia is indicated in adult patients with out-of-hospital cardiac arrests and who have an initial rhthym of ventricular fibrillation or nonperfusing ventricular tachycardia, that are comatose or have a Glasgow coma score < 8, that are hemodynamically stable, and lack a verbal response. Although these are the criteria for which hypothermia is recommended, there are other patients that may benefit from therapeutic hypothermia such as post-resuscitation patients having initial rhthyms other than ventricular fibrillation or nonperfusing ventricular tachycardia, as well as in-hospital cardiac arrest patients.

Survivors of witnessed out-of-hospital cardiac arrest of suspected cardiac origin

Persons with a Glasgow Coma Scale ≤ 8

Persons with ventricular fibrillation or non-perfusing ventricular tachycardia (those with other rhythyms such as asystole or electomechanical dissociatrion *may* also benefit although firm data is lacking)

Persons who are hemodynamically stable (those in cardiac shock *may* also benefit although firm data is lacking)

Consider for survivors of in-hospital cardiac arrest (although firm data is lacking)

* Adapted from Holzer 2010.

Table 2. Summary of indications for induced therapeutic hypothermia in comatose survivors of cardiac arrest.

5.2.2 Contraindications

Exclusion criteria for the use of therapeutic hypothermia are based upon increased risks to the patient. Studies have reported increased but non-significant increases in risk for the following patients: having major surgery within the previous 14 days; having systemic infections or sepsis, in a coma which is non-cardiac in origin, having active known bleeding or inherited bleeding disorder, being pregnant or terminally ill, those with a do-no-resuscitate (DNR) order, or having a tympanic temperature $< 30°C$ upon admission (Oommen & Menon, 2011).

6. Outcomes

Various methods have been used to try and determine the likelihood of neurologic recovery after cardiac arrest, but no single test is effective in accurately predicting neurologic outcome post-resuscitation. Clinical trials have established that combining examinations, laboratory tests and accounting for co-morbidities is often more accurate in determining neurologic outcome. Precise predictors of neurologic recovery are lacking and seriously limit the way clinicians assess patient prognosis, develop appropriate plans of care, and counsel family members. Therefore, more clinical studies are required to determine a uniform protocol for predicting neurologic outcome.

6.1 Modalities predicting neurological outcome
6.1.1 Neurologic examination

A neurologic examination is a fairly reliable predictor of neurological outcome after cardiac arrest. The presence of neurologic function during or immediately after return of spontaneous circulation (ROSC) roughly predicts a good neurologic outcome. Conversely, patients with a Glasgow Coma motor score of ≤ 2 or absent pupillary or corneal reflex at 72 hours can be predicted to have a poor neurologic outcome. The CPC Scale has also been classically used to predict patient outcome. Patients with a CPC scale score of 1 and 2 are likely to have good outcomes, while patients scoring 3, 4 or 5 have a significantly higher chance of having a poor neurologic outcome or death (Nolan et al, 2008). It is worth noting that the neurologic exam and CPC score can be influenced by the physiologic circumstances of the patient such as hypotension, shock, and severe metabolic dysfunction. Interventions such as paralytics, sedatives, and hypothermia also influence the findings of a neurologic examination and must be taken into account. Cranial nerve findings and motor response to pain are the best physical features estimating neurologic status and recovery.

1	Good cerebral performance: conscious, alert, able to work, might have mild neurologic or psychologic deficit.
2	Moderate cerebral disability: conscious, sufficient cerebral function for independent activities of daily life. Able to work in sheltered environment.
3	Severe cerebral disability: conscious, dependent on others for daily support because of impaired brain function. Ranges from ambulatory state to severe dementia or paralysis.
4	Coma or vegetative state: any degree of coma without the presence of all brain death criteria. Unawareness, even if appears awake (vegetative state) without interaction with environment; may have spontaneous eye opening and sleep/awake cycles. Cerebral unresponsiveness.
5	Brain death: apnea, areflexia, EEG silence, etc.

Note: If patient is anesthetized, paralyzed, or intubated, use "as is" clinical condition to calculate scores.

Table 3. Cerebral Performance Categories Scale (CPC Scale)

6.1.2 Neurophysiologic tests

Electroencephalography (EEG) has been used to characterize the degree of brain damage after cardiac arrest. Various EEG patterns have been associated with poor neurologic outcome such as generalized suppression, burst-suppression patterns with generalized epileptiform activity, and generalized periodic complexes on a flat background. Nevertheless, EEG alone is likely to be insufficient to prognosticate neurologic recovery. The EEG requires a physician with experience in its interpretation and knowledge of the influence of drugs and metabolic disorders on its results.

Madl & Holzer (2004) reviewed the literature on the pathophysiology of brain injury caused by cardiac arrest and the beneficial effect of therapeutic hypothermia on neurologic outcome. They summarized that electrophysiologic techniques and molecular markers of brain injury allow the accurate assessment and prognostication of long-term outcome in cardiac arrest survivors. In particular, somatosensory evoked potentials (SSEPs) appear to have the highest prognostic reliability; a systematic review of 18 studies analyzed the predictive ability of SSEPs performed early after onset of coma and found that absence of cortical SSEPs identify patients not returning from anoxic coma, with a specificity of 100%. Somatosensory-evoked potentials test the patency of the neuronal pathways, and are less affected by common drugs and metabolic disorders, making them a more reliable predictor of neurologic outcome than other modalities (Nolan et al, 2008). However, use of SSEPs in post-resuscitation patients requires advanced neurologic training which is usually restricted to specialized centers.

6.1.3 Neuroimaging

Neuroimaging is often performed to define structural brain injury related to cardiac arrest (either as a cause or consequence), including hemorrhage and cerebral vascular occlusion.

Most clinical studies evaluating neurologic outcome after use of therapeutic hypothermia do not make use of neuroimaging. The most common type of neuroimaging employed has been cranial computed tomography (CT), predominately because of the technical difficulties in performing magnetic resonance imaging (MRI) and positron emission tomography (PET) scans in the setting of arrest. Limited studies have shown that diffusion-weighted imaging (DWI), fluid attenuated inversion recovery (FLAIR), abnormalities in PET, and magnetic resonance spectroscopy can help predict poor neurologic outcome (Nolan et al, 2008).

6.1.4 Biochemical markers

Biochemical markers derived from the cerebrospinal fluid (CSF) and peripheral circulation, such as creatine phosphokinase (CPK) and neuron-specific enolase (NSE) respectively, have been used to predict neurologic outcome after cardiac arrest. The ease of obtaining blood compared to CSF has favored blood-based biochemical markers. Neuron-specific enolase is easily measured in the blood after injury to the brain and is, therefore, a good marker for neurologic outcome. Studies have shown that values of NSE > 33µg/L are predictor of poor neurologic outcome.

A calcium-binding protein from astroglia and Schwann cells, S100β, may also be a marker of neurologic outcome. An S100 β concentration > 1.2 µg/L, drawn between 24 and 48 hours after ROSC, is indicative of poor neurologic recovery (Nolan et al, 2008). Biomarker threshold values established in clinical trials vary based on the time blood and CSF are drawn after ROSC and the method for measuring the biomarker. Therefore, standardization must be applied in future clinical trials so that true threshold values can be elucidated and used to predict patient outcome.

6.1.5 Co-morbidities

We previously reported that the risk of poor neurologic outcome among patients treated with mild therapeutic hypothermia was related to the number of risk factors present (Table 4) (Vanston et al, 2010). A first rhythm of non-ventricular tachycardia/ventricular fibrillation after cardiac arrest, acute kidney injury within the first 72 hours of intensive care, and any treated cardiac arrhythmia were factors significantly associated with poor neurologic outcome and death (Table 4).

	No. patients		Risk of poor CPS (%)	No. risk factors[d] (95% CI)
	Good CPS (n = 17)	Poor CPS (n = 24)		
None	6	1	17	(0.3-52.6)
One	9	2	18	(2.3-51.8)
Any two	2	15	88[b]	(63.6-98.5)
All three	0	6	100[c]	(54.1-100)

[a] CPS. Pittsburgh Cerebral Performance Scale; C.I. = confidence intervals
[b] Significantly greater than the risk of poor neurologic outcome amongs patients with no predictive factors ($p = 0.004$).
[c] Significantly greater than the risk of poor neurologic outcome amongs patients with no predictive factors ($p = 0.002$).
[d] Include first rhythm other than ventricular fibrillation/ ventricular tachycardia, any arrhythmia, and acute kidney injury.

Table 4. Risk of poor neurologic outcome among patient treated with mild therapeutic hypothermia, according to number of risk factors present.[a]

6.2 Adverse effects

Adverse effects of mild induced therapeutic hypothermia are either directly related to the cooling device or due to hypothermia itself. In 41 clinical trials using therapeutic hypothermia the overall rate of adverse events related to a cooling device was 1% (Holzer, 2010). These adverse effects included three cases of bleeding, eight cases of infection, ten cases of deep venous thrombosis, and eight cases of pulmonary edema. The cases of deep venous thrombosis were seen in patients that were cooled with a catheter-based device, while the cases of pulmonary edema occurred in patients that were cooled with cold intravenous fluid.

Hypothermia causes a decrease in insulin secretion, as well as insulin resistance in many patients. This state of hyperglycemia requires administration of insulin to maintain glucose levels within an acceptable range. More importantly, during the re-warming phase patients can regain appropriate sensitivity to insulin rapidly, making them susceptible to hypoglycemia if insulin administration is not reduced accordingly. Glycemic lability is one of several reasons why re-warming rates after hypothermia are typically slow and controlled.

Some of the adverse effects most commonly associated with therapeutic hypothermia include pneumonia, shivering hyperglycemia, cardiac arrhythmias, seizures, and electrolyte disorders. Less frequently seen complications are sepsis, coagulopathy, and metabolic disturbances. Many of these effects can be easily managed by proper patient monitoring. In a study compiling data from major clinical trials on adverse effects unrelated to the cooling devices, such events occurred in 74% of patients who were treated with hypothermia (223 events in 300 patients) and in 71% of 285 patients given standard, normothermic treatment (Holzer, 2010). The incidences of cardiac arrhythmia, hemodynamic instability, bleeding, pneumonia, sepsis, renal failure, seizures, and pancreatitis were not significantly different between the two groups.

7. Slow implementation

Although its use is becoming more widespread, therapeutic hypothermia is still not appropriately initiated for a majority of eligible patients. Concerns with the ease of use, efficacy, and cost have limited use in the community setting. The current level of implementation of therapeutic hypothermia is difficult to measure, although hypothermia registries are attempting to bridge the gap. The AHA, along with some local communities, is advocating for the care of all patients with cardiac arrest at centers specializing in post-arrest care in order to provide the best possible outcomes. Such centers would have the capability to perform therapeutic hypothermia, perform percutaneous coronary intervention, and utilize standardized protocols for the treatment of cardiac arrest survivors, as well as pay close attention to related aspects of overall management including hemodynamic stability, ventilator support (with timely normalization of FiO_2 and pCO_2), thromboembolic prophylaxis, and glycemic control.

8. Ongoing and potential future research

8.1 Neurologic prognosis

In patients managed with therapeutic hypothermia clinical research is ongoing regarding clinical modeling and the use of aspects of the neurologic exam and acute and chronic medical co-morbidities in predicting neurologic recovery. We have previously found that several simple and reproducible clinical markers (i.e., first rhythm at cardiac arrest; the presence of acute kidney injury in the ICU; any treated cardiac arrhythmia after admission; and Glasgow Coma Score < 8 determined 12 hours after re-warming) can help predict neurologic prognosis during and after treatment, in patients managed with therapeutic hypothermia for cardiac arrest (Vanston, 2010). Additional investigation is neded to examine the potential role of other exam techniques, and electrophysiologic and neurobiochemical tests in reliably predicting neurologic outcomes, and to determine the correlation between laboratory values or exam scores and time after return of spontaneous circulation.

8.2 Non-shockable rhythms/ other cardiac

Small randomized trials and registries have begun to collect data on the use of therapeutic hypothermia in cardiac arrests with non-shockable rhythms and in-hospital cardiac arrests. Recently, in a retrospective cohort study treatment with mild therapeutic hypothermia at a temperature of 32-34°C for 24 hours was associated with improved neurologic outcome and a reduced risk of death following out-of-hospital cardiac arrest in 135 with non-shockable rhythms (Testori et al, 2011). To date, the level of evidence is inadequate to firmly recommend therapeutic hypothermia for these patients; nevertheless, many of these patients are treated with therapeutic hypothermia in the community if their arrest is thought to be of cardiac origin or if the initial rhythm after arrest is unknown. Further research is needed to determine the potential role of therapeutic hypothermia for these subsets of patients. The ILCOR currently advocates the use of therapeutic hypothermia following perinatal asphyxia-related cardiac arrest in term newborns.

At least one study (a retrospective analysis of the Hypothermia after Cardiac Arrest (HACA) trial) suggested that cooling after successful resuscitation for ventricular fibrillation cardiac arrest did not influence infarct size (Koreny et, 2009). The authors contended that cautious interpretation of the subgroup analysis may indicate a favorable trend for early cooling, and thus additional research is indicated.

8.3 Non-cardiac applications

Clinical trials are still revealing further application of therapeutic hypothermia. It is likely that recommendations and the use of therapeutic hypothermia will expand to encompass several other pathologies such as traumatic brain and spinal cord injury and acute ischemic stroke. Currently, therapeutic hypothermia is not approved by an advisory panel for any other use besides comatose patients after return of spontaneous circulation due to ventricular fibrillation or pulseless ventricular tachycardia (Adler et al, 2011).

8.4 Aspects of treatment

Current and potential future areas of clinical research on treatment aspects of therapeutic hypothermia include, among others:

- Optimal target temperature, duration, onset, cooling rates, and re-warming rates
- Use of external, internal, or mixed modality cooling techniques
- Pharmacologic uses and standardized drug protocols i.e. (analgesics, sedatives, paralytics, etc.)

9. Areas of uncertainty

Some persistent unexposed topics that relate to the pathophysiology of therapeutic hypothermia include the precise mechanism(s) of greatest importance for good neurologic recovery, the mechanism(s) through which hypothermia exerts the most influence, the effects of co-morbidities in reducing the efficacy of therapeutic hypothermia, and the time course of cellular cascades and the ability to attenuate these processes (Holzer, 2010).

10. Guidelines

Sedation, analgesia, and paralysis should be initiated prior to hypothermia to prevent shivering which can increase oxygen consumption, promote labored breathing, increase heart rate, delay hypothermic induction, and increase patient discomfort.

The ILCOR and the AHA recommend that core body temperature of unconscious adult patients with spontaneous circulation after an out-of- hospital ventricular fibrillation cardiac arrest should be lowered to 32-34°C. The cooling process should be started in the pre-hospital setting or as soon as possible and continued for 12-24 hours. Core temperature should be continuously monitored via the esophagus, rectum, trachea or bladder. General management of hypothermia patients includes concurrent measurement of mean arterial pressure, central venous pressure, urine output, arterial blood gases, central venous oxygen saturation, serum lactate, blood glucose, electrolytes, and complete blood count, and continuous ECG monitoring and stabilization.

After hypothermia, patients should be re-warmed at a rate of 0.5°C per hour with avoidance of hyperthermia. Potassium administraction should be stopped to avoid hyperkalemia during the re-warming phase. After re-warming to 36°C, sedation and paralytic agents should be discontinued and the patient should be weened off ventilator support (Jacobshagen et al, 2010). Neurologic recovery can take several hours after discontinuation of hypothermia. Therefore, it is important to wait until the patient is completely re-warmed and stabile before evaluating patients with prognositic neurologic exams like the Glasgow Coma Scale.

11. Conclusions

Mild therapeutic hypothermia is indicated for use in witnessed out-of-hospital cardiac arrest patients with a return of spontaneous circulation, for persons with an initial rhythm of ventricular fibrillation or non-perfusing ventricular tachycardia, for persons who are comatose or have a Glasgow coma score < 8, those who are hemodynamically stable, and those who lack a verbal response. Clinical evidence has shown that mild hypothermia decreases mortality and increases the proportion of patients with a favorable neurologic outcome (score of 1 or 2 on the CPC Scale) with mininimal risk of adverse effects. Therapeutic hypothermia is a relatively inexpensive treatment modality with an incremental cost-effectiveness ratio of $47,168 (Merchant et al, 2009) and can be implemented in a variety of settings from rural community-based hospitals to specialized cardiac and neurologic centers. The indications for mild therapeutic hypothermia will broaden in the future as more clinical trials are conducted. It is important to understand the pathophysiologic processes involved in the post-cardiac arrest syndrome, as well as the concominant changes in human physiology during induced mild therapeutic hypothermia.

12. References

Adler, J., Bessman, E., Talavera, F., Setnik, G., & Halamka, J.D.. Therapeutic hypothermia. (2011). (http://emedicine.medscape.com/article/812407-overview).

Arrich, J., Holzer, M., Herkner, H., Mullner, M. (2009). Hypothermia for neuroprotection in adults after cardiopulmonary resuscitation. *Cochrane Database of Systematic Reviews* Issue 4. Art. No.: CD004128. DOI: 10.1002/14651858.CD004128.pub2

Bernard, S.A. (2002). Treatment of comatose survivors of out-of-hospital cardiac aresst with induced hypothermia. *New England Journal of Medicine* 346(8):557-563

Bernard, S., Buist, M,, Monteiro, O., Smith, K. (2003). Induced hypothermia using large volume, ice-cold intravenous fluid in comatose survivors of out-of-hospital cardiac arrest: a preliminary report. *Resuscitation* 56(1):9-13.

Haugk M, Stratil P, Sterz F, et al (2010). Temperature monitored on the cuff surface of an endotracheal tube reflects body temperature. *Crit Care Med* 38(7):1569-1573

Haugk M, Testori C, Sterz F, et al (2011). Relationship between time to target temperature and outcome in patients treated with therapeutic hypothermia after cardiac arrest. *Crit Care* 15(2):R101

Holzer, M. (2010). Targeted temperature management for comatose survivors of cardiac arrest. *New England Journal of Medicine* 363(13):1256-1264

Holzer, M., Sterz, F., Hypothermia After Cardiac Arrest Study Group. (2002). Therapeutic hypothermia after cardiopulmonary resuscitation. *Expert Rev Cardiovasc Ther* 1(2):317-25.

Howes D, Ohley W, Dorian P, et al (2010). Rapid induction of therapeutic hypothermia using convective-immersion surface cooling: safety, efficacy and outcomes. *Resuscitation* 81(4):388-392.

Hypothermia after Cardiac Arrest Study Group.(2002). Mild therapeutic hypothermia to improve the neurologic outcome after cardiac arrest. *New England Journal of Medicine* 346(8):549-556

Jacobshagen, C., Pelster, T., Pax, A., et al. (2010). Effects of mild hypothermia on hemodynamics in cardiac arrest survivors and isolated failing human myocardium. *Clinical Research in Cardiology* 99(5):267-276

Koreny M, Sterz F, Uray T, et al (2009). Effect of cooling after human cardiac arrest on myocardial infarct size. *Resuscitation* 80(1):56-60

Merchant, R.M., Becker, L.B., Abella, B.S., Asch, D.A., Groeneveld, P.W. Cost-effectiveness of therapeutic hypothermia after cardiac arrest. *Circulation: Cardiovascular Quality Outcomes*. 2009 Sep;2(5):421-428

Nolan, J.P., Morley, P.T., Vanden Hoek, T.L., & Hickey, R.W. (2003). Therapeutic hypothermia after cardiac arrest.

An advisory statement by the Advanced Life Support Task Force of the International Liaison Committee on Resuscitation. *Resuscitation* 57(3):231-235

Nolan, J.P. (2008). Post-cardiac arrest syndrome: epidemiology, pathophysiology, treatment, and prognostication. *Resuscitation* 79(3):350-379

Oommen, S.S., & Menon V. (2011). Hypothermia after cardiac arrest: beneficial, but slow to be adopted. *Cleveland Clinic Journal of Medicine* 78 (7):441-448

Prior, J., Lawhon-Triano, M., Fedor, M., et al. (2010). Community-based application of mild therapeutic hypothermia for survivors of cardiac arrest. *Southern Medical Journal* 103(4):295-300

Polderman, K.H. Mechanisms of action, physiological effects, and complications of hypothermia. (2009). *Crit Care Med* ;37(7 Suppl):S186-202

Safar, P.J., & Kochanek, P.M. (2002). Therapeutic hypothermia after cardiac arrest. *New England Journal of Medicine* 346(8):612-613

Sinclair, H.L., & Andrews, P.J.D. (2010). Bench-to-bedside review: hypothermia in traumatic brain injury. *Critical Care* 14(1):204

Testori, C., Sterz, F., Behringer, W., et al. (2011). Mild therapeutic hypothermia is associated with favourable outcome in patients after cardiac arrest with non-shockable rhythms. *Resuscitation* 82(9):1162-1167

Vanston, V.J., Lawhon-Triano, M., Getts, R., et al. (2010). Predictors of poor neurologic outcome in patients undergoing therapeutic hypothermia after cardiac arrest. *Southern Medical Journal* 103(4):301-306

Wandaller, C., Holzer, M., Sterz, F., et al. (2009). Head and neck cooling after cardiac arrest results in lower jugular bulb than esophageal temperature. *American Journal of Emergency Medicine* 27(4):460-465

Weihs, W., Schratter, A., Sterz, F., et al. (2011). The importance of surface area for the cooling efficacy of mild therapeutic hypothermia. *Resuscitation* 82(1):74-78

Zeiner, A., Klewer, J., Sterz, F., et al. (2010). Non-invasive continuous cerebral temperature monitoring in patients treated with mild therapeutic hypothermia: an observational pilot study. *Resuscitation* 81(7):861-866

11

Development of Computer Aided Prediction Technology for Paroxysmal Atrial Fibrillation in Mobile Healthcare

Desok Kim[1], Jae-Hyeong Park[2] and Jun Hyung Kim[2]
*[1]Departments of Electrical Engineering and
Information Communication Engineering, KAIST, Daejeon,
[2]Chungnam National University, School of Medicine and Hospital,
Department of Cardiology, Daejeon,
Korea*

1. Introduction

Atrial fibrillation (AF) is one of the major health risks for strokes, and has been found to increase the risk of ischemic stroke fivefold (Wolf et al., 1987). Strokes with AF are more severe, cause greater disability and have worse outcomes than those without (Jørgensen et al., 1996; Lin et al., 1996). Approximately 15–20% of all strokes are due to AF but the percentage increases up to 40% for patients over the age of 90 (Marini et al., 2005). As the risk of initial strokes in these patients can be reduced up to 64% by long-term treatment with anti-coagulants (Hart et al., 2007), accurate and timely detection of AF is essential in high-risk elderly populations. Paroxysmal AF (PAF) is defined as an AF episode that lasts longer than 2 min but less than 7 days. Most PAF episodes terminate spontaneously within 24 h. Although PAF is short-lived, it shares similar stroke risks with long-lasting persistent AF (Friberg et al., 2010). Furthermore, the rare and asymptomatic manifestation of AF episodes makes a definitive diagnosis of PAF even harder to provide. Holter or event recorder devices are used conventionally to capture actual episodes of AF. Using 24-h Holter monitoring, only 23% of cases were detected among PAF patients whose diagnosis was confirmed by continuous bedside electrocardiograph (ECG) monitoring (Rizos et al., 2010), which indicates an underestimated detection of PAF leading to inadequate treatment. Using 7-day event-loop recording, 5.7% of cases that were missed by 24-h Holter monitoring were revealed to be PAF (Jabaudon et al., 2004). Thus, prolonged ECG monitoring by event recorders improves the detection rates of PAF cases. However, event recorders may not be appropriate for all patients, and depend on patient compliance. The extended use of Holter monitors is not commonly practiced in clinics, and few technical guidelines are currently available for the improvement of PAF detection by a short-term use of Holter monitors.

Prediction methods have been studied in order to suppress PAF episodes through atrial pacing techniques and to provide the clinical benefit of maintaining normal sinus rhythm (NSR) in, for example, drug-refractory AF patients (Delfaut et al., 1998). Most of the methods developed were inspired by earlier physiological findings that were associated with the triggering mechanisms of PAF, namely, activated ectopic nodes in abnormal atrial tissue and the imbalance of the autonomic nervous system (ANS) via increased sympathetic or parasympathetic tone. A hypothetical transition period has been proposed during which the triggering mechanisms are activated, forcing NSR to change to PAF. During the transition, the number of premature atrial complexes (PAC), runs of atrial bigeminy and trigeminy, and length of paroxysmal atrial tachycardia were increased before PAF onset (Thong et al., 2004). Spectral analysis revealed a significant increase in ANS activity in both the sympathetic and parasympathetic branches, which were represented by increased low-frequency (LF) and high-frequency (HF) components in the power spectrum density of the heartbeat intervals (RR intervals) (Chesnokov et al., 2008; Kim et al., 2008a). Heart rate variability (HRV) features in time domain analysis were also significantly changed during the transition (Kim et al., 2008a), again indicating a change in ANS activity. The complexity of RR interval dynamics decreased before the onset of PAF episodes (Chesnokov, 2008; Vikman et al., 1999). Poincaré plots depicting the correlation between two successive RR intervals in a two-dimensional diagram were also found to be closely related to ANS activity and to exhibit highly heterogeneous patterns during the transition (Duong et al., 2009). Recently, recurrence plots representing the frequency of two RR intervals in close proximity were investigated to discover dynamic behaviors during the transition that were not uncovered by earlier methods (Mohebbi & Ghassemian, 2011). In these studies, prediction models were derived by running pattern classification algorithms on learning sets that consisted of two types of ECG data: one distant and the other immediately before the onsets, representing NSR and the transition period, respectively (available from the PhysioBank's MIT-BIH AF Prediction Database as 30-min ECG data sets). These prediction models were able to detect the transition to PAF events at rates of 70-97%. Some of PAF prediction reports are summarized in Table 1. Recent reviews of these techniques and their performance are also available (Sahoo et al., 2011; Mohebbi & Ghassemian, 2011). To apply these methods to atrial pacing techniques, ECG data need to be sampled continuously.

Authors	Feature sets	Accuracy (%)	Sensitivity (%)	Specificity (%)	Duration of ECG learning sets	Databases and their usage
Thong et al. (2004)	Number of PACs, bigeminy, and trigeminy	90	89	91	30 min	MIT-BIH AF Prediction Database as learning and test sets
Mohebbi & Ghassemi (2011)	Recurrent plots (recurrence rate, L_{max}, L_{mean}, entropy, and trapping time)		97	100	30 min	
Hickey et al. (2004)	LF, HF, and power spectral density, PAC	80.5	43.0	99.3	30 min	MIT-BIH AF Prediction Database as learning sets
	Empirical rule	100	100	100	All 30-min segments	MIT-BIH AF and NSR Database as test sets
Kikillus et al. (2008)	Poincaré plot image, SDSD	94.4	91.5	96.9	60 min	MIT-BIH AF and NSR Database as learning and test sets
Kim et al. (2008a)	HRV features		90	95	3 min	MIT-BIH AF and NSR Database as learning and test sets

Table 1. Summary of previous studies for the prediction of AF onsets and PAF subjects

Due to the low detection rates of PAF events provided by Holter devices, alternative approaches have been motivated by the physiological findings of different dynamics of heart rate controls in PAF subjects, even when AF is not actually occurring. Thus, instead of relying on the capture of PAF episodes, prediction methods have been developed to provide a diagnostic assessment of PAF cases that display either no episodes of AF or a small number of episodes (Hickey et al., 2004; Kikillus et al., 2008; Kim et al., 2008a). Although these prediction models were motivated by the similar findings and methods explained above, they were evaluated against public databases that provide long-term ECG data from PAF and NSR subjects (available from the PhysioBank's MIT-BIH AF and NSR Databases). The AF Database provides 25 ECG data sets of 10-h recordings obtained from patients with PAF. The NSR Database provides 18 ECG data sets of 24-h recordings obtained from healthy persons with no arrhythmias. Numerous approaches have been reported because multiple representations of heart rate dynamics were feasible at different time-points of the day or night. Each short segment was classified by a first-stage classifier who relied on the detection of abnormal HRV features and PAC. To incorporate prediction results made at different time-points into one assessment, a second-stage classifier inquired whether an empirical rule was satisfied. For example, a subject was classified as PAF if at least 10% of the segments were classified as PAF segments and the average probability of PAF was at least 0.35 (Hickey et al., 2004). For this approach, finding the empirical rule was critical to evaluate the performance of the classifier. The performance of this prediction model may be directly related to not only how often a PAF patient experiences a physiological condition resembling the transition period, but also how often actual PAF episodes occur immediately after the presumed transition period. However, no information is available on the frequency of a transition period being followed by an actual PAF event. Furthermore, the performance of these prediction models over a long-term monitoring period has not yet been investigated.

In contrast, if the sampling of ECG data as learning sets is not confined to the transition period, then a prediction model may be less sensitive to whether a subject experiences the transition period or not and still performs as anticipated. Instead of confining learning set samples to the transition period, 1-h ECG segments were sampled from all available time-points and evaluated by a classifier based on a risk assessment of HRV analysis and Poincaré plot analysis performed on all samples (Kikillus et al., 2008). Because the test sets included the AF episodes, the classification performance was sensitive to the length of AF episodes included in the data. Alternatively, multiple ultra-short 3-min segments were sampled from different time periods of the day and classified using two different formulas designed for day or evening time (Kim et al., 2008a, 2008b). This method did not contain AF episodes in the test data, and thus the prediction accuracy relates exclusively to detecting the transition period. In addition, transition periods were treated differently depending on the time of their occurrence (Kim et al., 2008b), which resulted in two time-dependent classifiers performing better than one classifier disregarding the occurrence time of transitions. These methods require ECG data to be continuously analyzed, that may demand some extraordinary functional capabilities from wireless devices and data networks in mobile healthcare systems. For instance, a limited battery time is common in potable wireless gateway devices such as personal data assistant (PDA) or cellular phones. Network congestion and loss should be avoided or reliably handled in a medical sensor network (MSN) (Hu & Xiao, 2009) that may monitors large number of mobile subjects. As a strategy that alleviates these requirements of future mobile healthcare devices and networks, an intermittent data sampling and its relevance to clinical decision makings could be considered. Thus, we propose that intermittently sampled ECG data (but devoid of any arrhythmic episodes) may be used as learning sets for calculating a PAF prediction model. Our driving hypothesis remains the same as that stated in previous reports: the non-episodic state of PAF subjects is different to that of NSR subjects (Kikillus et al., 2008; Kim et al., 2008a).

The recurrence rate of silent AF is high even when the patient has undergone apparently successful ablation or drug therapy. Patients who had been treated with atrial ablation and circumferential pulmonary vein ablation were reported to have a 26.7% recurrence rate after 13 months and a rate of 31% after 19 months, respectively (Berruezo et al., 2007; Grubitzsch et al., 2008). Patients who underwent chemical or electrical cardioversion also showed high recurrence rates of 30–43% after 0.5–42 months (Aytemir et al., 1999; Lombardi et al., 2001). The recurrence of silent AF in stroke victims can also be as high as the percentage reported in these earlier studies. If clinicians and patients can be alarmed by the early diagnosis of AF to take appropriate measures and avoid the recurrence of ischemic strokes, tens of thousands of recurrent stroke victims can be saved each year. In this study, we first sought to develop a detection method for PAF subjects using HRV patterns obtained from intermittently sampled ECG. Based on this model, we then sought to predict recurrent PAF subjects among patients who had been successfully treated for AF previously and were currently under anti-arrhythmic medication. In addition, we have implemented our algorithms to a remote real-time heartbeat analysis system that consists of a portable ECG sensor with a three-axis accelerometer, a smart phone, and a data analysis server. This internet-based system should provide a developmental platform to investigate the detection of PAF further through the use of long-term monitoring.

2. Methods and subjects

2.1 Subjects and data acquisition

The 24-h ECG data of 50 cases were obtained from the archive storage in Chungnam National University Hospital, Department of Cardiology. Subjects visited the clinic due for a variety of complaints with symptoms that might have been related to underlying cardiac diseases. Data were included if the subject was older than 35 years, had visited the clinic during the past 2 years, and were free of any cardiovascular disease. All ECG data were obtained by using the same type of Holter monitors for 24 h. The use of patient ECG data was approved by the internal review board of the hospital.

Thirty-nine patients with previously diagnosed AF were recruited for 48-h Holter monitoring in the same department. Patients completed the consent form for the use of experimental data and a stress questionnaire (Koh et al., 2001). Six patients were excluded due to the failure of 48-h Holter monitoring (n = 3) and the loss of ECG data during data handling (n = 3). A total of 33 patients had been under AF management for the past 1.5 years on average (15 women: age range, 39–82 years, median age, 66 years; and 18 men: age range, 43–78 years, median age, 66 years). This experiment was approved by the internal review board of the hospital.

2.2 Data processing
2.2.1 Preparation of ECG data

ECG signals were sampled at 125 samples per second by Holter recorders (Marquette MARS PC Holter monitor, GE Healthcare) and screened for arrhythmic events first by the computer software and then by two cardiologists. A 24-h binary record (in .bin format) was transformed into four 6-h text-based records using a software tool called "rdsamp.exe" available at the Physionet. Each record represented four different time periods of the day (namely morning from 6 am to 12 noon, afternoon from noon to 6 pm, evening from 6 pm to 12 midnight, and night from midnight to 6 am). ECG segments that contained arrhythmic episodes were also removed based on medical records. Noisy parts of ECG data were automatically removed by a cut-off value that represented the maximum value of local heterogeneity of ECG signals (data not shown). The percentage of ECG signals detected as noise was also recorded.

2.2.2 RR interval detection

Time intervals between two successive QRS complexes (RR intervals) were obtained using the previous ECG analysis software for a mobile application (Salahuddin & Kim, 2006). Java-based analysis software was developed to detect RR intervals and calculate the HRV features. The analysis algorithm was mainly adapted from a derivative method (Pan & Tompkins, 1985) but several modifications had to be added to ensure the detection of true RR intervals in noisy ECG signals. Briefly, a tophat operation was performed on the band-pass waveforms to suppress noisy peaks and remove the baseline shift. A set of rules was applied to avoid detecting R peaks from unusually high or low amplitude parts and noisy parts of ECG signals. After detecting R peaks, another set of rules was applied to avoid extracting RR intervals that were too short or too long compared with average RR intervals calculated from accumulated RR intervals. The analysis algorithm was divided into three phases: a pre-processing, an R peak decision and a post-processing. During the pre-processing phase, the ECG signal (Figure 1a) was passed through a band-pass filter — a 60th order finite impulse response digital filter using a Hamming window — with a cut-off frequency ranging from 8 to 12 Hz (Figure 1b). The band-passed signal was then filtered through a tophat operation that consisted of a series of minimum and maximum operations and a subtraction operation (Figure 1c). Since the size of the tophat filter was set to equal the average width at half maximum of the R peaks (seven time-points), tophat filtering preferentially enhanced RR intervals and suppressed noisy small peaks and large T peaks. The subtraction of the minimum-maximum filtered waveforms from the original waveforms eliminated baseline drifts completely. The tophat-processed ECG signal was differentiated so that RR interval signals resulted in two wave peaks with relatively larger amplitudes (Figure 1d). The resultant signal was squared to amplify the part of the signal with larger amplitude to a greater extent (Figure 1e). An integral waveform was generated by a moving window of 30 time-points in width (Figure 1f). The integral waveform was compared with the adaptive thresholds that were continuously updated estimates of the peak signal level (Figure 1g) and the peak noise level (data not shown) (Pan & Tompkins, 1985). In our algorithm, the search back (or dual thresholds) technique (Pan & Tompkins, 1985) was not used since it did not seem to contribute significantly to the detection of the RR intervals of our ECG signals. The adaptive threshold produced a series of time-point ranges (rectangular wave tops), representing possible locations of R peak candidates (Figure 1h). The local maximum of band-passed waveform within each range was found to be an R peak candidate (shown as arrowheads in Figure 1i). During the R peak decision phase, a true R peak was found if the following two conditions were satisfied at the time-point of the R peak candidate: 1) if the amplitude of the raw signal was less than 1000; and 2) if the amplitude of tophat-filtered signal was greater than 30. During the post-processing phase, some RR intervals were often found to be unreasonably short or long due to errors such as detecting spurious peaks or missing true peaks. An RR interval was considered as valid if it satisfied the following two conditions: 1) if the RR interval was longer than 0.75 times; and 2) if the RR interval was shorter than 1.5 times the accumulated RR interval average to avoid unusually short or long RR intervals caused by noisy signals or missing R peaks, respectively.

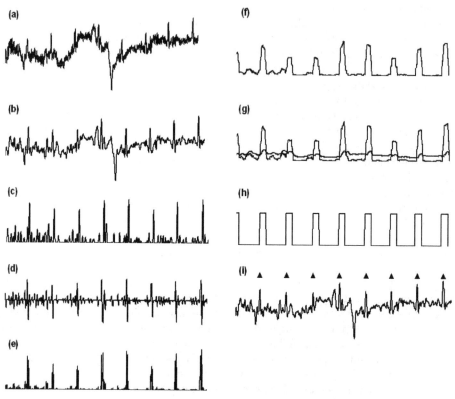

Fig. 1. Processing steps of R peak detection algorithm. (a) the input signal, (b) the output of bandpass filtering, (c) tophat, (d) differentiator, (e) squaring; (f) moving-window integration, (g) locally adaptive thresholding, (h) possible QRS complex ranges, (i) QRS complex candidates detected from band-passed waveform. (Permission from Salahuddin & Kim, 2006).

2.2.3 HRV calculation

From each 6-h RR interval record, four 30-min RR records were randomly selected. The baseline trend in heart rates introduced by postural change or movement was removed using a linear curve-fitting method. Detrended time series were cubically interpolated and re-sampled at 4 Hz, and the fast Fourier transform was windowed with 256-sample-width Hamming windows with 50% overlap. All HRV features were calculated from the detrended RR interval series.

In each RR interval set, the following HRV features were calculated using the ECG analysis software (also available at http://mhealth.kaist.ac.kr/afdectection): mean heart rate (mean HR), mean heartbeat intervals (mean RR), standard deviation of NN interval (SDNN), coefficient of variation (CV), root mean square of successive differences (RMSSD), and percentage heartbeat intervals with difference in successive heartbeat intervals greater than 50 ms (PNN50) as time domain features; HRV index (bin width of 8.0 ms), triangular interpolation of heartbeat interval histogram (TINN), and stress index (SI) (Lednev et al., 2008) as geometrical analysis features; and LF (LF 0.04-0.09 Hz), HF (HF >0.1 Hz), the ratio of LF to HF (LF/HF), normalized LF (LFnu) and normalized HF (HFnu) components as frequency domain features (Task Force, 1996). Among the HRV features, the RMSSD is worthy of further mention because it has been used to indicate the levels of mental or physical stress of a subject (Task Force, 1996). In preparing the learning sets, RMSSD was used as basis to estimate the activity level of a subject during daily activity.

2.2.4 Poincaré plot pattern analysis

The Poincaré plot is a two-dimensional scatter plot of each heartbeat interval plotted against the subsequent interval, and thus depicts the correlation between successive heartbeat intervals (Woo et al., 1992). Recently, Poincaré plots of arrhythmic ECG data were systematically investigated to discover 10 distinctive prototypical patterns that represent different kinds of arrhythmias from 24-h Holter ECG data (Esperer et al., 2008). For example, fan-shaped Poincaré plots were typical in subjects with AF; multiple side lobe patterns specified the presence of atrial premature beats or ventricular premature beats; while an island pattern was highly correlated with atrial flutter or atrial tachycardia (Esperer et al., 2008). Poincaré plots were generated to calculate Poincaré plot features and classify them into different patterns such as torped, island, multiple side lobes, and fan pattern (Duong et al., 2009). Finally, standard deviations of the minor axis (SD_1) and major axis (SD_2), the ratio of SD_1 to SD_2 (SD_1/SD_2), standard deviation of the RR intervals (SDRR), standard deviation of the successive differences of the RR intervals (SDSD), and autocorrelation function of the RR intervals (rRR) were calculated from the Poincaré plot (Brennan et al., 2001). In addition to the previously reported conventional descriptors, new cluster descriptors were calculated by analyzing the Poincaré plots as an image (Duong et al., 2009). In brief, Poincaré plot images (Figure 2A) were thresholded at the gray level of 0 (Figure 2B). Second, binary plot images were eroded once with the 3×3 structuring element, reconstructed with respect to the binary plot, and seed-filled (Figure 2C) (Serra, 1984). A cluster was defined as an isolated group of connected points containing more than 12 points that effectively represented highly correlated heartbeat interval events. Then, the cluster was described by using shape attributes, such as form factor and minor to major axis ratio; texture attributes, such as entropy and contrast; and location attributes, such as the number of clusters on the diagonal line. Torpedo, island, and multi-sided lobe patterns were classified at the accuracy of 99% using the combined set of conventional and new Poincaré plot features.

2.2.5 Circadian rhythm analysis

Circadian rhythm (CR) represents physiological phenomena repeatedly occurring during a time period of approximately 24 h. In humans, almost every physiological function displays CR to some degree and the mechanism can be endogenous, exogenous or a combination of both. The cardiovascular system also exhibits a pronounced CR which is influenced by both external stimuli and endogenous homoeostatic control mechanism with the latter playing a more important role than the former (Guo & Stein, 2002). Circadian variations are found in a number of electrophysiological parameters such as heart rate, QT interval, sinus node recovery time, and atrial refractory periods (Guo & Stein, 2002). Although detailed genetic or epigenetic mechanisms are not fully understood, numerous cardiovascular and cerebrovascular diseases show circadian variations. For example, paroxysmal and persistent atrial arrhythmia occurs more frequently during the evening time (Mitchell et al., 2002), whereas sudden cardiac death (Savopoulos et al., 2006) and myocardial ischemia (Li, 2003) occur predominantly in the morning. In previous studies, we reported circadian variations of HRV features in NSR and PAF subjects (Kim et al., 2008a) and CR parameters such as amplitudes, phase, and shift obtained from a least square fitting of sinusoidal functions to various HRV features. On the day of onset of PAF, CR of PAF subjects were affected and significantly different from those of NSR subjects. The CR parameters obtained from the non-episodic data for that day were used to detect PAF patients with an accuracy of 84.6% (Olemann & Kim, 2011).

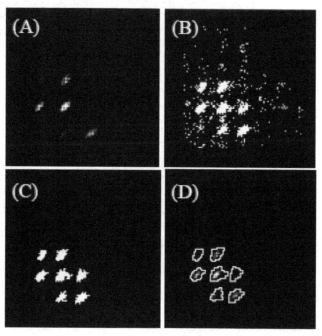

Fig. 2. The Poincaré plot of island pattern (A), its binary plot (B), opening by reconstruction and closing (C), and cluster boundary overlaid onto the binary plot (D). (Permission from Duong et al., 2009).

To obtain CR parameter patterns of HRV features, a non-linear curve-fitting method known as the Levenberg-Marquardt algorithm (Levenberg, 1944) was applied (Statgraphics Plus V4.1 Professional System®, Manugistics, Inc., Rockville, MD, USA) to each HRV feature set that consisted of at least six time-points which represents a time span of at least 6 h. The initial values for the regression were set by trial and error and were maintained constant for both the NSR and PAF group. The CR parameters obtained were the amplitude, the shift and the phase, from the following sinusoidal equation used for the curve fitting:

$$H(t) = b \times cosine\,(w\,t + p) + a \tag{1}$$

where $H(t)$ represents the HRV feature, b represents amplitude, p represents phase (in degrees), a represents shift, t represents time of the day (in hours), and w represents 15°/h. The final amplitude was obtained by taking the absolute value. The final phase was modified to restrict its phase value between 0 and 180 using the following formula:

$$Phase = 180/phi \times cosine^{-1}(b \times cosine\ (p \times phi/180\ )/\ /b\ /) \qquad (2)$$

While performing the sinusoidal curve fitting, time-points that showed unusual residuals (Studentized residual > |3.0|) were removed from the analysis.

2.3 Data analysis
2.3.1 Preparation of learning sets

Before preparing the learning sets, based on the pattern recognition algorithms of Poincaré plots, feature sets showing noisy plots that consist of most of events out of the clusters were also removed since these were caused by the poor contact of electrodes (Figure 3). Feature sets showing island, multi-sided lobe, and fan patterns were removed from learning sets of NSR group since they represent arrhythmic events (Esperer et al., 2006). However, only records showing fan shapes were removed from learning sets of PAF group. To divide learning sets according to the level of physical or mental activity, an arbitrary cut-off value of RMSSD (in sec) was selected to assign each 30-min RR interval to two types of ANS conditions: one representing the activated state of the vagal nervous system (RMSSD > 0.040 sec) and the other representing the suppressed state of the vagal nervous system due to mental or physical activity (RMSSD <0.040 sec) experienced by the subject during daily activity. HRV feature sets from different subject groups were compared by Mann-Whitney signed rank test (Statgraphics Plus V 4.1). Test results were considered significant if the p-value was less than 0.05 (95% confidence level).

From the prepared learning sets, the CR curve fittings were performed according to the procedure described in the section above. The calculated CR parameters were compared between NSR and PAF groups based on median values by the Mann-Whitney test (Statgraphics Plus V 4.1). The results were considered significantly different if p-values were less than 0.05.

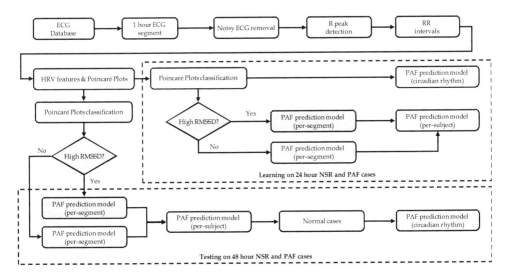

Fig. 3. Flow diagram for data processing and analysis used in the study.

2.3.2 Derivation of prediction models

Significant HRV and Poincaré plot features were selected from the learning sets by evaluating the worth of a feature based on the value of the chi-squared statistic with respect to the class (Weka 6.1, The University of Waikato, Hamilton, New Zealand). Naïve Bayesian, logistic regression, and support vector machine (SVM) analyses were performed to derive classification models that detect 30-min RR intervals of PAF subjects (Weka 6.1). Because this first classification was based on 30-min segments of RR interval data, it was called the segment-based classification. Once each 30-min segment was annotated, a second phase of classification was derived from a heuristic rule. Because annotation results for each subject were used, it was called the subject-based classification. A similar approach of two-phase classification has been reported previously (Hickey et al., 2006). According to the clinical definition of PAF, a subject would be diagnosed with PAF if at least one 30-min segment contained AF episodes. However, because our learning sets did not contain any segments with AF episodes (fan-shaped plots were removed), the empirical rule in this study was modified to classify subjects as PAF if any of four time periods had two or more segments annotated as PAF within the same time period.

Significant CR features were selected from the learning sets by the chi-squared test (Weka 6.1). Naïve Bayesian, logistic regression, and SVM analyses were performed to derive classification models that detect PAF subjects using CR features (Weka 6.1).

2.3.3 Preparation of test sets

Before preparing the test sets, the records showing noisy Poincaré plots were removed from further analysis. Testing sets were divided according to the RMSSD cut-off. The segment-based classification was performed using the classification algorithm that produced the best accuracy. These outputs were further tested using the subject-based classification rule with different segment sampling methods: two, three, or four 30-min samples per time period to determine the dependence of classification accuracy on the number of sample segments. Cases classified as NSR were tested using the CR classification (Figure 3).

3. Results

3.1 Establishment of PAF prediction models using data from the 24-h study
3.1.1 Segment-based model and subject-based model

A total of 299 and 319 items of RR interval data were obtained from 20 NSR and 24 PAF patients, respectively, and were processed for HRV calculation. HRV features that differed significantly between two types of data were initially screened by the Mann-Whitney test at a significance level of $p = 0.05$. Most HRV features were higher in the PAF groups except for SD_2, SI, and HFnu, which were lower (*data not shown*, $p<0.01$). Similar outcomes have also been reported in previous studies (Kim et al., 2008a, 2008b) using NSR and AF databases available at Physionet. These HRV features were further ranked based on their contribution to a prediction model (chi-squared feature selection method, Weka 6.1). The top nine HRV features (RMSSD, SDSD, SD_1, SDRatio, rRR, %Cluster, SDNN, CV, and PNN50) were then used to generate a prediction model that represented the segment-based classification model. The accuracy of each classification method is summarized in Table 2. The logistic regression analysis produced the highest accuracy among three classification algorithms (71.4%) and was selected for the testing.

Based on this observation, a simple heuristic rule was applied to generate the subject-based classification. Two of 24 PAF cases were misclassified as NSR (false negative) and four of 20 NSR cases (false positive) were misclassified (Table 3). False-negative cases showed only one record classified as PAF. All false-positive cases showed fan-shaped Poincaré plots.

Classification methods	Sensitivity	Specificity	Accuracy
Naïve Bayesian	39.5%	96.0%	66.8%
Logistic regression analysis	58.3%	85.3%	71.4%
Support vector machine	49.5%	89.6%	68.9%

Table 2. Performance of different classification algorithms for the segment based classification using 30-min ECG records.

Observed \ Predicted	NSR	PAF
NSR ($n=20$)	16 (80%)	4 (20%)
PAF ($n=24$)	2 (8%)	22 (92%)

Table 3. Performance of the subject based classification using the results from the segment-based classification by logistic regression analysis

3.1.2 The CR model

The phases of the HRV features of the two groups did not show significant differences (data not shown; $p > 0.05$), thereby suggesting that there was no significant difference in the time-point of HRV peak occurrence. The CR amplitudes and shifts of rRR, HF, LF, HR and RMSSD showed significant differences between the two groups (data not shown; Mann-Whitney test, $p < 0.05$). These CR features were further ranked based on their contribution to a prediction model (chi-squared feature selection method, Weka 6.1). The top three CR features (rRR shift, LF amplitude, and HR amplitude) were then used to generate a prediction model that represented the segment-based classification model. These three HRV features were curve-fitted and plotted to determine the circadian change in individual subjects (Figure 4). Logistic regression analysis was performed with the three CR features and produced an accuracy of 86% in predicting PAF cases (sensitivity of 79% classifying 19/24 PAF cases and specificity of 95% classifying 19/20 NSR cases). The false-positive subject (n=1) seemed to show greater fluctuations, whereas false-negative subjects (n=5) showed fewer fluctuations in CR amplitudes.

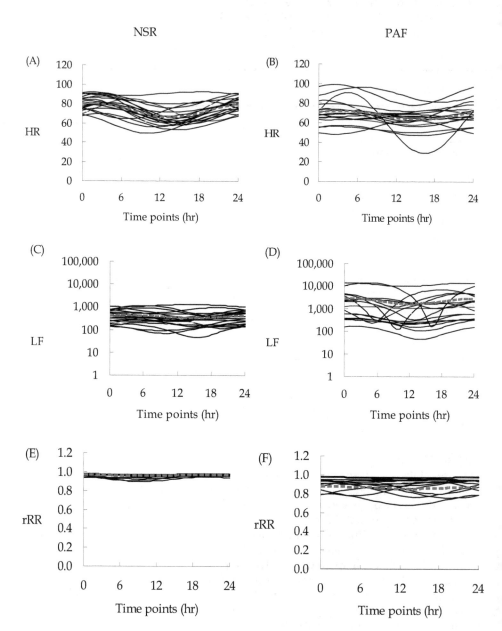

Fig. 4. Circadian rhythms of selected HRV features were significantly different between NSR and PAF cases. HR: heart rates per min, LF: low frequency area (msec^2) after logarithmic transform, and rRR: autocorrelation function of the RR intervals.

3.2 Prediction of AF recurrence using 48-h recordings

ECG data from 48-h Holter monitoring were first screened for AF episodes using the software in the Holter system and software findings for AF were confirmed by two cardiologists (JHP, JHK). Nineteen of 33 subjects were diagnosed as NSR whose heart rhythms were successfully maintained for 48 h under drug treatment (normal group). Ten subjects were diagnosed as PAF and four as persistent AF (recurrent group; recurrence rate of 42%). Normal and recurrent groups did not differ significantly different in terms of age (Mann-Whitney test, $p > 0.05$), gender, or other diseases such as diabetes, hypertension, or past strokes (chi-squared test, $p > 0.05$).

The noise detection algorithm detected four NSR cases and showed that more than 30% of the total ECG data were corrupted by noise possibly due to poor electrode contacts; these were removed from the test sets to avoid misinterpretation. When four ECG segments were sampled from each time period of ECG data, a total of 350 and 270 segments were obtained from 15 normal and 14 recurrent cases, respectively, and were processed for the calculation of HRV and Poincaré plot features. Using the segment-based classification and subject-based rule, 9/10 recurrent PAF patients were correctly identified, whereas 13/15 normal subjects were correctly identified (data not shown). In addition, four persistent AF cases were all correctly identified. An illustrative example for the subject-based rule is described in Figure 5, in which a data point represents the probability density value of the segment based model at a given time-point. Data points for an NSR case remain higher than the empirical cut-off at all time-points, whereas those for a PAF case often fall below the cut-off even during the days when no episodes were evident (Figure 5). Subjects classified as normal cases by the subject-based rule (n = 14) were further tested with the CR-based model. One false-negative case was correctly identified as recurrent and all normal cases were correctly confirmed as normal cases. Therefore, the final classification resulted in a sensitivity of 100% (14/14 recurrent cases) and a specificity of 86% (13/15 normal cases) (Table 4). The same classification procedure was applied to the data sets obtained by sampling two or three segments per time period and classification results are summarized in Table 4. The number of sampled segments did not change the classification outcomes drastically.

4. Conclusion and discussion

In this study, we have developed a new method for predicting PAF subjects using intermittently sampled ECG data and applied it to the identification of recurrent AF cases. The proposed method consists of an empirical rule and a CR-based classification. The empirical rule alone identified nearly 93% of recurrent cases (13/14 cases) and 86% of normal cases (13/15 cases). Because our aim was not to miss any recurrent cases, normal cases classified by the empirical rule were re-tested using the CR-based prediction model. The false-negative case was correctly identified as a recurrent case thus achieving a 100% sensitivity and no false-positive cases were generated thus maintaining the 86% specificity. Our results suggest that intermittently sampled ECG data could be used to detect the increased likelihood of PAF episodes. Since previous PAF prediction methods relied on the change during the transition from NSR to PAF, ECG needs to be analyzed continuously not to miss transition periods. Furthermore, somewhat higher degree of false positive errors may be expected in an actual implementation of long term ECG analysis since the likelihood of not having subsequent PAF episodes following a transition period is not known.

Contrary to previous prediction methods, our classification models were not designed to detect the transition period prior to PAF episodes exclusively. Instead, they were aimed to evaluate the likelihood of a 24 hour period when PAF episodes may occur. Thus, the performance of our proposed method can be less sensitive to the continuity of ECG data but allows ECG recordings to be sampled over the whole day. Two samples gave results that were as accurate as those of four samples taken during four 6-h time periods (Table 4). Furthermore, our results indicated that the proposed methods tended to show an increased likelihood of detecting PAF cases even during the days when no PAF episodes were evident (Figure 5). Therefore, we conclude that our intermittent sampling strategy is as accurate for predicting recurrent PAF as previously reported methods.

CLASS	NSR	PAF	NSR	PAF	NSR	PAF
NSR ($n = 15$)	14 (93%)	1 (7%)	13 (86%)	2 (14%)	13 (86%)	2 (14%)
PAF ($n = 10$)	0 (0%)	10 (100%)	0 (0%)	10 (100%)	0 (0%)	10 (100%)
No. of samples taken in each time period (6 hrs)	2		3		4	

Table 4. Performance of proposed methods for predicting PAF subjects using a subject-based rule and a CR-based classification algorithm. Performance results were obtained when two, three, or four 30-min ECG records were sampled from each of four time periods during a day.

The intermittent sampling approach might be more effective in mobile healthcare settings because the sensor may not need to be worn all day, which could effectively reduce many problems caused by poor sensor tolerance, limited battery life, and high data transmission costs of current technology. In general, mobile healthcare technology offers many attractive features such as convenient wearable ECG sensors, real-time feedback of abnormal heart rhythms, and timely intervention in the case of adverse events. However, the continuous measurement of ECG signals might not be ideal as a long-term monitoring solution in mobile healthcare settings because it requires long hours of wearing a sensor that may stigmatize a majority of patients and eventually influence the quality of the data. For example, Holter monitoring was regarded as inconvenient because of hygienic aspects, physical activity, night sleep, and skin reactions (Fensli & Boisen, 2009). Based on our understanding of current advances in low-power bioelectronics (Sarpeshkar, 2010), the proposed intermittent sampling of ECG signals is believed to provide an attractive alternative strategy to long-term monitoring in mobile healthcare settings. It could be specially adapted to work with wireless devices such as wearable sensors and gateway devices that consume battery power at high rates. In addition, the amount of data traffic would be minimized, which is also attractive in countries where wireless data transfer is costly. Thus, in developing a computer-aided prediction method for mobile healthcare settings, it seems important to consider human factors, such as patient acceptance of procedures, or device factors, such as battery time or data transfer costs.

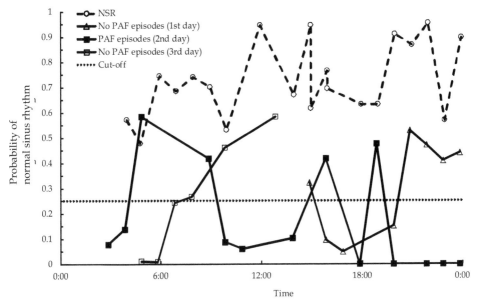

Fig. 5. Distribution of probability values from the segment-based model applied to two patient cases. Data points in the hollow circle are from a normal case (NSR). Data points in the solid square are from a PAF case on the day when PAF episodes were recorded, whereas those in the hollow square and triangle are from the same case during the previous and following days when no PAF episodes were recorded. The points in the area under the cut-off at 0.25 (broken line) were classified as PAF.

It is becoming evident that a significant proportion of cryptogenic stroke is due to intermittent AF. By using 30-day cardiac event monitors, 20% of such strokes was found to be related to AF (Elijovich et al., 2009). Warfarin treatment was given to patients after the detection of intermittent AF (despite no detection of AF on ECG or in-patient telemetry monitoring in the majority of patients). Similarly to the detection of recurrent PAF, prevention of recurrent strokes related to PAF in particular may require long-term ECG monitoring. For these applications, our proposed intermittent sampling method should also be suitable as an initial screening method that generates a real-time alarm or trend report that enables timely intervention. For example, if the incidence of abnormal segments increases, then the ECG sampling strategy may be changed to a continuous monitoring mode to capture the PAF episodes. In this way, patients can be monitored in the long term to determine recurrence after conversion treatment or the origin of strokes, so that conventional Holter monitoring can be complemented or improved. For initial screening purposes, the ECG sensor used in this study can be replaced by a heartbeat sensor because all analytic features were calculated from RR interval data rather than the morphology of ECG signals. Current advances in microelectronics have provided a variety of heartbeat sensors ranging from conventional chest belt type to Doppler radar-based non-contact types. These sensors are usually equipped with a module of wireless data communication so they can transmit the signals to the gateway device that is connected to the internet.

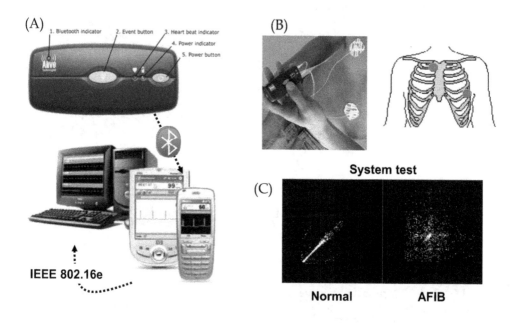

Fig. 6. (A) System components of web-based heartbeat analysis system. (B) Electrode attachment. (C) Poincaré plots were generated from wirelessly transmitted ECG data obtained from an NSR and an AF subject (Pictures in (A) and (B) were kindly provided by Alivetec Technologies Pty. Ltd.).

4.1 Development of web-based real-time heartbeat analysis

Currently, we are actively developing a remote real-time heartbeat analysis system that consists of a wearable ECG sensor (AliveECG monitor, Alive Technologies Pty. Ltd, Ashmore, Queensland, Australia) with a three-axis accelerometer, a smart phone (HD2, HTC Corporation, Taoyuan, Taiwan ROC), and a data analysis server (Microsoft Windows XP; Figure 6). The original server software (Cardiomobile, Alive Technologies) displays ECG, activity features, and global positioning system-based location in a web-based map in real time or in review mode. In addition to these functions, HRV features and outputs from a PAF prediction model are also calculated and displayed in our current version (Figure 7). A feasible scenario of using our system is that a wireless ECG sensor worn by a patient, and communicating to the smart phone through the near field Bluetooth, transmits ECG signals to the remote server through a wireless data streaming service. The remote server performs real-time analysis of transmitted ECG data and detects abnormal events (or trends). In the case of PAF prediction, a cardiology specialist at the hospital may be notified to interpret the remote monitoring and confirm the diagnosis. Compared with conventional Holter monitoring systems, a mobile healthcare solution can be designed to enable the patient to carry out normal daily activities, while still being under continuous monitoring.

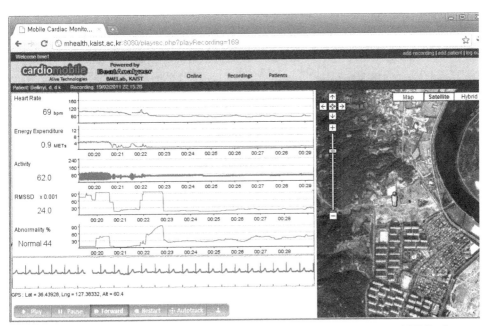

Fig. 7. Real-time heartbeat analysis system for remote monitoring of ECG and HRV of patients. Heart rates, energy expenditure, physical activity, HRV (RMSSD), and abnormal heartbeats (Abnormality %) can be monitored by remote clinical staff in real time while a patient is exercising outdoors during daily activity. In the case of advent events, user location data from the global positioning system can be provided to paramedic staff (user's current position is indicated by the avatar on the web-based map) (Cardiomobile is the trademark of Alivetec Technologies Pty. Ltd. The server software was kindly provided to be modified by us.)

Since the patient may experience an arrhythmic episode during physical activity, mobile solutions may enhance the quality of data measured by enabling the patient to carry out normal daily routines. Currently, we are also implementing the CR analysis of HRV features and its related PAF prediction. This prototype system should help us to discover the "real problem" and the users' requirements, demonstrate the actual functionality of a device, and provide many insights on how to design and build a more advanced system that should enable long-term ECG monitoring. The future system is being designed to provide additional benefits for stroke or heart disease rehabilitation patients.

5. Acknowledgement

We would like to express sincere gratitude to Mrs. Young Mi Choi who participated in patient recruitment and data retrieval, Ms. Yoon Ju Na who developed a batch run software, and Dr. Seung Hwan Kim who initially suggested this collaboration. This work was partly supported by Science and Technology Fundamental Frontier Research fund at KAIST ICC, Korea.

6. References

Aytemir, K., Aksoyek, S., Yildirir, A., Ozer, N., & Oto, A. (1999). Prediction of Atrial Fibrillation Recurrence After Cardioversion by P Wave Signal-averaged Electrocardiography. *International Journal of Cardiology*, Vol. 70, No. 1, pp. 15.

Berruezo, A., Tamborero, D., Mont, L., Benito, B., Tolosana, J.M., Sitges, M., Vidal, B., Arriagada, G., Méndez, F., Matiello, M., Molina, I., & Brugada, J. (2007). Pre-procedural Predictors of Atrial Fibrillation Recurrence After Circumferential Pulmonary Vein Ablation. *European Heart Journal*, Vol. 28, No. 7, pp. 836.

Brennan, M., Palaniswami, M., & Kamen, P. (2001). Do existing Measures of Poincaré Plot Geometry Reflect Nonlinear Features of Heart rate Variability? *IEEE Transactions on Biomedical Engineering*, Vol. 48, No. 11, pp. 1342.

Chesnokov, Y.V. (2008). Complexity and Spectral Analysis of the Heart Rate Variability Dynamics for Distant Prediction of Paroxysmal Atrial Fibrillation with Artificial Intelligence Methods. *Artificial Intelligence in Medicine*, Vol. 43, No. 2, pp. 151.

Delfaut, P., Saksena, S., Prakash, A., & Krol, R.B. (1998). Long-term Outcome of Patients with Drug-refractory Atrial Flutter and Fibrillation after Single- and Dual-site Right Atrial Pacing for Arrhythmia Prevention. *Journal of the American College of Cardiology*, Vol. 32, No. 7, pp. 1900.

Duong, N.D., Jeong, H., Youn, C.-H. & Kim, D. (2009). Development of New Cluster Descriptors for Image Analysis of Poincare Plots In: *World Congress on Medical Physics and Biomedical Engineering*, Vol. 25/IV Image Processing, Biosignal Processing, Modelling and Simulation, Biomechanics, pp. 1661, Munich, Germany.

Elijovich, L., Josephson. S.A., Fung, G.L., & Smith, W.S. (2009). Intermittent Atrial Fibrillation May Account for a Large Proportion of Otherwise Cryptogenic Stroke: A Study of 30-day Cardiac Event Monitors. *Journal of Stroke Cerebrovascular Disease*, Vol. 18, No. 3, pp. 185.

Esperer, H.D., Esperer, C., & Cohen, R.J. (2008). Cardiac Arrhythmias Imprint Specific Signatures on Lorenz Plots. *Annals of Noninvasive Electrocardiology*, Vol. 13, No. 1, pp. 44.

Fensli, R. & Boisen, E. (2009). Human Factors Affecting the Patient's Acceptance of Wireless Biomedical Sensors, Biomedical Engineering Systems and Technologies. *Communications in Computer and Information Science*, Vol. 25, No. 4, pp. 402.

Friberg, L., Hammar, N., & Rosenqvist, M. (2010). Stroke in Paroxysmal Atrial Fibrillation: Report from the Stockholm Cohort of Atrial Fibrillation. *Eurorpean Heart Journal*, Vol. 31, No. 8, pp. 967.

Grubitzsch, H., Grabow, C., Orawa, H., & Konertz, W. (2008). Factors Predicting the Time until Atrial Fibrillation Recurrence After Concomitant Left Atrial Ablation. *European Journal of Cardiothoracic Surgery*, Vol. 34, No. 1, pp. 67.

Guo, Y.F. & Stein, P.K. (2002). Circadian Rhythm in the Cardiovascular System: Considerations in Non-invasive Electrophysiology. *Cardiac Electrophysiology Review*, Vol. 6, No. 3, pp. 267.

Hu, F. & Xiao, Y. (2009). Congestion Aware, Loss-Resilient Bio-Monitoring Sensor Networking for Mobile Health Applications. *IEEE Journal on Selected Areas in Communications*, Vol. 27, No. 4, pp. 450.

Hart, R.G., Pearce, L.A., & Aguilar, M.I. (2007). Meta-analysis: antithrombotic therapy to prevent stroke in patients who have nonvalvular atrial fibrillation. *Ann Intern Med.* Vol. 146, No. 12, pp. 857.

Hickey, B., Heneghan, C., & De Chazal, P. (2004). Non-episode-dependent Assessment of Paroxysmal Atrial Fibrillation Through Measurement of RR Interval Dynamics and Atrial Premature Contractions. *Annals of Biomedical Engineering,* Vol. 32, No. 5, pp. 677.

Jabaudon, D., Sztajzel, J., Sievert, K., Landis, T., Sztajzel, R. (2004). Usefulness of ambulatory 7-day ECG monitoring for the detection of atrial fibrillation and flutter after acute stroke and transient ischemic attack. *Stroke,* Vol. 35, No. 7, pp. 1647.

Jørgensen, H.S., Nakayama, H., Reith, J., Raaschou, H.O., & Olsen, T.S. (1996) Acute Stroke with Atrial Fibrillation. The Copenhagen Stroke Study. *Stroke,* Vol. 27, pp. 1765.

Kikillus, N. , Schweikert, M., & Bolz, A. (2008). Identifying Patients Suffering from Atrial Fibrillation During Atrial Fibrillation and Non-atrial Fibrillation Episodes. In: *4th European Conference of the International Federation for Medical and Biological Engineering 2008,* Vol. 22, pp. 1349–1352, Antwerp, Belgium.

Kim, D., Seo, Y., Jung, W., & Youn, C.-H. (2008a). Detection of Long Term Variations of Heart Rate Variability in Normal Sinus Rhythm and Atrial Fibrillation ECG Data. In: *Biomedical Engineering and Informatics 2008,* Sanya, Hainan, China.

Kim, D., Seo, Y., & Youn, C.-H. (2008b). Prediction of Atrial Fibrillation Onsets by Multiple Formulas Based on Long Term Variation of Heart Rate Variability. In: *Healthcom 2008,* Singapore.

Koh, K.B., Park, J.K., Kim, C.H., & Cho, S. (2001). Development of the Stress Response Inventory and Its Application in Clinical Practice. *Psychosomatic Medicine,* Vol. 63, pp. 668.

Lednev, V.V., Belova, N.A., Ermakov, A.M., Akimov, E.B., & Tonevitsky, A.G. (2008). Modulation of Cardiac Rhythm in the Humans Exposed to Extremely Weak Alternating Magnetic Fields. *Biophysics,* Vol. 53, No. 6, pp. 648.

Levenberg, K. (1944). A Method for the Solution of Certan Non-linear Problems in Least Squares. *The Quarterly of Applied Mathematics,* Vol. 2, pp. 164.

Li, J.J. (2003). Circadian Variation in Myocardial Ischemia: The Possible Mechanisms Involving in This Phenomenon. *Medical Hypotheses,* Vol. 61, No. 2, pp. 240.

Lin, H.J., Wolf, P.A., Kelly-Hayes, M., Beiser, A.S., Kase, C.S., Benjamin, E.J., & D'Agostino, R.B. (1996). Stroke Severity in Atrial Fibrillation: The Framingham study. *Stroke,* Vol. 6, No. 27, pp. 1760.

Lombardi, F., Colombo, A., Basilico, B., Ravaglia, R., Garbin, M., Vergani, D., Battezzati, P.M., & Fiorentini, C.J. (2001). Heart Rate Variability and Early Recurrence of Atrial Fibrillation after Electrical Cardioversion. *Journal of the American College of Cardiology,* Vol. 37, No. 1, pp. 157.

Marini, C., De Santis, F., Sacco, S., Russo, T., Olivieri, L., Totaro, R., & Carolei, A. (2005). Contribution of Atrial Fibrillation to Incidence and Outcome of Ischemic Stroke: Results from a Population Based Study. *Stroke,* Vol. 36, pp. 1115.

Mitchell, A.R., Spurrell, P.A., & Sulke, N. (2002). Circadian Variation of Arrhythmia Onset Patterns in Patients with Persistent Atrial Fibrillation. *American Heart Journal,* Vol. 6, No. 3, pp. 262.

Mohebbi, M. & Ghassemian, H. (2011). Prediction of Paroxysmal Atrial Fibrillation Using Recurrence Plot-based Features of the RR-interval Signal. *Physiological Measurement,* Vol. 32, pp. 1147.

Olemann, A. & Kim, D. (2011). Detection of Paroxysmal Atrial Fibrillation Subjects based on Circadian Rhythm Parameters of Heart Rate Variability. In: IEEE International Conference on Bioinformatics and Biomedicine, Atlanta, GA (2011) *(in press).*

Pan, J. & Tompkins, W.J. (1985). A Real-time QRS Detection Algorithm. *IEEE Transactions on Biomedical Engineering,* Vol. 32, No. 3, pp. 230.

Rizos, T., Rasch, C., Jenetzky, E., Hametner, C., Kathoefer, S., Reinhardt, R., Hepp, T., Hacke, W., & Veltkamp, R. (2010). Detection of Paroxysmal Atrial Fibrillation in Acute Stroke Patients. *Cerebrovascular Diseases,* Vol. 30, No. 4, pp. 410.

Sahoo, S.K., Lu, W., Teddy, S.D., Kim, D. & Feng, M. (2011). Detection of Atrial Fibrillation from Non-Episodic ECG Data: A Review of Methods. In: *33rd Annual International IEEE EMBS Conference,* Boston, MA, USA (in press).

Salahuddin, L. & Kim, D. (2006). Detection of Acute Stress by Heart Rate Variability Using a Prototype Mobile ECG Sensor. In: *Hybrid Information Technology, ICHIT' 06,* Vol. 2, pp. 453-459, Jeju, Korea.

Sarpeshkar, R. (2010). *Ultra Low Power Bioelectronics: Fundamentals, Biomedical Applications, and Bio-Inspired Systems.* Cambridge University Press, New York, NY, USA.

Savopoulos, C., Ziakis, A., Hatzitolios, A., Delivoria, C., Kournanis, A., Mylonas, S., Tsougas, M. & Psaroulis, D. (2006). Circadian Rhythm in Sudden Cardiac Death : A Retrospective Study of 2,665 Cases. *Angiology,* Vol. 57, No. 2, pp. 197.

Serra, J. (1984) *Image Analysis and Mathematical Morphology.* Academic Press, New York, NY, USA.

Task Force (Task Force of the European Society of Cardiology and the North American Society of Pacing and Electrophysiology) (1996) Heart Rate Variability: Standards of Measurement, Physiological Interpretation and Clinical Use. *European Heart Journal,* Vol. 17, pp. 1043.

Thong, T., McNames, J., Aboy, M. & Goldstein, B. (2004). Prediction of Paroxysmal Atrial Fibrillation by Analysis of Atrial Premature Complexes. *IEEE Transactions on Biomedical Engineering,* Vol. 51, pp. 561.

Vikman, S., Mäkikallio, T.H., Yli-Mäyry, S., Pikkujämsä, S., Koivisto, A.-M., Reinikainen, P., Airaksinen, K.E.J. & Huikuri, H.V. (1999). Altered Complexity and Correlation Properties of R-R Interval Dynamics Before the Spontaneous Onset of Paroxysmal Atrial Fibrillation. *Circulation,* Vol. 100, pp. 2079.

Wolf, P.A., Abbott, R.D., & Kannel, W.B. (1987). Atrial Fibrillation: A Major Contributor to Stroke in the Elderly. The Framingham Study. *Archhives of Internal Medicine,* Vol. 147, pp. 1561.

Woo, M.A., Stevenson, W.G., Moser, D.K., Trelease, R.B., & Haper, R.M. (1992). Patterns of Beat to Beat Heart Rate Variability in Advanced Heart Failure. *American Heart Journal,* Vol. 123, No. 3, pp. 704.

Permissions

The contributors of this book come from diverse backgrounds, making this book a truly international effort. This book will bring forth new frontiers with its revolutionizing research information and detailed analysis of the nascent developments around the world.

We would like to thank Prof. Dr. F. R. Breijo-Marquez, for lending his expertise to make the book truly unique. He has played a crucial role in the development of this book. Without his invaluable contribution this book wouldn't have been possible. He has made vital efforts to compile up to date information on the varied aspects of this subject to make this book a valuable addition to the collection of many professionals and students.

This book was conceptualized with the vision of imparting up-to-date information and advanced data in this field. To ensure the same, a matchless editorial board was set up. Every individual on the board went through rigorous rounds of assessment to prove their worth. After which they invested a large part of their time researching and compiling the most relevant data for our readers. Conferences and sessions were held from time to time between the editorial board and the contributing authors to present the data in the most comprehensible form. The editorial team has worked tirelessly to provide valuable and valid information to help people across the globe.

Every chapter published in this book has been scrutinized by our experts. Their significance has been extensively debated. The topics covered herein carry significant findings which will fuel the growth of the discipline. They may even be implemented as practical applications or may be referred to as a beginning point for another development. Chapters in this book were first published by InTech; hereby published with permission under the Creative Commons Attribution License or equivalent.

The editorial board has been involved in producing this book since its inception. They have spent rigorous hours researching and exploring the diverse topics which have resulted in the successful publishing of this book. They have passed on their knowledge of decades through this book. To expedite this challenging task, the publisher supported the team at every step. A small team of assistant editors was also appointed to further simplify the editing procedure and attain best results for the readers.

Our editorial team has been hand-picked from every corner of the world. Their multi-ethnicity adds dynamic inputs to the discussions which result in innovative outcomes. These outcomes are then further discussed with the researchers and contributors who give their valuable feedback and opinion regarding the same. The feedback is then collaborated with the researches and they are edited in a comprehensive manner to aid the understanding of the subject.

Apart from the editorial board, the designing team has also invested a significant amount of their time in understanding the subject and creating the most relevant covers. They scrutinized every image to scout for the most suitable representation of the subject and create an appropriate cover for the book.

The publishing team has been involved in this book since its early stages. They were actively engaged in every process, be it collecting the data, connecting with the contributors or procuring relevant information. The team has been an ardent support to the editorial, designing and production team. Their endless efforts to recruit the best for this project, has resulted in the accomplishment of this book. They are a veteran in the field of academics and their pool of knowledge is as vast as their experience in printing. Their expertise and guidance has proved useful at every step. Their uncompromising quality standards have made this book an exceptional effort. Their encouragement from time to time has been an inspiration for everyone.

The publisher and the editorial board hope that this book will prove to be a valuable piece of knowledge for researchers, students, practitioners and scholars across the globe.

List of Contributors

Judith A. Lens, Jeroen Hermanides and Peter L. Houweling
Diakonessenhuis Utrecht, Departments of Anesthesiology, the Netherlands

Jasper J. Quak and David R. Colnot
Otolaryngology/Head and Neck Surgery, the Netherlands

F. R. Breijo-Marquez
Clinical and Experimental Cardiology, School of Medicine, Commemorative Hospital, Boston, Massachusetts, USA

M. Pardo Ríos
School of Medicine and Dentistry, University Research Institute on Aging, University of Murcia, Spain

Daniel Olmos-Liceaga
University of Sonora, México

Federico Guerra, Matilda Shkoza, Marco Flori and Alessandro Capucci
Cardiology Clinic, Marche Polytechnic University, Italy

Farid Sadaka and Christopher Veremakis
St John's Mercy Medical Center, St Louis University, USA

Shahnaz Jamil-Copley, Louisa Malcolme-Lawes and Prapa Kanagaratnam
Imperial College Healthcare NHS Trust, St Mary's Hospital, London, National Heart and Lung Institute, Imperial College London, UK

Pascal Fallavollita
Chair for Computer Aided Medical Procedures & Augmented Reality, Technische Universität München, Germany

Shimon Rosenheck, Jeffrey Banker, Alexey Weiss and Zehava Sharon
Hadassah Hebrew University Medical Center, Jerusalem, Israel

Marius Craina, Răzvan Nițu, Lavinia Stelea, Dan Ancuşa, Corina Şerban, Rodica Mihăescu and Ioana Mozoş
"Victor Babeş" University of Medicine and Pharmacy, Timişoara, Romania

Gheorghe Furău
"Vasile Goldiş" Western University of Arad, Romania

Kevin Baker, John Prior, Karthik Sheka and Raymond A. Smego, Jr.
The Commonwealth Medical College, USA

Desok Kim
Departments of Electrical Engineering and Information Communication Engineering, KAIST, Daejeon, Korea

Jae-Hyeong Park and Jun Hyung Kim
Chungnam National University, School of Medicine and Hospital, Department of Cardiology, Daejeon, Korea

Printed in the USA
CPSIA information can be obtained
at www.ICGtesting.com
JSHW011412221024
72173JS00003B/514

9 781632 412973